THE *Pioneer Woman Cooks*
DINNERTIME

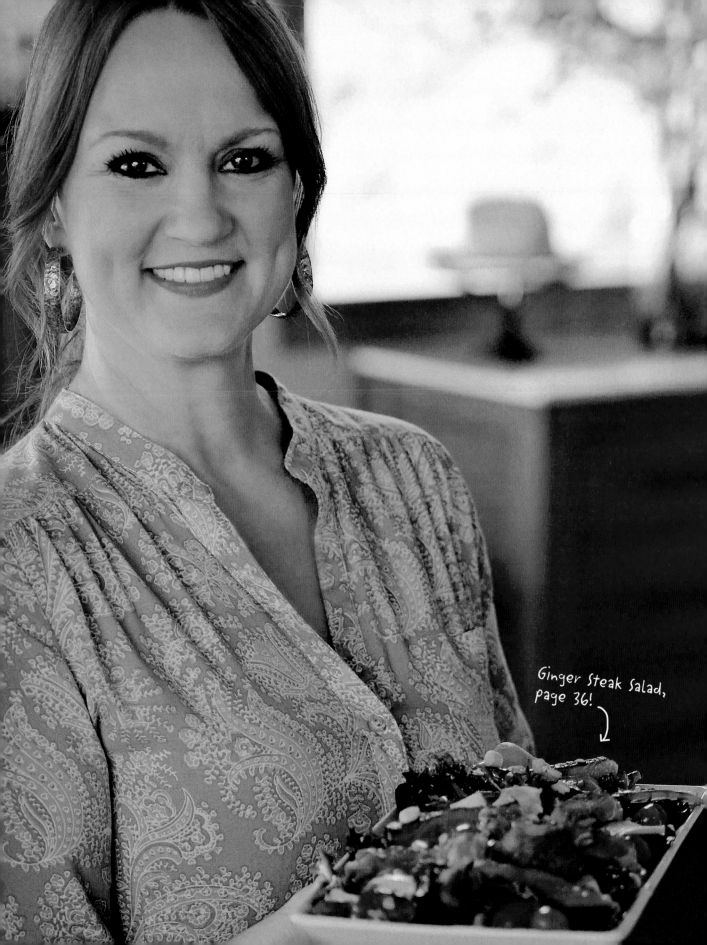

Ginger Steak Salad, page 36!

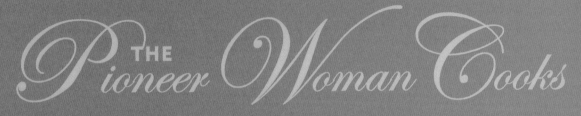

THE Pioneer Woman Cooks

DINNERTIME

COMFORT CLASSICS, FREEZER FOOD, 16-MINUTE MEALS, AND OTHER DELICIOUS WAYS TO SOLVE SUPPER!

REE DRUMMOND

WM
WILLIAM MORROW
An Imprint of HarperCollinsPublishers

ALSO BY REE DRUMMOND

The Pioneer Woman Cooks: Recipes from an Accidental Country Girl

The Pioneer Woman Cooks: Food from My Frontier

The Pioneer Woman Cooks: A Year of Holidays

The Pioneer Woman: Black Heels to Tractor Wheels—A Love Story

Charlie the Ranch Dog

Charlie and the Christmas Kitty

Charlie Goes to School

Charlie and the New Baby

Charlie Plays Ball

FIRST EDITION

Designed by Kris Tobiassen of Matchbook Digital

All photographs by Ree Drummond, except pages ii, vii, 350, Matt Ball; pages x, 151: Paige Drummond; page 15, Missy Drummond; pages 48-49, 73, 175, 202–203, 221, 316, 334–335, 369, Ladd Drummond; page 295, Rachel Purnell

Library of Congress Cataloging-in-Publication Data has been applied for.

ISBN 978-0-06-222524-5 (hardcover)
ISBN 978-0-06-242435-8 (Target edition)
ISBN 978-0-06-241926-2 (Walmart edition)
ISBN 978-0-06-244168-3 (B&N signed edition)
ISBN 978-0-06-244169-0 (BAM signed edition)

15 16 17 18 19 ID/QG 10 9 8 7 6 5 4 3 2 1

TO MY FAMILY.

You're my favorite.

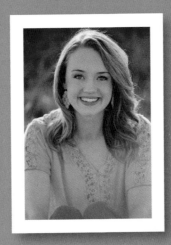

AND TO ALEX.

(If you're reading this for the first time, you're in college.
Our dinnertime isn't the same without you!)

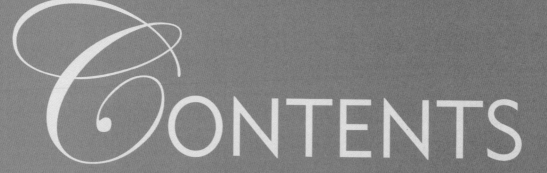

CONTENTS

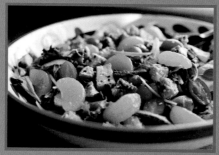

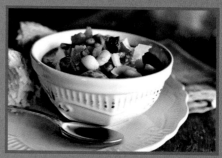

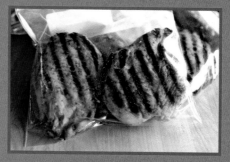

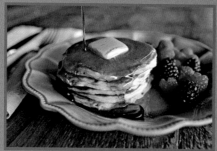

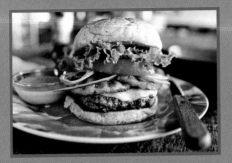

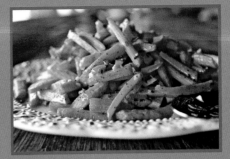

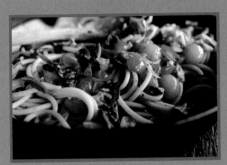

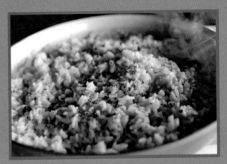

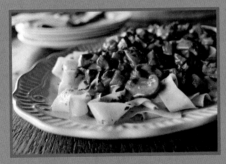

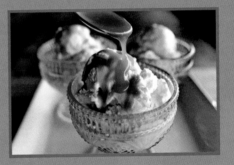

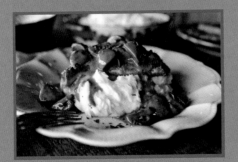

INTRODUCTION

Dinnertime is my life.
Dinnertime is my religion.
There's no time like dinnertime.
Dinnertime . . . because you're worth it!

I could go on and on! The truth is, in case you haven't gleaned this already, I *love* dinnertime. It's the time of day when the work, school, and grind are coming to a close and you can reward your loved ones (and yourself!) for a job well done. It's the time of day when you gather around the dining room table (or the kitchen table . . . or the patio table . . . or, heck, the coffee table!) and enjoy delicious food while touching base with one another about how your respective days have shaped up.

Dinnertime also happens to be the one time of day that home cooks struggle with the most! I mean, we can always rustle up some eggs for breakfast. Slap together a sandwich for lunch. Snack on fruits and nuts and Twinkies and raw vegetables all day long. But when it comes to churning out dinner several nights a week, I've learned through the years that I just can't fake it till I make it, or things start to get boring and lifeless really fast.

(Did I just say *Twinkies* out loud? Oops.)

Anyway, that's why I was so very excited to write this cookbook: I've determined that as a wife, mother, woman, and citizen of this planet, all I really want and need on a daily basis is something to make for dinner tonight. *Tonight.* Not a party I'm having next summer. Not a luncheon I'm hosting next millennium. Not a dinner I'm hosting on the eve of my baby's graduation from college. Not a cocktail hour I'm hosting on the fifth of never. But dinner. Tonight. Tonight, tonight, *tonight*! Because before long, and I literally mean here in about two hours, my family members are going to be banging their forks on the table and looking at me with longing (read: ravenous) eyes, and the only way I'm going to be able to get them out of my hair (and okay, spend some quality time with the cuties), will be to whip up something simple, scrumptious, and absolutely satisfying.

In this cookbook, I show you how to attack the greatest meal of the day, using lots of different

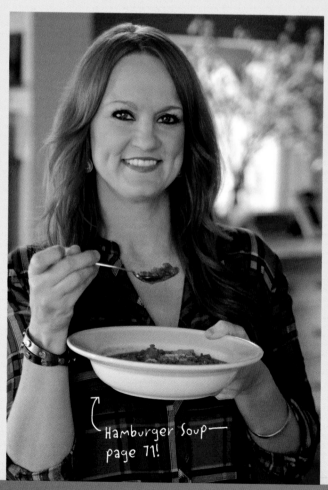

Hamburger Soup—
page 71!

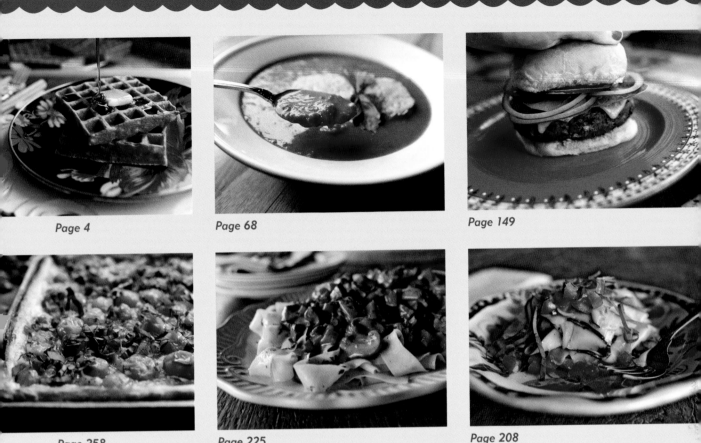

Page 4

Page 68

Page 149

Page 258

Page 225

Page 208

angles to suit what's going on in your life on any given evening. I kick things off with Breakfast for Dinner, highlighting some of my family's favorite "brinner" recipes. (Who says you can't eat pancakes for supper?) Main-dish salads and soups are some of my girls' favorite dinners, so you'll have plenty of those to add to your arsenal. Also, because life is crazy and unpredictable, I've found that having ready-to-go meals and recipe components in the freezer has been a lifesaver through my years of raising kids, so the Freezer Food section is chock-full of my favorites!

For years, I've had fun creating tongue-in-cheek (and delicious-in-mouth) 16-Minute Meals, and they've become a well-loved feature on my cooking blog. You'll love how quick and easy they are. And there's so much more in the book: irresistible pastas, classic comfort foods, new favorites for my family . . . not to mention amazing sides and super-quick desserts that will top off your family's dinnertime in sweet style. I also share my favorite fridge, pantry, and freezer staples so you'll be all stocked up and ready to start cooking!

I hope you love the recipes in this cookbook, friends. I hope you dive in and start cooking them right away. And I especially hope they become a part of your dinner table for years and years to come.

Lots of love,

Ree

A TYPICAL WEEK

I laughed as I typed that headline, because there is no such thing as a typical week in our house, unless I were allowed to use a one-word descriptor, in which case I'd probably just type *chaotic*.

Well, maybe chaotic isn't the right word. *Unpredictable* might be more like it. On any given day, there might be a grass fire to put out, fence to fix, a flat tire to tend to, or a calf to bottle-feed, not to mention all the normal things that happen in a family of six: football practice, soccer practice, cattle working, homeschooling co-op, cows in the yard, dogs on the porch, and a five-mile stretch of gravel road before we even get to the highway. And once we get to the highway, the journey has just barely begun.

So, yeah . . . eating dinner on a set schedule. It isn't going to be a reality for me for a very long time. As such, here's a peek at how a week of dinners in our house might look.

Monday night: Hamburger Soup (page 71) at 6:00, which I started mid-afternoon, and Cheese Biscuits (page 332), which are always a quick-and-easy (and cheesy) dinner roll recipe. (After getting the soup to the point of simmering, I browned the rest of the raw hamburger meat in a separate pot and added seasoning to make Ready-to-Go Beef Taco Filling [page 124] to store in individual bags in the freezer. I can never have too much of the stuff, and when I need to use up ground beef quickly, that's one of my go-to things to make.)

Tuesday night: I find out mid-afternoon that Ladd won't be finished working calves in time to take Paige an hour away to her soccer practice, so at 3:00 I pull three mini pans of Lasagna Roll-Ups (page 141) out of the freezer and put them on a baking sheet in the oven to thaw and bake, low and slow, for two hours. Paige and I leave at 4:00, and I tell Alex to pull out the roll-ups at 5:00, so they'll be ready for chowing down, and to grab the Raw Veggies and Creamy Chipotle Dip (page 304) I have in containers in the fridge and serve them on the side. I leave a plate of Chocolate Chunk Cookies (page 357), made earlier that evening, for dessert.

Wednesday night: Hallelujah! We're all home together again! It's a make-it-and-serve-it kind of evening, so at 6:30 I whip out one of my family's favorite quick pasta dishes, Cajun Chicken Pasta (page 188), along with a simple green salad and a batch of The Bread (page 336), which couldn't be easier to make. We all go to bed very, very happy. And very full!

Thursday night: The boys and Ladd have pizza night with their football team in town, so the girls and I opt for Chicken Taco Salad (page 53), one of our favorite main-dish salads these days. Instead of making the chicken on the spot, though, I use the Ready-to-Go Grilled Chicken (page 110) I pulled out of the freezer that morning once I confirmed the boys would be gone. When they get home after pizza, we each enjoy a Mason jar of Pudding (page 340)—four chocolates, two vanillas—that I made and chilled Wednesday morning.

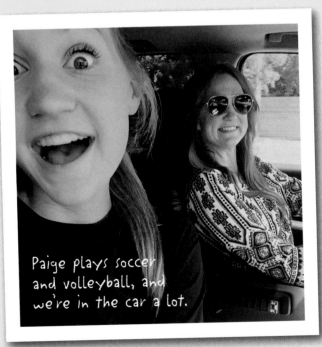

Paige plays soccer and volleyball, and we're in the car a lot.

Friday night: It's been one of those days, and by the time the kids and I get home from homeschool co-op in Tulsa, academically exhausted, there's only one thing that sounds good to all of us: Waffles (page 4)! I fry up some link sausage to serve on the side, and we inhale it all. (While in Tulsa, I grabbed a bunch more ground beef in bulk so I could make a huge batch of Ready-to-Go Freezer Meatballs [page 102] for the freezer the next morning.)

Saturday night: After my morning of making meatballs, I take a few minutes to bask in the glory of the future meals they'll be a part of, then I kick into gear for dinner that night: We haven't gotten together recently with Ladd's brother Tim, his wife, Missy, and their two kids, so we invite them over for a bountiful spread: Oven-Barbecued Chicken (page 234), Quick Shells and Cheese (page 214; Alex's request), and Lemony Green Beans (page 292; they're a last-minute veggie, and Missy helps me). For dessert it's vanilla ice cream with reheated Hot Fudge Sauce (page 348) that I made earlier in the day and chilled. And here's the fun part: Because Tim's getting ready for a huge week of work on his ranch, I send Missy home with a frozen pan of Mexican Tortilla Casserole (page 130) to bake at her discretion throughout the week. Nothing says "I love you" like a delicious, hearty freezer casserole.

Sunday night: After church I have little spare time, so I season a pork butt, wrap it in plastic wrap, and stick it in the fridge to season overnight. It'll go in the oven Monday morning and become Classic Pulled Pork (page 228) by dinnertime. For Sunday night dinner, it's a little bit of a mash-up in order to use up some ingredients in the fridge: Orange Chicken (page 160; I had leftover uncooked bone-in chicken thighs from the night before; I just removed the bones) for Alex and Paige; Chili Dogs (page 118; using the thawed Ready-to-Go Chili Packets on page 115) for Ladd, the boys, and me; and a big pan of Roasted Asparagus (page 280). (A crazy combination, and we loved every bite.)

Monday morning: The pork goes in the oven . . . and suddenly I look up, and it's a new week!

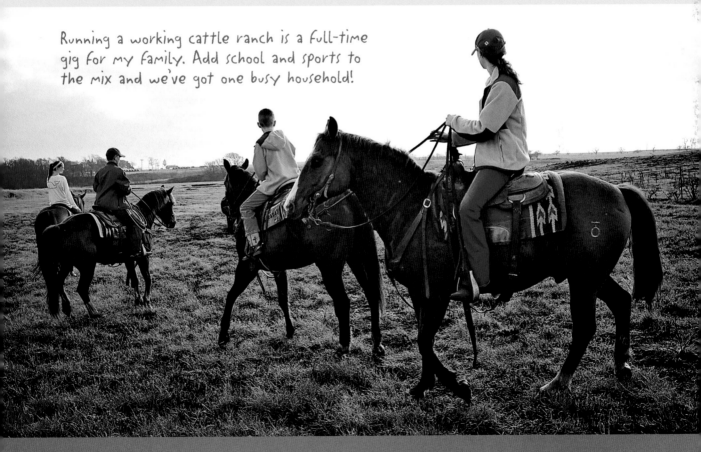

Running a working cattle ranch is a full-time gig for my family. Add school and sports to the mix and we've got one busy household!

PREP TIPS

**PREPPING'S NATURAL, PREPPING'S GOOD!
NOT EVERYBODY DOES IT, BUT EVERYBODY SHOULD . . .**

When it comes to dinner, I feel like I'm always in prep mode. Oh, of course there are plenty of dinners that I prep and cook up on the spot . . . but in general, anything I can think of to do ahead of time to save my sanity, you can bet I'm going to do it. When I'm in the kitchen working on one meal, I'm usually running through the coming days' meals and trying to figure out something I can prep early. It's the kind of gal I am.

Here are some of my favorite prep tips:

Clean veggies: As soon as my mother-in-law's aunt Dot got home from the market with veggies, she would always clean them (and, if applicable, peel them) before they ever made it into the fridge. She'd peel carrots, clean celery, wash cauliflower and broccoli and break them into florets, and so on. Just eliminating the prep step invited healthy snacking and made dinnertime so much easier.

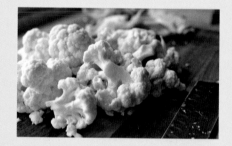

Dice veggies: If you're going to dice an onion, peel a carrot, or chop a stalk of celery . . . go ahead and knock out a bunch! Get all your tears out at once, stink up the cutting board in one session—however you want to think about it. Diced onion stays in the fridge, stored in a zipper bag, for five to seven days. So dice away, then just grab as much as you need at a time. (I store them in separate bags to keep the flavors pure.)

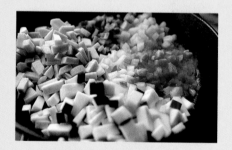

Prep lettuce and other greens: As soon as you get home from the grocery store, rinse, tear, and spin salad greens and heartier greens such as kale. Line large zipper bags with three or four paper towels and store the lettuce/greens inside with the zipper open. Makes salads (and/or recipes containing greens) throughout the week so easy!

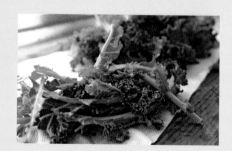

Mix dressings and marinades: Mincing garlic and finding bottles of olive oil and vinegars and jars of spices and seasonings can add a lot of activity right before a meal. Mix up dressings ahead of time and store them in the fridge in small jars. Whether it's a simple vinaigrette or a creamy Caesar, make all the dressings on Sunday night for the week ahead. Done!

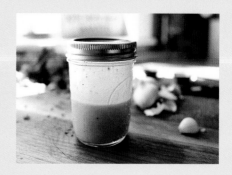

Brown ground meats: If you're browning hamburger, sausage, or ground turkey for chili, tacos, or soup, double (or triple! or quadruple!) the meat and brown it in a big batch. Let it cool, then store it in storage bags for the freezer or fridge. To use, just thaw and heat it in a skillet and proceed with the sauce, meat mixture, or soup you have in mind. (For recipes that call for browning onions with the beef, simply cook the onions in a little olive oil first, then add the meat.) So handy to have on standby!

Mise en place: It's a fancy term, but it's one of the best get-ahead tricks any home cook can have. In my cooking life, *mise en place* can manifest itself in two different ways: The first is simply taking a few minutes to measure and assemble ingredients before I start cooking a meal—it makes the cooking process more efficient because I'm not stopping and starting every time I have to retrieve and measure ingredients.

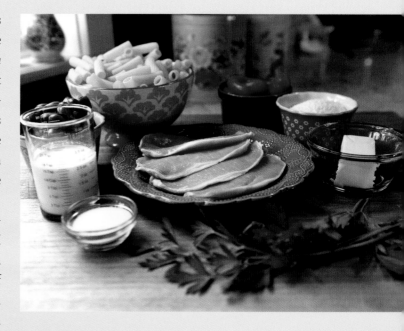

The second is what I like to call "make-ahead *mise en place*." Using this method, I prepare the entire array of ingredients for a recipe one, two, even three nights ahead (if the ingredients hold well), then store them on a rimmed baking sheet in the fridge. On the baking sheet, I place small Pyrex bowls with lids, various sizes of zipper bags, ceramic bowls and ramekins, and foil packets to store the grated cheese, diced onion, chopped vegetables, measured meat, butter—heck, even Mason jars with a dressing or stir-fry sauce all mixed and ready. Place a label on the baking sheet identifying the recipe the ingredients are for and, if necessary, have a corresponding nonperishable tray set aside on the countertop with the pantry items for that recipe (rice, beans, flour, cornmeal, canned tomatoes, and so on).

These make-ahead meal "kits" are exciting because they give me the promise of a super-quick homemade meal in the coming days. Have your kids help you put these together at the start of the week. It really does make dinnertime fun.

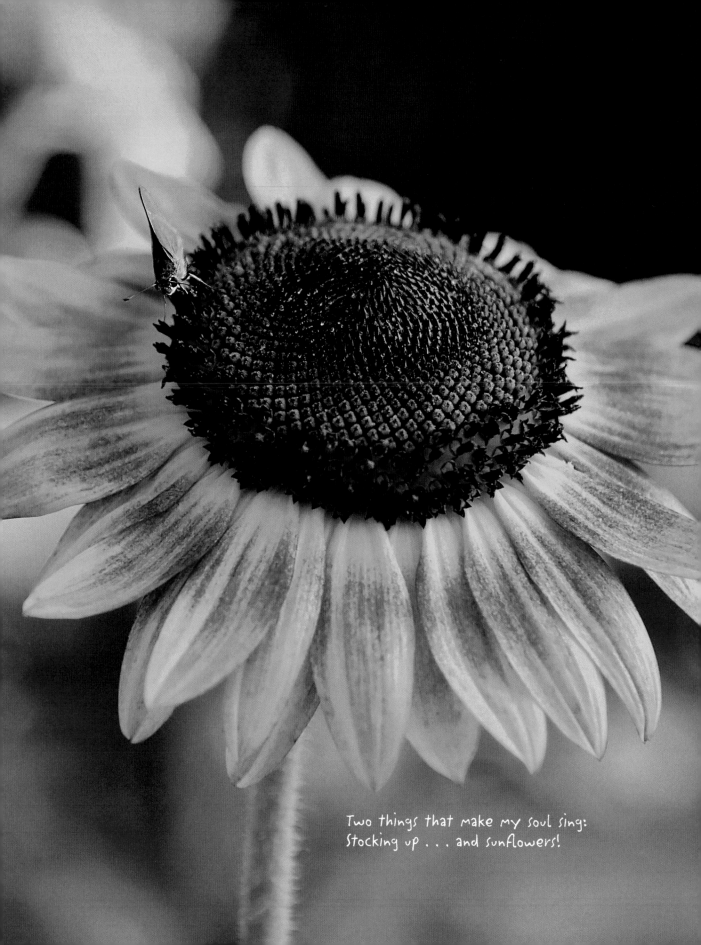

Two things that make my soul sing:
Stocking up . . . and sunflowers!

STOCKING UP

I'm going to tell you something that perhaps a cookbook author shouldn't necessarily say out loud, but here goes: *I really don't like going to the grocery store.* I'm not saying that to freak anyone out; I just felt I should be honest. Now, don't get me wrong: I love having all the ingredients I need in order to cook, which, just to reassure you, I absolutely love doing. If I ever tell you in a cookbook that I don't enjoy cooking, please send help immediately.

Back to my true confession: Yep. It's true. I just don't derive a substantial amount of joy from the act of grocery shopping. Throw in the fact that I would be 100 percent happy if I never had to get in my car and leave our homestead, and you've got a hot mess on your hands. But here's how I deal with it: I try my best to structure things so that I have a stockpile of basic essentials that I buy in bulk once, twice, three times a year . . . then I just fill in the fresh things (milk, bread, eggs, fresh produce, meat) as needed.

Here's the complete, comprehensive list of what I must have in my pantry, fridge, and freezer at all times or else I get twitchy and start to have disturbing dreams. Or, to put it positively, having a nicely stocked pantry, fridge, and freezer makes me smile! Big time.

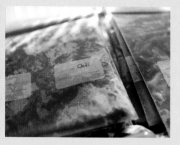 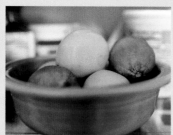 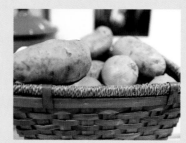 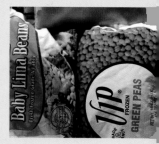

FRIDGE

Apples and oranges: for snacking, salads, and sauces

Assorted berries: blueberries, raspberries, strawberries, blackberries—for muffins, cobblers, salads, and snacking

Bacon: make BLTs, top burgers, cut into bits and fry with onion as the basis for some pasta sauces and soups

Basic vegetables: bell peppers, cucumbers, carrots, celery, zucchini, yellow squash

Butter: salted and unsalted

Cheese: blocks of long-lasting varieties such as Cheddar, Parmesan, blue, and feta

Corn and flour tortillas: stored properly, they seem to last forever in the fridge

Cream cheese: use in desserts, as a dip with pesto or chutney poured over, or in baked artichoke and spinach dips

Greek yogurt: for dips and dressings, and to serve with berries drizzled with honey

Greens: iceberg lettuce, romaine, green-leaf lettuce, mixed greens, kale, cabbage

Heavy cream: for desserts, sauces . . . and coffee!

Lemons and limes: for dressings, marinades, and sweet drinks

Sour cream: for baking and to dollop on top of baked potatoes and Mexican dishes

PANTRY

Assorted olives: pimiento-stuffed, black, Kalamata

Baking ingredients: bulk flour (all-purpose, whole wheat, self-rising), yeast, granulated sugar, brown sugar (store in an airtight container), powdered sugar, baking powder, baking soda, salt, cinnamon, nutmeg, allspice, cloves, flavored extracts, and so on

Canned artichoke hearts: throw into a pantry pasta sauce, make baked artichoke dip, etc.

Canned tomatoes: Crushed, whole, diced, tomato paste, tomatoes with chiles (such as Ro-Tel), sauce

Chipotle peppers in adobo sauce: Add to soups. Add to roasts. Puree with mayonnaise for a great salad dressing or veggie dip.

Chocolate chips and other forms of baking chocolate: semisweet, bittersweet, and unsweetened

Cornmeal: use in baking, of course, but also dissolve a little in water and stir into soups and chilis for a little thickening and flavor

Dried beans: Put 'em in soups. Put 'em in stews. Cook 'em in a pot with a ham hock. Make refried beans.

Dried pastas: in every shape and size imaginable

Evaporated milk and sweetened condensed milk: for baking and dessert sauces

Honey: for sweetening yogurt smoothies, adding a hint of sweet to recipes . . . and drizzling on hot biscuits

Jalapeños, pepperoncini, and other peppers: for sandwiches, salads, and snacking

Jarred marinara: in bulk!

Jarred pesto, specialty relishes, chutneys, and so on: Jarred pesto is an easy way to inject big flavor into soups, pasta, quiches, chicken salads, dips, and dressings when you don't have access to fresh basil.

Jarred salsas: traditional, peach, chipotle

Ketchup, mustards, and barbecue sauce

Masa harina: corn flour, sold in the Hispanic foods aisle. Use in similar ways as cornmeal.

Mayonnaise: real mayo, please!

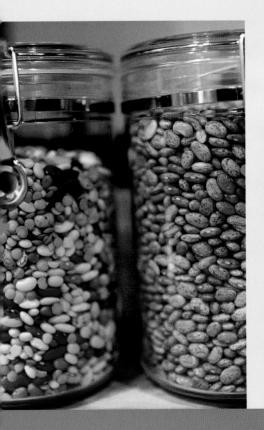
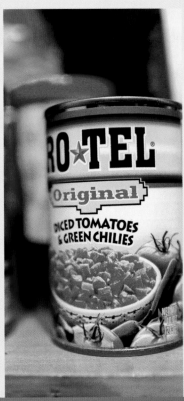
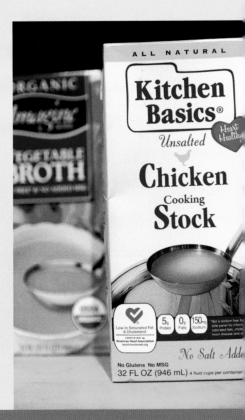

Oatmeal: for breakfast, for cookies, for adding to meatloaf and meatball mixtures

Oils: olive, vegetable, peanut

Panko breadcrumbs: Top casseroles. Coat mozzarella for frying. Mix them into meatballs and meatloaf. Bread chicken breasts.

Peanut butter: crunchy and creamy, for sandwiches, sauces, and sweets

Potatoes, onions, and garlic: Store 'em in separate baskets so air can circulate.

Quinoa and other grains

Real maple syrup: for topping pancakes and waffles, and sweetening sauces and dressings

Rice: long grain, medium grain, wild, brown, and Arborio for risotto

Roasted red peppers: Place them on paninis, cut them into strips and put them in frittatas, puree them and make a soup or pasta sauce, chop them and make bruschetta.

Seasonings, herbs, and spices: kosher salt, seasoned salt, black pepper, dried thyme, oregano, parsley, turmeric, Worcestershire sauce, Tabasco sauce, and so on

Shortening: for frying and baking

Stocks and broths: chicken, beef, vegetable . . . for soups, brisket, pot roasts, and so on

Various jellies: strawberry, apricot, jalapeño, peach, plum

Vinegars: distilled white, white wine, apple cider, red wine, rice

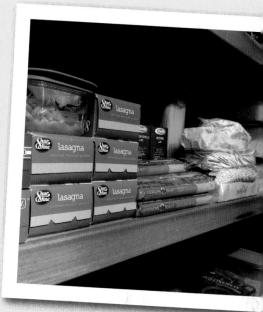

FREEZER

Beef: wrapped in butcher paper or vacuum sealed

Bread: crusty artisan loaves, plus a couple of back-up loaves of sandwich breads

Chicken breasts, wings, legs, and thighs: either flash frozen and stored in zipper bags or vacuum sealed

"Fresh" vegetables: The freezer is where I stock the veggies that aren't great in canned form: green beans, peas, spinach, Brussels sprouts, lima beans, carrots, corn. These nonacidic vegetables stay so much more delicious, nutritious, and fresh in the freezer. (Freeze your own veggies out of the garden by blanching, then cooling them in ice water, drying, flash freezing, and adding them to larger zipper bags.)

Frozen dinner rolls: I love the (store-bought!) unrisen, unbaked little round balls of dough. They rise and bake up so beautifully, and you can slather them with butter and chopped rosemary and turn them into something entirely different. And you can roll them out and use them to make calzones or mini pizzas.

Frozen fruits: Peaches, berries, cherries, and so on. These are awesome stand-ins for pies, crisps, and cobblers when the fresh fruits aren't in season. And you throw the frozen fruit right into the blender for smoothies whenever you want.

Pecans and walnuts: shelled and packed in plastic bags

Pie crust: Formed into disks and stored in zipper bags. To use, just remove, let thaw for 30 minutes or so, then roll out. For savory and sweet pies.

Pizza dough: unrisen, stored in zipper bags

Raw shrimp: deveined, in plastic bags, for pastas, soups, salads, and appetizers

Sausage: breakfast sausage, Italian sausage, chorizo, etc.

And **weird ingredients** such as homemade pumpkin puree—measure them into 1- or 2-cup quantities so you can easily use them in holiday recipes

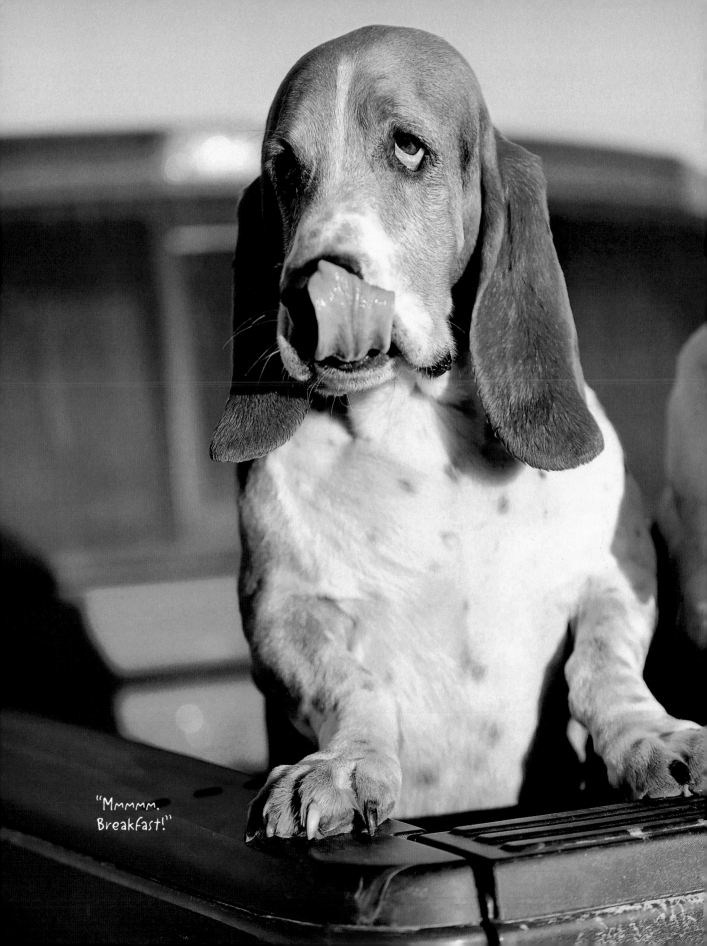

"Mmmmm.
Breakfast!"

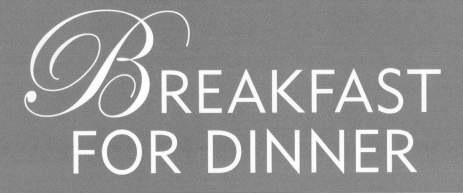BREAKFAST FOR DINNER

Whether you call it brupper, brinner, or just come right out and call it breakfast for dinner, these usually-seen-in-the-morning recipes are even better in the evening. From pancakes and waffles to frittatas and scrambles, these dishes will cause you to proclaim from the rooftops, "Breakfast! It's not just for breakfast anymore!"

GREEK YOGURT PANCAKES

MAKES 9 OR 10 PANCAKES

My husband's sweet and beautiful grandmother Edna Mae has made a sour cream pancake recipe for years that has knocked approximately 93,440,921 socks off. (Don't ask me where that missing sock is. It will never be found!) They're light and airy and utterly divine, and while they could never be improved, I made this Greek yogurt version once when I had no sour cream in my fridge.

I can only report the result using one word: *Oh my*.

And okay, that was two words. But you get the point. These are a-ma-zing.

7 tablespoons all-purpose flour

2 tablespoons sugar

1 teaspoon baking soda

½ teaspoon kosher salt

1 cup Greek yogurt

2 large eggs

½ teaspoon vanilla extract

Butter, for frying and serving

Warm maple or pancake syrup, for serving

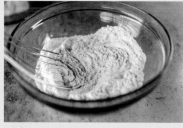

1. In a medium bowl, whisk together the flour, sugar, baking soda, and salt.

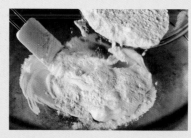

2. Place the yogurt in a large bowl and sprinkle in the dry ingredients. Stir until just combined.

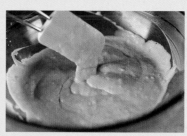

4. Fold until the batter is just barely combined.

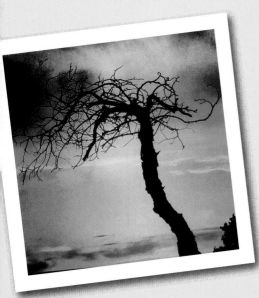

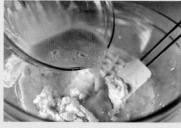

3. In a medium bowl, whisk together the eggs and vanilla, then pour them into the bowl with the yogurt mixture.

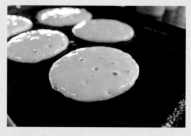

5. Heat a griddle or skillet over medium-low heat and smear a little butter over the surface. Drop the batter onto the griddle in ¼-cup portions and cook until bubbles form on top, about 2 minutes.

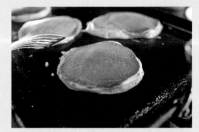

6. Flip the pancakes and cook for another minute or so.

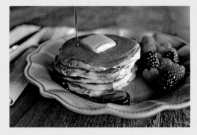

7. Serve with softened butter and warm syrup.

Ⓜ MAKE AHEAD

Pancake batter can be mixed up to 2 hours before frying and kept in the fridge. (Thin with a little milk, if needed.)

Ⓥ VARIATIONS

Substitute any kind of flavored Greek yogurt you'd like (strawberry, blueberry, and so on) for the plain Greek yogurt.

Add blueberries or chocolate chips to the pancake batter.

Top the pancakes with a dollop of whipped cream to make them extra decadent!

Ⓢ SERVE WITH

Fresh fruit

Fried bacon, sausage, or ham

Breakfast Potatoes (page 312)

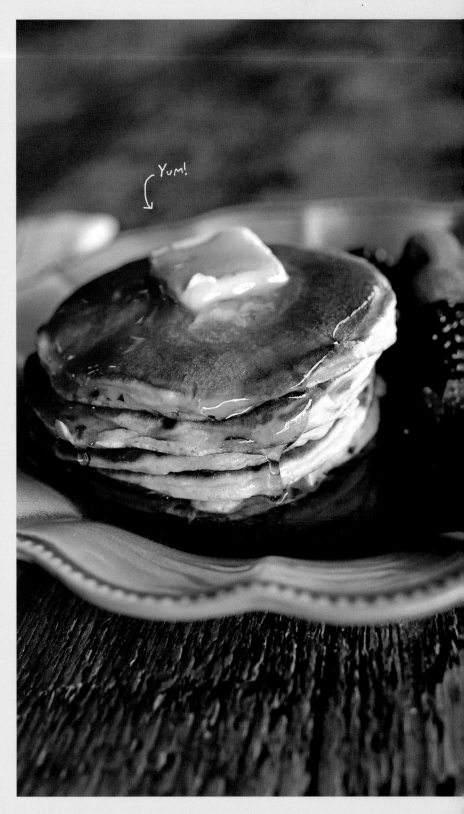

Yum!

WAFFLES

MAKES 8 SQUARE BELGIAN WAFFLES OR
20 THIN WAFFLES, TO SERVE 4 TO 6

Who doesn't love waffles, I ask you? I can't think of a single soul! And while they're normally associated with breakfast, waffles actually make the most satisfying dinner, and they ensure that when you go to bed later that night, you'll dream about only good things. So the next time you have a hankering for waffles, fire up the waffle iron and give these beautiful babies a try. (*Pssst*. If you don't have a waffle iron, you can thin the batter with just a little milk and make pancakes. This light and lovely batter works both ways.)

2 cups all-purpose flour

1 tablespoon baking powder

½ teaspoon kosher salt

¼ cup sugar

1½ cups milk

2 egg yolks

1 tablespoon plus 1 teaspoon vanilla extract

4 egg whites

½ cup (1 stick) butter

Butter and warm maple or pancake syrup, for serving

1. Heat a waffle iron to medium heat.

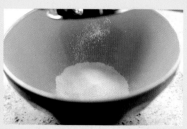

2. Into a large bowl, sift together the flour, baking powder, salt, and sugar.

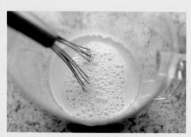

3. In a small pitcher, whisk together the milk, egg yolks, and vanilla.

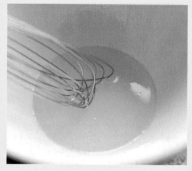

4. In a separate bowl, begin whisking the egg whites . . .

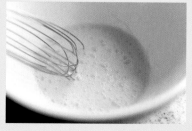

5. And keep going until they're thick and slightly stiff. Note that this will make your arm feel like it's going to fall off, so feel free to use a mixer with a whisk attachment if you want to take the easy road! I usually do; I'm just showing off for these photos.

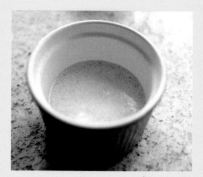

6. Finally, melt the butter in a small bowl or ramekin in the microwave.

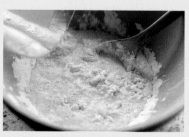

7. Now it's time to make the batter! Pour the milk mixture into the dry mixture, stirring gently to combine.

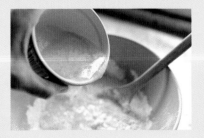

8. Stir in the melted butter . . .

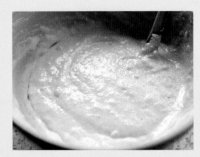

9. Then pour in the beaten egg whites . . .

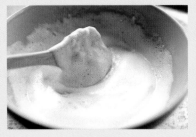

10. And gently fold them in just until they're combined.

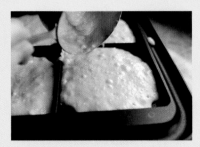

11. Scoop the batter into the waffle iron and cook for several minutes . . .

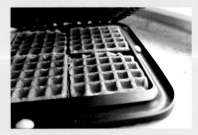

12. Until the waffles are deep golden brown and crisp. Repeat to make the rest of the waffles.

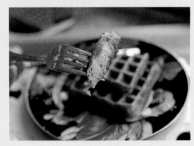

13. Serve the waffles warm, with butter and syrup.

They'll make your dreams extra sweet! I promise.

M MAKE AHEAD

If needed, you can make the batter up to 2 hours before cooking the waffles. Just keep it in the fridge until waffle time.

To freeze waffles, allow them to cool completely, then package them in freezer storage bags. Pop them into the toaster to defrost and reheat!

V VARIATIONS

Add mini chocolate chips to the batter before you cook the waffles.

Add ground cinnamon, nutmeg, and cloves to the batter for a little spice.

S SERVE WITH

Pork or chicken sausage, bacon, or diced ham

A mix of berries or other fresh fruit

Cold applesauce

Breakfast Potatoes (page 312)

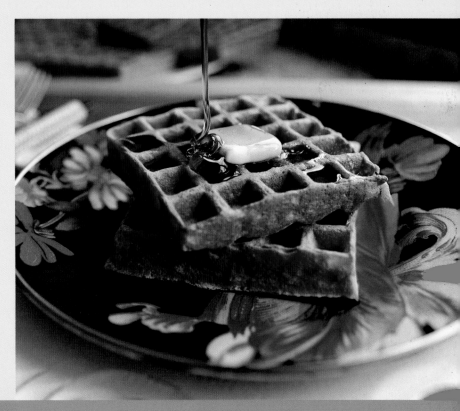

HUEVOS RANCHEROS

MAKES 1 OR 2 SERVINGS

Confession: I really don't know what "Huevos Rancheros" is. All I know is that it's some combination of eggs and tortillas and sauce. So I'm going to hold my figurative breath—figuratively hold my breath? Hold my breath figuratively? I never know the order of these things—and post the following, which, authentic Huevos Rancheros or not, is a delicious plateful of wonder.

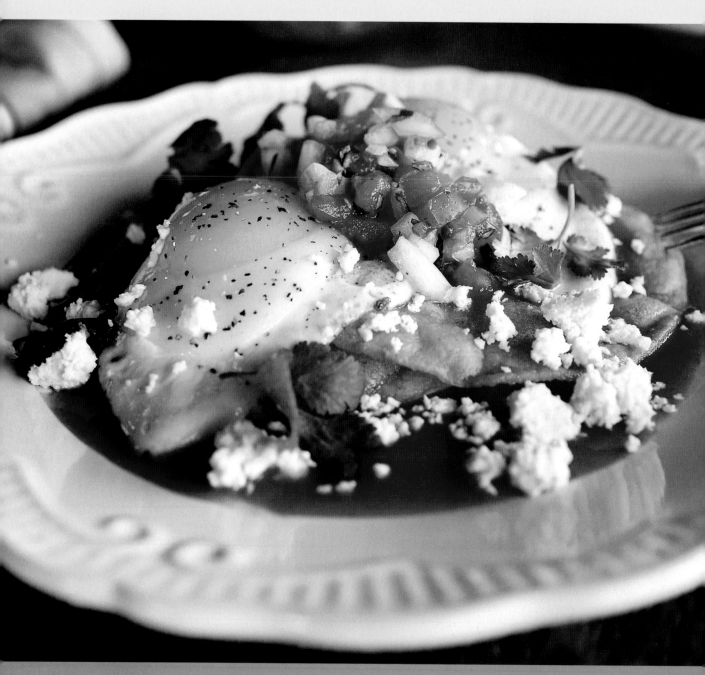

1 tablespoon butter

2 large eggs

Kosher salt and black pepper to taste

Vegetable oil, for frying

2 corn tortillas

½ cup Homemade Enchilada Sauce (page 8, or use canned), warmed

¼ cup crumbled Cotija cheese

2 tablespoons salsa or pico de gallo (see page 23)

Cilantro leaves, for garnish

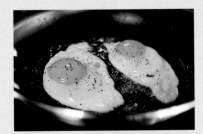

1. Melt the butter in a nonstick skillet over medium heat. Crack in the eggs, then turn the heat to low. Sprinkle with salt and pepper and cook until the whites are mostly set and the yolks are still very soft, about 3 to 4 minutes. You can place a lid on the skillet for the final minute of cooking to help set the whites on top. (If you prefer them cooked more fully, fry them 2 minutes per side.) Keep warm.

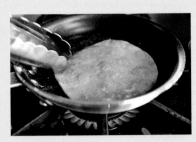

2. In a separate small skillet, heat ¼ inch of oil over medium heat and fry the tortillas one at a time until light brown and crisp, about 45 seconds, flipping them halfway through. Transfer them to paper towels to drain.

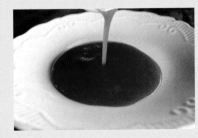

3. To serve, spoon half the enchilada sauce onto a plate.

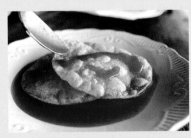

4. Overlap the tortillas on top of the sauce, then spoon the rest of the sauce over the top.

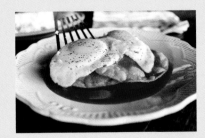

5. Add the eggs . . .

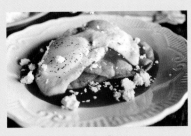

6. Sprinkle on the Cotija cheese . . .

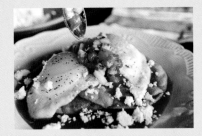

7. And add salsa or pico de gallo.

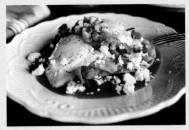

8. Finish with a sprinkling of cilantro leaves, then share it with a loved one . . . or just dig in by yourself! You'll absolutely love it.

V VARIATIONS

Warm the tortillas in the microwave for 20 seconds instead of frying them.

Use green enchilada sauce instead of red (or use both!).

Add a dollop of sour cream on top of the salsa or pico de gallo (see page 23).

S SERVE WITH

Cooked chorizo sausage

Diced sautéed ham

Breakfast Potatoes (page 312)

HOMEMADE ENCHILADA SAUCE

MAKES 3 CUPS

I don't have the slightest thing against canned enchilada sauce, and I always have plenty of it in my pantry. But whenever I get a chance, I make a batch or two of this homemade stuff. The secret really *is* in the sauce!

2 tablespoons vegetable oil

¼ cup finely chopped onion

1 tablespoon finely chopped garlic

¼ cup finely chopped red bell pepper

2 teaspoons chili powder

1 teaspoon ground cumin

¼ teaspoon cayenne pepper

¼ teaspoon kosher salt

¼ teaspoon black pepper

1 bouillon cube
(beef, chicken, or tomato)

1 tablespoon all-purpose flour

½ cup chicken broth

One 15-ounce can tomato sauce

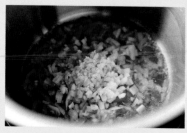

1. Heat the oil in a medium saucepan over medium heat. Add the onion, garlic, and bell pepper and cook until soft, about 2 minutes.

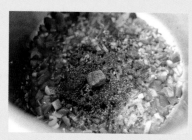

2. Add the chili powder, cumin, cayenne, salt, black pepper, and bouillon cube . . .

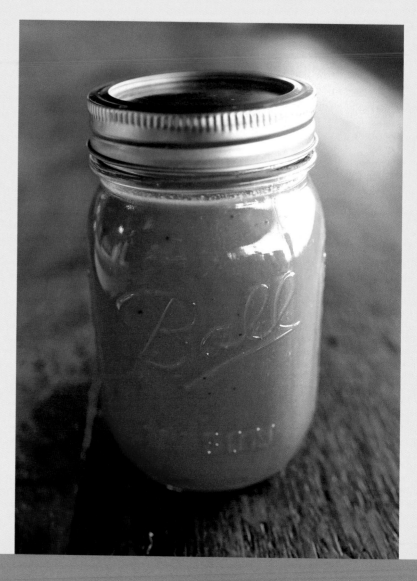

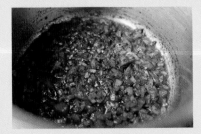

3. And cook for 2 minutes, until the spices darken and their flavors are released.

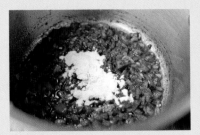

4. Sprinkle in the flour, stir to combine, and cook the mixture for another minute.

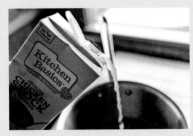

5. Add the broth and stir to combine . . .

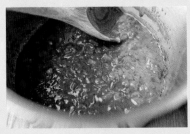

6. Then cook, stirring, until the liquid thickens, 2 to 3 minutes.

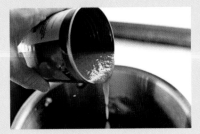

7. Add the tomato sauce . . .

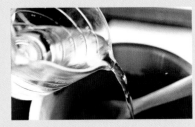

8. And 1½ cups water and bring to a boil.

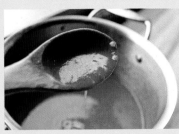

9. Cook the sauce until it has reduced by about a third and is nice and thick, 4 to 5 minutes.

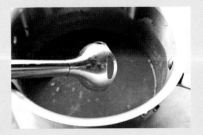

10. Let it cool slightly, then use an immersion blender to puree the sauce until completely smooth. (Alternatively, you can transfer it to a blender to puree it; just make sure the sauce is cooled, as blending hot liquids is dangerous!)

Ⓜ MAKE AHEAD

The sauce will keep in the refrigerator for up to a week and can also be frozen! Just reheat the sauce in a saucepan or skillet and use as the recipe calls for it.

Ⓤ USE IN

Huevos Rancheros (page 6)

Mexican Tortilla Casserole (page 130)

Ready-to-Go Beef Taco Filling (page 124)

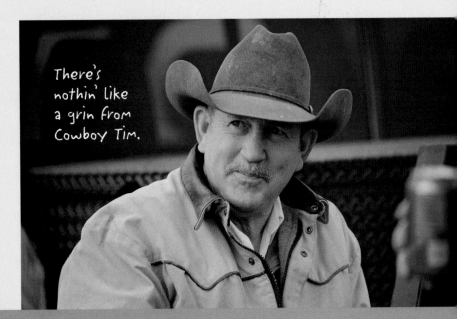

There's nothin' like a grin from Cowboy Tim.

FRITTATA

MAKES 8 SERVINGS

A frittata, my friends, is basically a crustless quiche, and one of the glorious things about it is that you cook the filling ingredients and bake the frittata in the same skillet. Super-simple, super-easy, and it's one of those fabulous dishes that works for breakfast, lunch, or dinner. I love that in a recipe!

Another huge advantage to frittatas is that you can use up a whole bunch of random leftover ingredients that might be languishing in your fridge, begging to be used. There's really no limit to what you can throw in, so just use this recipe as a general guide. Change up the cheeses and veggies, add meats . . . have some frittata fun!

Equipment note: While you could fight with a regular skillet and try to get the frittata not to stick, a good, *ovenproof nonstick skillet* really is essential when it comes to making frittatas. Being able to slide it neatly out of the pan and slice it up is the key to happiness.

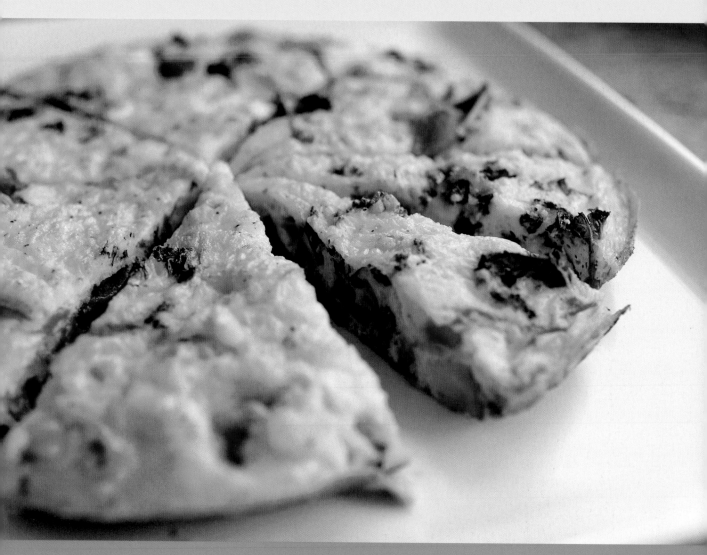

12 large eggs

Kosher salt and black pepper to taste

¼ cup grated Parmesan or Pecorino Romano cheese

½ cup grated Cheddar or Monterey Jack cheese

Several dashes of hot sauce (optional)

2 tablespoons butter

1 medium onion, halved and thinly sliced

1 russet potato, baked until tender (45 minutes at 375°F) and cut into cubes

2 cups torn kale leaves or whole spinach leaves

2 large jarred roasted red peppers, thinly sliced

¼ cup green or Kalamata olives, chopped

Fresh fruit, for serving

1. Preheat the oven to 375°F.

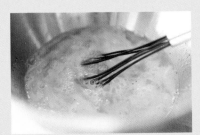

2. In a large bowl, whisk the eggs with salt and pepper.

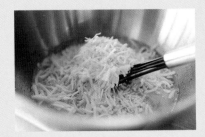

3. Add the grated cheeses and stir to mix them in with the eggs. Stir in the hot sauce, if using. Set it aside.

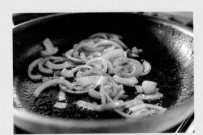

4. In a large ovenproof nonstick skillet, melt the butter over medium-high heat. Add the onion and cook for several minutes, stirring frequently, until the onion is soft and gorgeously golden.

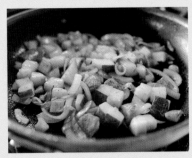

5. Add the potato, sprinkle with salt and pepper, and stir. Cook with the onion for a couple of minutes.

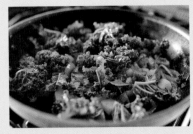

6. Add the kale and stir. Cook for a minute or so.

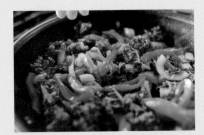

7. Finally, add the roasted red peppers and olives, stir them in, and arrange all the veggies evenly in the pan.

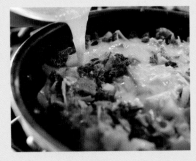

8. Slowly pour the egg mixture over the veggies, making sure it's evenly distributed in the middle and around the edge of the pan.

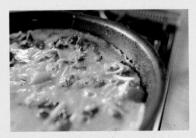

9. Keep the frittata on the burner for 30 to 45 seconds to set the edges, then put the skillet in the oven.

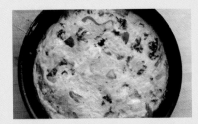

10. Bake the frittata for 10 to 12 minutes, or until the eggs are set. Keep an eye on it, though, and make sure it doesn't get too brown on top!

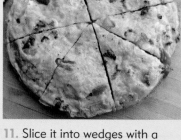

11. Slice it into wedges with a long, serrated knife . . .

V VARIATIONS

Sub in mushrooms, spinach, bell pepper, carrots, asparagus, or lots of other veggies.

Sub in pepper Jack, goat cheese, Fontina, or lots of other cheeses.

Add cooked, crumbled sausage, bacon, or finely diced ham.

S SERVE WITH

Kale Citrus Salad (page 40)

Roasted Grape Tomatoes (281)

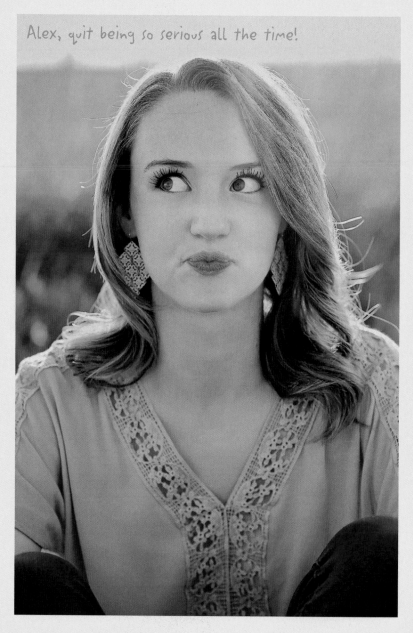

Alex, quit being so serious all the time!

12. And serve it with cool fresh fruit. I always want fruit with my frittata.

A fruit . . . and a frittata.

A fruit a frittata.

Afruita frittata.

Hakuna frittata.

HAKUNA MATATA. Sing it with me, everyone!

This is how my mind works.

(Enjoy the frittata!)

Note: Leftover frittata can be kept in the fridge and reheated!

CROISSANT FRENCH TOAST

MAKES 8 SERVINGS

Rather than subject you to a detailed description of how positively sublime this delectable dish is, I'll spare you all the adjectives and launch right into the recipe . . . but just trust me on this: You're gonna want to make it sometime this week. This lovely breakfast dish actually makes a pretty elegant dinner!

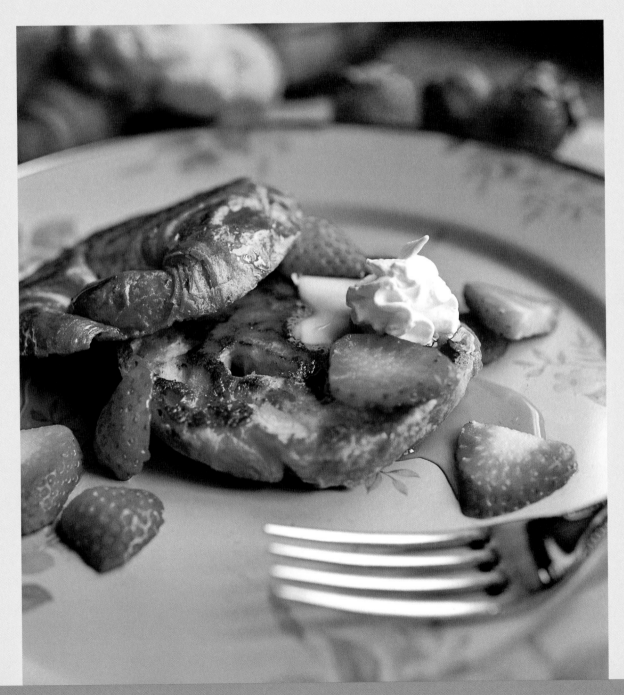

5 large eggs

¼ cup half-and-half

2 tablespoons sugar

1 teaspoon ground cinnamon

2 teaspoons vanilla extract

8 croissants (if they're a little stale, that's great!)

Butter, for frying and serving

Warm maple or pancake syrup, for serving

Strawberries, for serving

Whipped cream, for serving (optional)

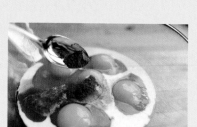

1. In a medium bowl, combine the eggs, half-and-half, sugar, cinnamon, and vanilla.

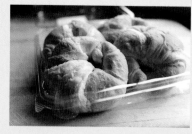

3. Grab the croissants . . .

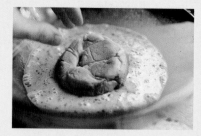

5. One by one, drop the croissants into the egg mixture . . .

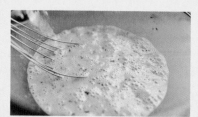

2. Whisk until totally combined.

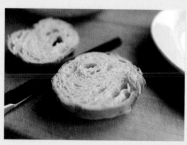

4. And use a serrated knife to slice them in half.

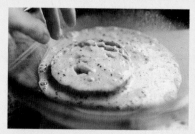

6. Flip them over . . .

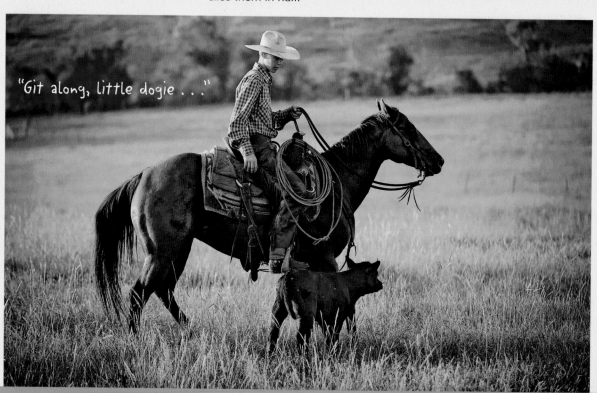

"Git along, little dogie . . ."

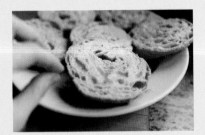

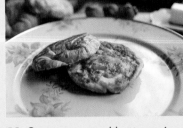

7. And set them on a plate while you dunk the rest!

10. Serve a top and bottom piece together on a pretty plate . . .

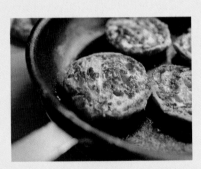

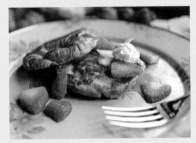

8. Heat a large skillet (nonstick works great!) over medium-low heat, then melt a small amount of butter in the pan. Add as many croissant halves as will fit, cut side down. Let the croissants cook for 3 to 4 minutes, moving them around the skillet to make sure they don't burn.

With butter, warm syrup, strawberries, and whipped cream, if you'd like.

9. Flip the croissants to the other side and cook for another 2 minutes or so. Transfer to a plate and repeat with the remaining croissants!

V VARIATIONS

Spread a small amount of cream cheese on the finished French toast before adding syrup, berries, and whipped cream.

Spoon applesauce on top of the finished French toast.

Drizzle French toast with a little caramel sauce for a decadent treat.

Use the same French toast recipe and procedure on banana bread or other quick bread.

S SERVE WITH

Regular or turkey bacon

Diced sautéed ham

Pork or chicken sausage links

Mixed berries, melon chunks, or other fruit

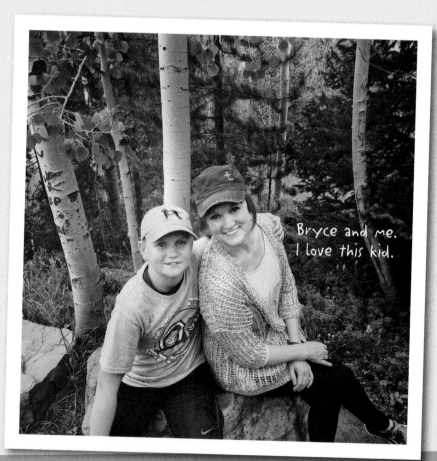

Bryce and me. I love this kid.

SCRAMBLES

EACH VARIETY MAKES 2 OR 3 SERVINGS

There's nothing quicker or easier than whipping up a big skillet of scrambled eggs, and if you throw in a bunch of simple add-ins, you can turn it into a delicious dinner in no time at all!

Unless you live on an isolated ranch and run out of eggs, in which case you will have to add the time it takes to find your shoes, put them on, drive to town, buy eggs, and drive back to the ranch.

Or, alternatively, you will have to add the time to convince your husband to build a chicken coop, procure some chickens, and wait for them to lay some eggs.

And at that point, the whole "quick and easy" angle to this recipe is pretty much shot. (But I'd encourage you to make it anyway!)

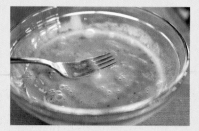

6 large eggs

¼ cup half-and-half

Kosher salt and black pepper to taste

To make each variety, mix together the eggs, half-and-half, and salt and pepper until combined. Then move on with the scramble you'd like to make.

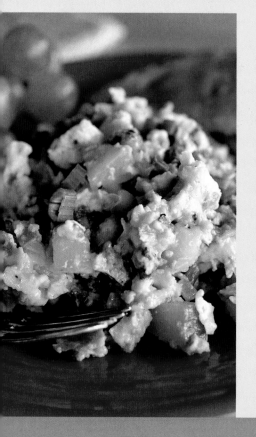
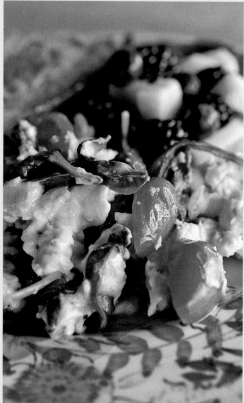
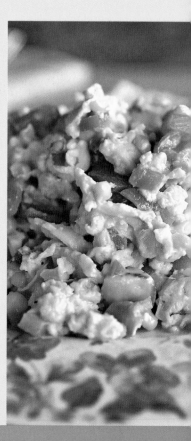

SANTA FE SCRAMBLE

Zesty flavor with warm chunks of creamy avocado. One of my faves!

2 tablespoons butter

½ cup fresh or frozen corn kernels

1 jalapeño, seeded and finely chopped

Scramble Mix (page 16)

½ cup diced green chiles (canned, or use fresh and roast them as on page 273)

1 avocado, pitted, peeled, and diced

 VARIATION

Add grated Monterey Jack cheese, diced tomatoes, and/or torn chunks of corn tortilla to the egg mixture.

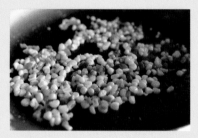

1. Melt the butter in a large skillet (I use nonstick) over medium-high heat. Add the corn and jalapeño and sauté for 1 to 2 minutes to soften.

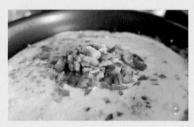

2. Lower the heat to medium-low. Pour in the egg mixture and add the chiles.

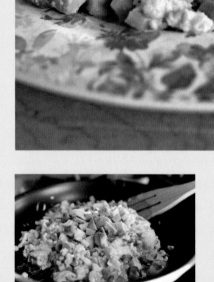

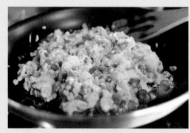

3. Stir and cook slowly until soft, creamy curds form and the mixture starts to come together.

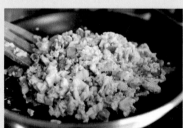

4. Add the diced avocado.

5. Stir in the avocado and continue cooking until the eggs are cooked.

MEAT AND POTATO SCRAMBLE

For the dudes (or dudettes) in your house who won't eat anything—even scrambled eggs—without meat.

2 tablespoons butter

½ onion, diced

4 slices bacon, cut into small pieces

½ pound breakfast sausage

1 small russet potato, baked until tender (45 minutes at 375°F) and diced

Kosher salt and black pepper to taste

Scramble Mix (page 16)

½ cup small-cubed Cheddar cheese

4 green onions, sliced

Ⓥ VARIATION

Add hot sauce to the egg mixture. Yum!

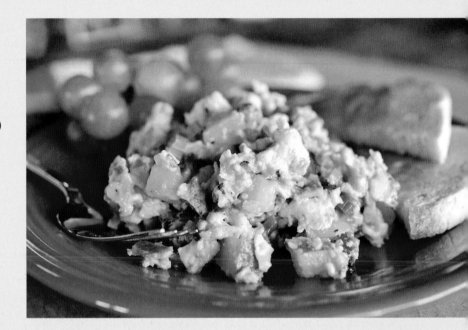

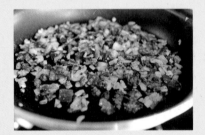

1. Melt the butter in a large skillet over medium-high heat. Add the onion, bacon, and sausage and sauté until the meats are cooked through and the onion is golden. Drain off the fat.

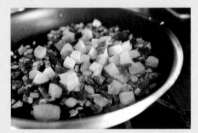

2. Add the potato, sprinkle with salt and pepper, and cook to warm the potato, about 3 minutes.

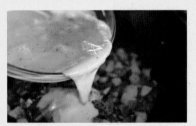

3. Lower the heat to medium-low. Pour in the egg mixture . . .

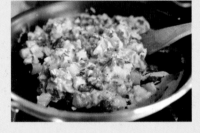

4. And cook until soft, creamy curds begin to form.

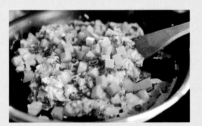

5. Add the cheese and green onions and stir until the eggs are cooked and the cheese is almost totally melted.

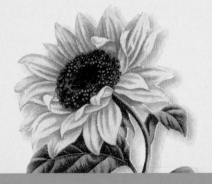

FLORENTINE SCRAMBLE

My very favorite kind of scramble, loaded with color, flavor, and goodness!

2 tablespoons butter
½ onion, diced
1 cup cherry tomatoes, halved

1 cup fresh baby spinach
Scramble Mix (page 16)
½ cup grated Swiss cheese

V VARIATIONS

Add crumbled goat cheese instead of (or along with!) the Swiss cheese.

Add chopped olives with the spinach and tomatoes!

S SERVE WITH

Wheat, white, rye, or sourdough toast

Warm corn tortillas

Fresh fruit

Breakfast Potatoes (page 312)

Sweet Potato Fries (page 308)

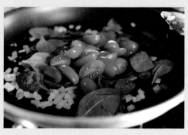

1. In a large skillet, melt the butter and sauté the onion until light golden brown, 3 to 4 minutes. Add the tomatoes and spinach and cook for 1 minute, until the spinach wilts slightly.

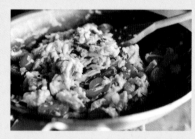

4. And stir until the cheese melts.

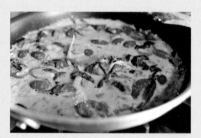

2. Pour in the egg mixture.

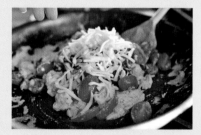

3. Stir and cook the eggs until they're almost completely set, then add the Swiss cheese . . .

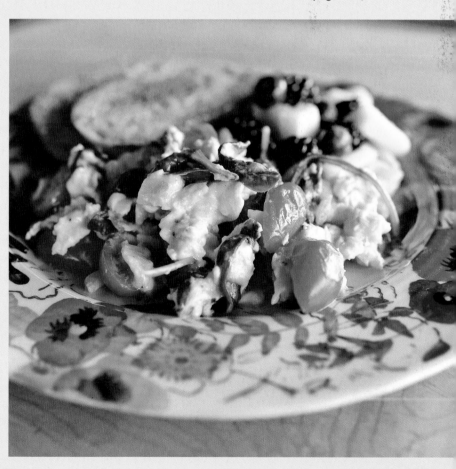

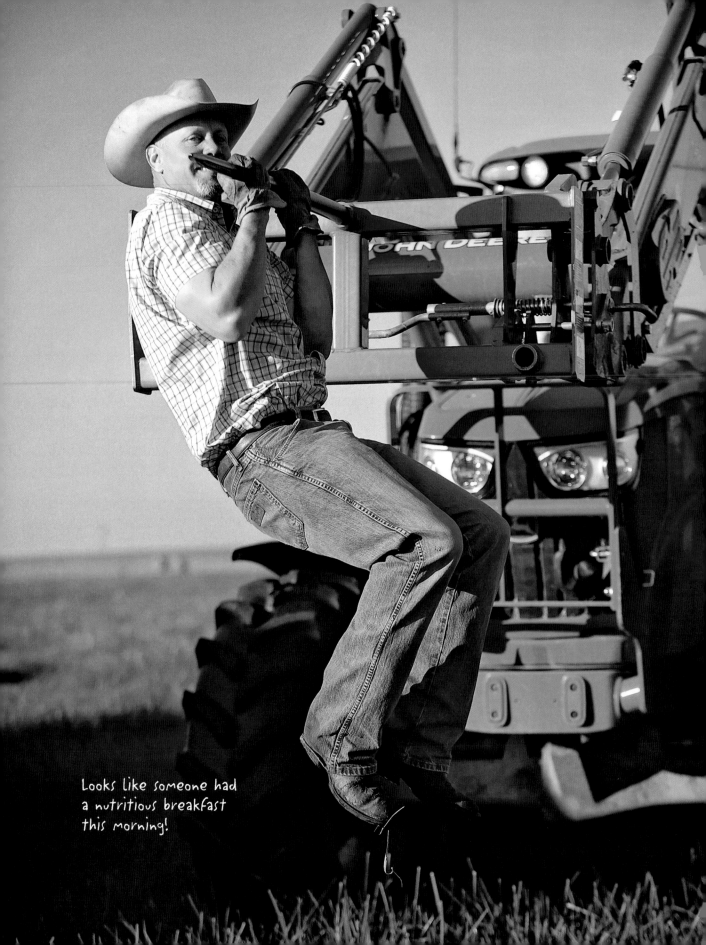

Looks like someone had a nutritious breakfast this morning!

BREAKFAST QUESADILLAS

MAKES 3 LARGE QUESADILLAS, TO SERVE ABOUT 6

"Knock it off, Napoleon! Make yourself a dang quesaDILLA!"

If you haven't seen the fine film *Napoleon Dynamite,* this quote might be a little confusing. And also, please go watch it today. The secrets of the universe are contained within.

Now, back to the recipe at hand: These are all that's wonderful, good, and holy about quesadillas, but with a breakfast twist, which, of course, is perfect for dinner! (Ha.) And you can serve 'em up on a plate with sour cream and pico de gallo as you would regular quesadillas . . . or you can just throw wedges at your loved ones as they head out the door on the way to a soccer game.

Let's go make ourselves a dang quesadilla! Napoleon's grandma would have wanted it that way.

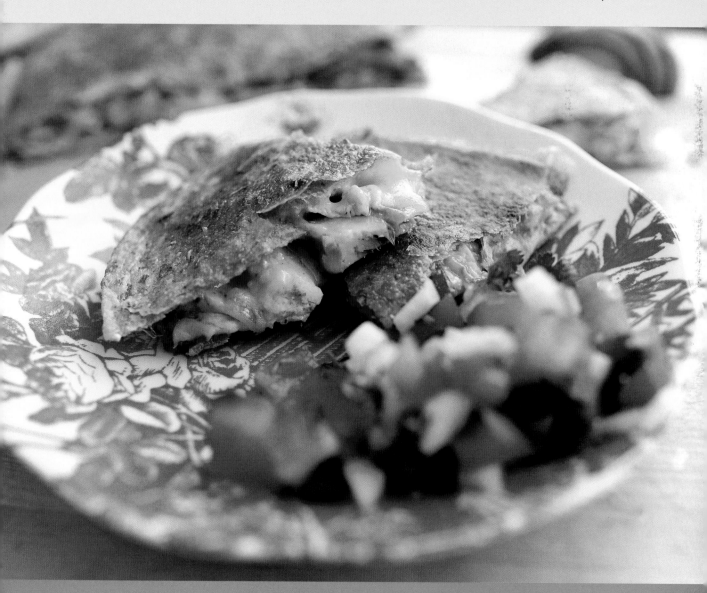

1 pound bacon

1 medium onion, diced

1 bell pepper (any color), seeded and diced

1 jalapeño, seeded and finely diced

1 tablespoon butter, plus more for frying the quesadillas

8 large eggs

¼ cup half-and-half

Kosher salt and black pepper to taste

6 large whole wheat tortillas

1½ cups grated Cheddar or Monterey Jack cheese

2 avocados, pitted, peeled, and sliced

Pico de gallo, (see opposite) for serving

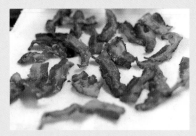

1. In a large skillet, fry the bacon over medium-high heat until crisp. Drain it on a paper towel . . .

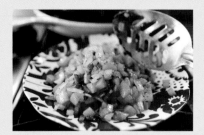

4. Remove them to a plate and set them aside. Reduce the heat to medium-low and add 1 tablespoon of butter to the pan.

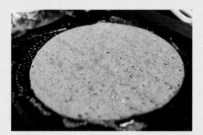

7. Now it's time to build the quesadillas! Melt some butter on a griddle or in a clean skillet and lay a tortilla on the butter.

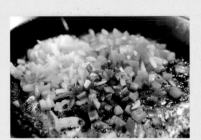

2. Then pour the excess grease out of the skillet (but don't clean the skillet!) and return it to the stove over medium-high heat. Throw in the onion, bell pepper, and jalapeño . . .

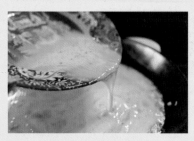

5. In a medium bowl, whisk together the eggs, half-and-half, and salt and black pepper. Pour the mixture into the pan.

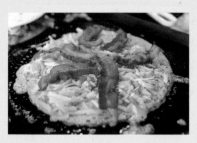

8. Add a generous layer of cheese, followed by several slices of bacon.

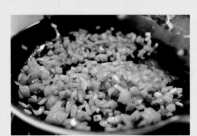

3. And cook them for several minutes, until the veggies start to soften and turn golden brown.

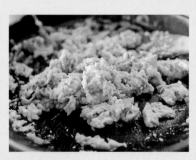

6. Cook the eggs, stirring them around the pan, until they're set. Remove them to a plate.

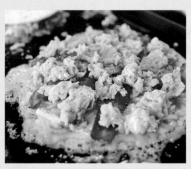

9. Top with a generous layer of eggs . . .

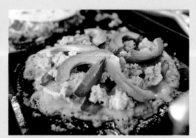

10. A few slices of avocado . . .

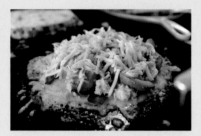

11. Another layer of cheese . . .

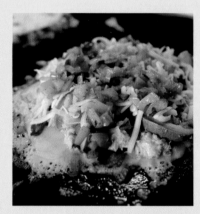

12. And, finally, the gorgeous sautéed veggies! (I'm a little worried this quesadilla isn't going to have enough filling. What about you?)

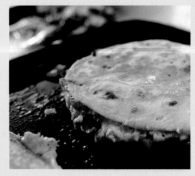

13. Top with a second tortilla, then flip to the other side once the cheese starts to melt. Things will calm down in there in no time!

V VARIATIONS

Use regular flour or corn tortillas.

Add chopped mushrooms to the veggie mixture.

Spoon salsa inside the quesadilla when assembling.

Serve with a dollop of sour cream.

S SERVE WITH

Fresh fruit salad

Breakfast Potatoes (page 312)

Black Bean Soup (page 77)

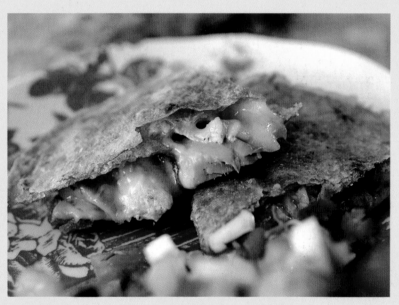

14. When the cheese has melted and the tortilla is as crispy as you want it, cut the quesadillas into wedges and serve with pico de gallo!

So darn delicious.

A QUICK PICO DE GALLO LESSON!

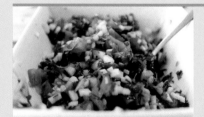

Combine equal amounts diced onion, tomato, and chopped cilantro in a bowl with finely diced jalapeño, lime juice, and salt to taste. Stir it together. Done! (Or you can buy good store-bought pico, if you prefer.)

LAZY CHILES RELLENOS

MAKES 8 TO 10 SERVINGS

This dish ain't fancy.

This dish ain't difficult to make.

This dish ain't . . . not delicious.

(Sorry. But I'm fluent in both Bad Grammar and Double Negative and I like to use them both occasionally so I won't get rusty.)

My mom used to make a dish like this, and it always goes over well no matter who I serve it to! It's a versatile, flavorful combination, and just like a good pair of jeans, it goes with everything.

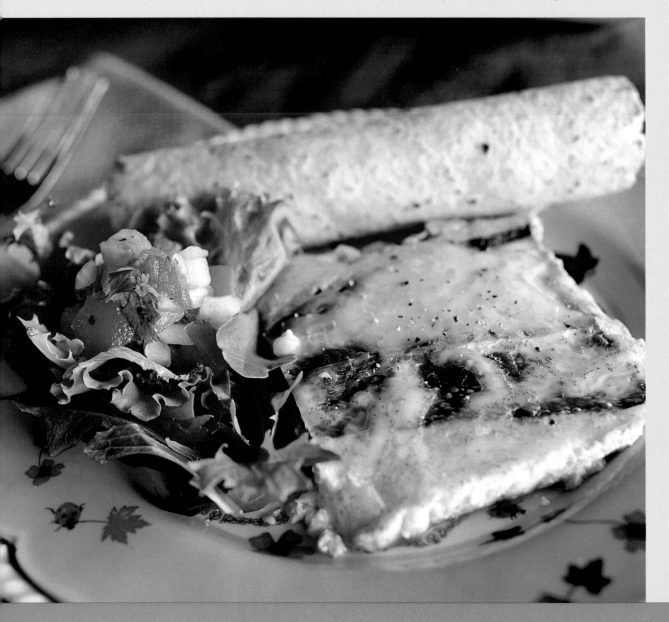

6 fresh poblano chile peppers (or you may use canned roasted green chiles)

5 large eggs

2 cups whole milk

Kosher salt and black pepper to taste

½ teaspoon paprika

¼ teaspoon cayenne pepper

1½ cups grated Monterey Jack cheese

Warm tortillas, for serving

1. Preheat the oven to 325°F.

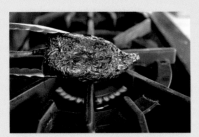

2. If you're using fresh poblanos, begin by roasting the peppers (if using canned, skip to step 5): Use tongs to hold the peppers over an open flame until the skin is completely charred. (If you don't have a gas burner, you can grill them or place them under the broiler in the oven.)

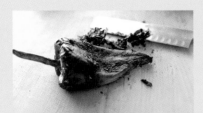

3. Place the charred peppers in a plastic bag and seal it to trap in the heat. Let the peppers stay in the plastic bag for 15 to 20 minutes to steam the skin off.

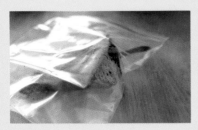

4. Use a knife to scrape the blackened skin off the peppers. (You can leave little bits behind for flavor.)

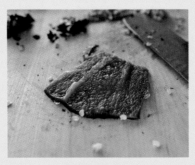

5. Slice open the peppers and scrape out the seeds.

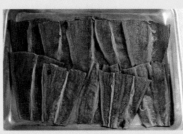

6. Cut each pepper in half.

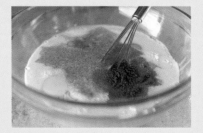

7. Next, in a large bowl, combine the eggs, milk, salt and black pepper, paprika, and cayenne.

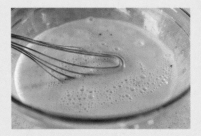

8. Whisk until totally combined.

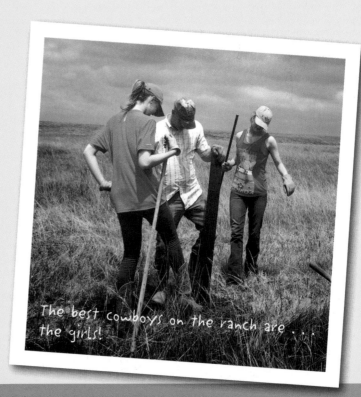

The best cowboys on the ranch are the girls!

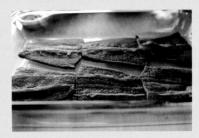

9. Now, to assemble the dish, arrange half the peppers in a single layer in a 9 x 13-inch baking pan.

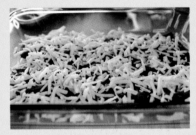

10. Sprinkle on half the cheese . . .

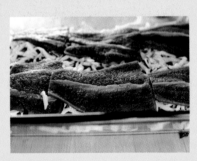

11. Then layer on the rest of the peppers . . .

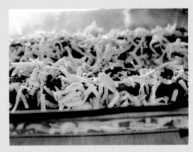

12. And the rest of the cheese.

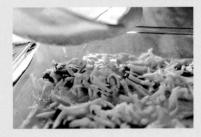

13. Pour the egg mixture evenly over the top.

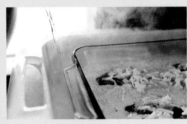

14. Finally, place the pan into a larger pan and pour hot water into the larger pan so that the level of the water reaches the level of the eggs. This helps the eggs cook evenly and keeps them from getting overcooked around the edges.

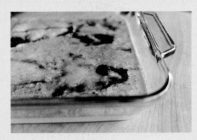

15. Carefully transfer the pan setup to the oven and bake for 35 to 40 minutes, or until the eggs are completely set. Watch to make sure the top doesn't get too brown.

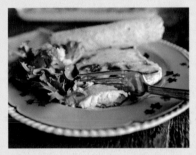

16. Let the casserole sit for 10 minutes, then slice it into squares and serve with warm tortillas.

Ⓜ MAKE AHEAD

The peppers can be roasted and peeled up to 3 days in advance, then stored in the fridge in a large zipper bag.

Several hours before, make the egg mixture, grate the cheese, roast the peppers, and keep them all in separate containers in the fridge. When you're ready, simply assemble the casserole and bake. Saves lots of last-minute time!

The casserole can be assembled up to 2 hours before baking and kept in the fridge.

Ⓥ VARIATIONS

Use sharp Cheddar or pepper Jack cheese instead of Monterey Jack.

Add diced fresh tomatoes to the egg mixture.

Top with pico de gallo (see page 23) and a dollop of sour cream.

Ⓢ SERVE WITH

Green salad

Fruit salad

Grilled chicken or steak as a side dish alongside

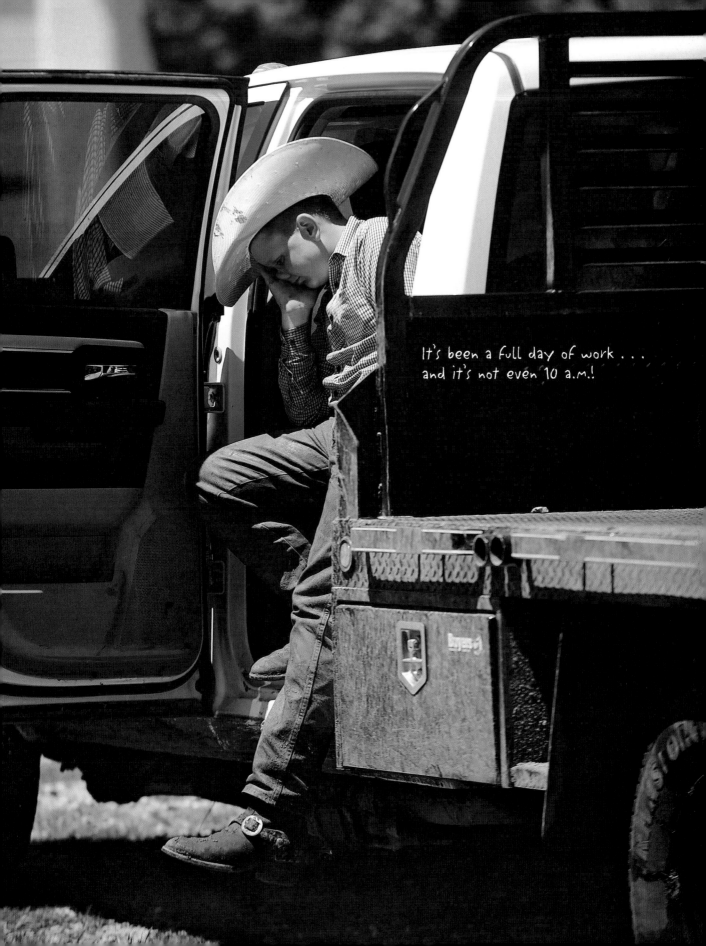

It's been a full day of work . . .
and it's not even 10 a.m.!

BREAKFAST HASH

MAKES 4 SERVINGS

I love hash, because first of all, the name is so fun to say, especially when you're telling your kids what's for dinner.

"Mom!!!!!!!! What's for dinner???????"

"Hash."

"Hash?"

"Hash."

"Hash?"

"Hash."

"Okay . . . thanks?"

I don't know, there's just something so final about it. Nobody has any clever replies!

Also, it reminds me of *The Little Rascals,* when the kids would often eat mush for dinner. And while hash isn't really anything like mush, this gave me the opportunity to mention one of my favorite TV shows of all time.

I miss you, Spanky.

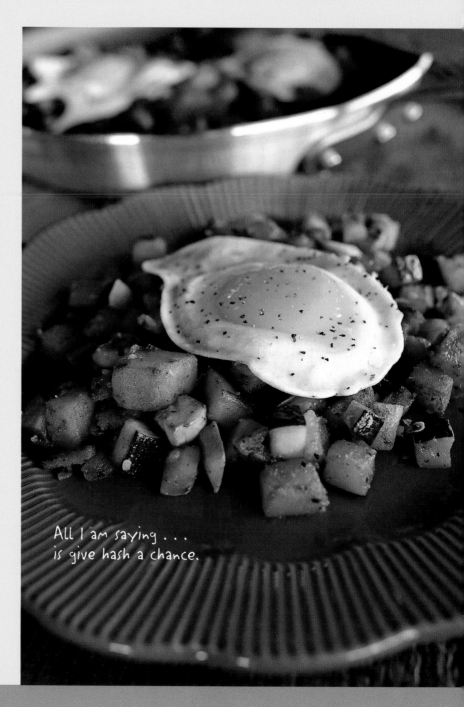

All I am saying . . .
is give hash a chance.

4 tablespoons (½ stick) butter

½ red onion, chopped

1 cup chopped zucchini

1 cup chopped red bell pepper

1 cup chopped yellow squash

**Kosher salt and black pepper
to taste**

**1 russet potato, baked until
tender (45 minutes at 375°F),
peeled, and diced**

**1 sweet potato, baked until tender
(45 minutes at 375°F), peeled,
and diced**

4 fried eggs (see page 7)

Hot sauce, for serving

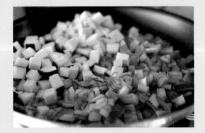

1. Melt 2 tablespoons of the butter in a large skillet over medium-high heat. Add the onion, zucchini, bell pepper, and squash.

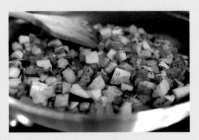

2. Sprinkle the mixture with salt and pepper and cook until the veggies are golden brown, 4 to 5 minutes.

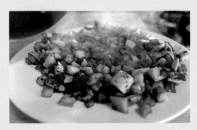

3. Remove the veggies to a plate. Try not to eat them—they're good!

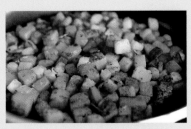

4. Add the remaining 2 tablespoons butter and the potatoes and sweet potatoes. Stir them around and cook for about 5 minutes, until golden.

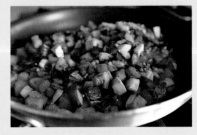

5. Add the veggies back in . . .

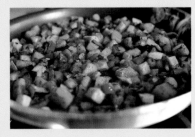

6. And stir everything together.

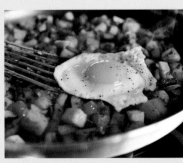

7. Add the eggs to the skillet and serve the skillet on the table!

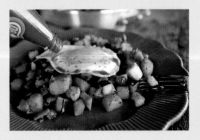

(*Pssst*. A little hot sauce makes it perfect.)

Ⓜ MAKE AHEAD

Bake the potatoes ahead of time and store in the fridge for up to 3 days.

Ⓥ VARIATIONS

Add chopped mushrooms to the veggie mixture.

Use diced green or yellow bell pepper in the veggie mixture instead of the red bell pepper.

Add diced ham to the veggie mixture.

Serve the hash without the eggs as a side dish for any main course.

Ⓢ SERVE WITH

Green salad

Warm corn or flour tortillas

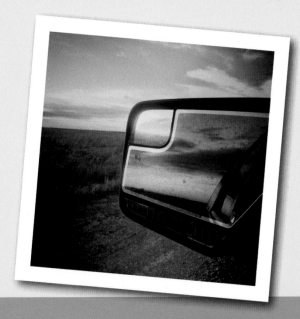

WILD RICE PANCAKES

MAKES 6 SERVINGS

Before I begin explaining this uniquely delicious recipe, I need to state for the record that I love the state of Minnesota. I've visited four times now, and I want to marry it for the following reasons:

1. The climate. I don't sweat there. And that translates to Heaven in my book.

2. The people. What's in the water up there? Everyone is seriously lovely and so kind.

Another reason I love Minnesota is that wild rice is everywhere. Seriously everywhere. You look out the window? You see wild rice. You shake hands with someone? There's a package of wild rice in his hands. You order pancakes from room service? They have wild rice in 'em! I found this out firsthand during one of my stays, and my life has never, ever been the same. The texture . . . the slightly nutty flavor . . . they're unforgettable! And they make a nice, hearty dinner.

1 cup uncooked wild rice

3 cups all-purpose flour

¼ cup ground flaxseed meal* (optional! But good.)

½ teaspoon kosher salt

2 tablespoons baking powder

¼ cup sugar

3½ cups whole milk, more as needed

2 large eggs

1 tablespoon vanilla extract

2 tablespoons butter, melted, plus more for frying and serving

Warm maple or pancake syrup, for serving

*Ground flaxseed meal can be found in most major supermarkets and specialty markets.

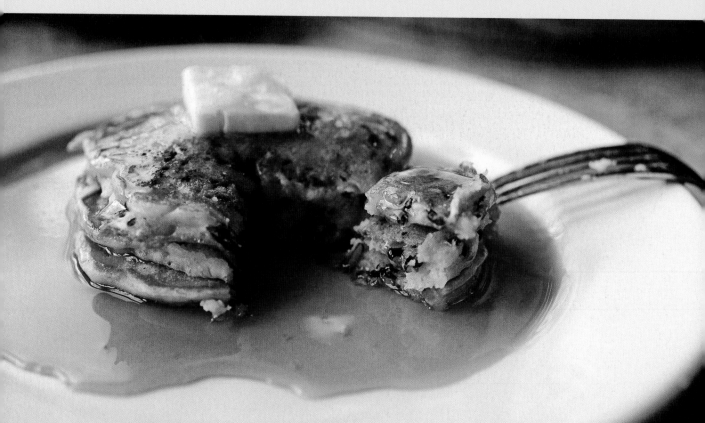

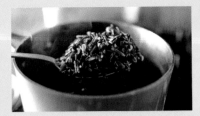

1. Cook the wild rice in water according to the package directions. (Keep in mind that this could take up to 45 minutes!) Set it aside to cool slightly.

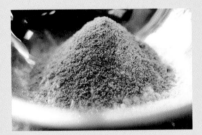

2. In a large bowl, combine the flour, flaxseed meal, salt, baking powder, and sugar. Stir it together.

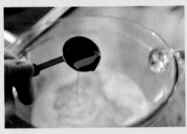

3. In a pitcher, whisk together the milk, eggs, and vanilla.

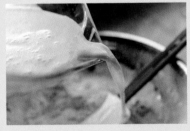

4. Pour the wet mixture into the dry mixture, stir it until halfway combined, then pour in the melted butter . . .

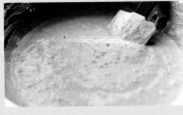

5. And stir the batter until it just comes together. If the batter seems too thick, stir in a little more milk until the consistency is right. It should be thick but still pourable.

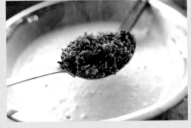

6. Add half the wild rice . . .

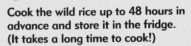

7. Then stir it in and take a gander. Keep adding more rice until the batter contains the amount you'd like. (I added all the rice myself; other folks may prefer slightly less rice.)

M MAKE AHEAD

Cook the wild rice up to 48 hours in advance and store it in the fridge. (It takes a long time to cook!)

V VARIATION

Add ⅓ cup chopped pecans or walnuts to the pancake batter.

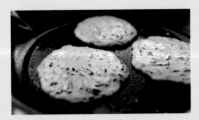

8. Heat a skillet or griddle over medium-low heat and coat it with butter. Drop ¼-cup scoops of batter onto the pan and cook the pancakes on both sides until deep golden brown. Repeat with the rest of the batter.

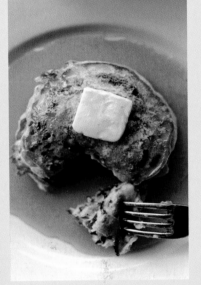

9. Serve the pancakes with a generous amount (that means a heckuva lot) of softened butter and warm syrup!

S SERVE WITH

Regular or turkey bacon

Sautéed diced ham

Pork or chicken sausage links

Fresh fruit

THE CARB BUSTER

MAKES 1 OR 2 SERVINGS

I ordered a dish similar to this when I was staying in a hotel in New York, and I re-create it at home from time to time, whether it's for breakfast, lunch, or dinner! It's chock-full of veggies and topped with perfect poached eggs, and it makes a lovely, satisfying supper any day of the week.

1 tablespoon butter or olive oil

½ medium onion, cut into chunks

½ zucchini, cut into chunks

½ yellow squash, cut into chunks

Kosher salt and black pepper to taste

1 tomato, sliced thick

1 teaspoon vinegar

2 large eggs

1 thin cheese slice (Monterey Jack, mozzarella, Cheddar—whatever you like!)

1. Bring a medium saucepan of water to a gentle boil over medium heat.

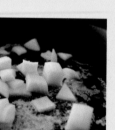

2. Melt the butter (or heat the olive oil) in a large skillet over medium heat. Add the onion . . .

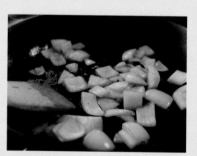

3. And cook it for 2 to 3 minutes, or until it's turning golden and starting to soften.

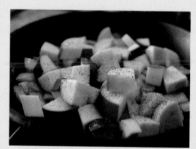

4. Add the zucchini and squash and sprinkle it with salt and pepper . . .

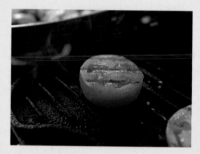

5. And stir. Cook for 3 to 4 minutes, until the veggies are cooked but still somewhat firm. Remove them from the heat and set them aside.

6. In a grill pan or skillet, grill or sauté the tomato slices for a couple of minutes on each side, just to slightly soften them and give them some nice color on the outside. Remove them from the pan and set them aside.

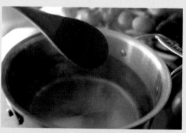

7. To poach the eggs, add the vinegar to the pan of boiling water. Use a wooden spoon to carefully stir the water into a circular "whirlpool."

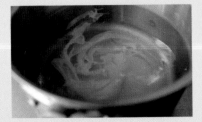

8. Once the whirlpool is swirling, crack in one of the eggs. The egg will swirl around itself and eventually begin to set. Let it stay in the water for about 1 minute (or longer, if you'd like a more set yolk) . . .

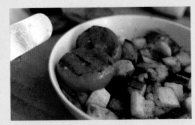

9. Then remove it from the pan with a slotted spoon and set it on a plate while you poach the second egg. (Note: You can do both at once if you're feeling adventurous!)

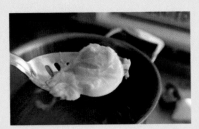

10. To assemble the dish, pile the veggies in a bowl and add the tomato slices.

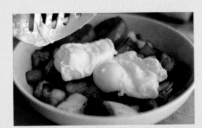

11. Add the eggs . . .

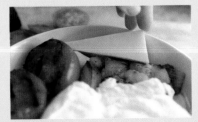

12. Then cut the cheese in half and lay the slices on the side. The warmth of the veggies will immediately start to soften the cheese, and oh . . . the bliss.

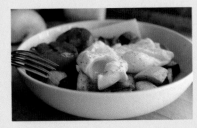

13. Sprinkle the eggs with a little salt and pepper, then break into the yolk and dig in. You will be a very happy human!

V VARIATIONS

Scramble or fry the eggs rather than poach them.

Add mushrooms, bell peppers, carrots—any vegetable you'd like.

Add diced ham to the veggie mixture as you cook it.

Top the eggs with a little hot sauce.

For a decadent twist, spoon warm hollandaise sauce over the eggs. Wow!

S SERVE WITH

Pork or chicken sausage links

Fresh fruit

Doughnuts. Of course, we'll then need to change the name of this recipe.

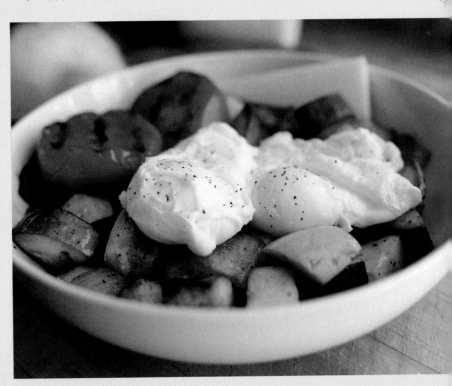

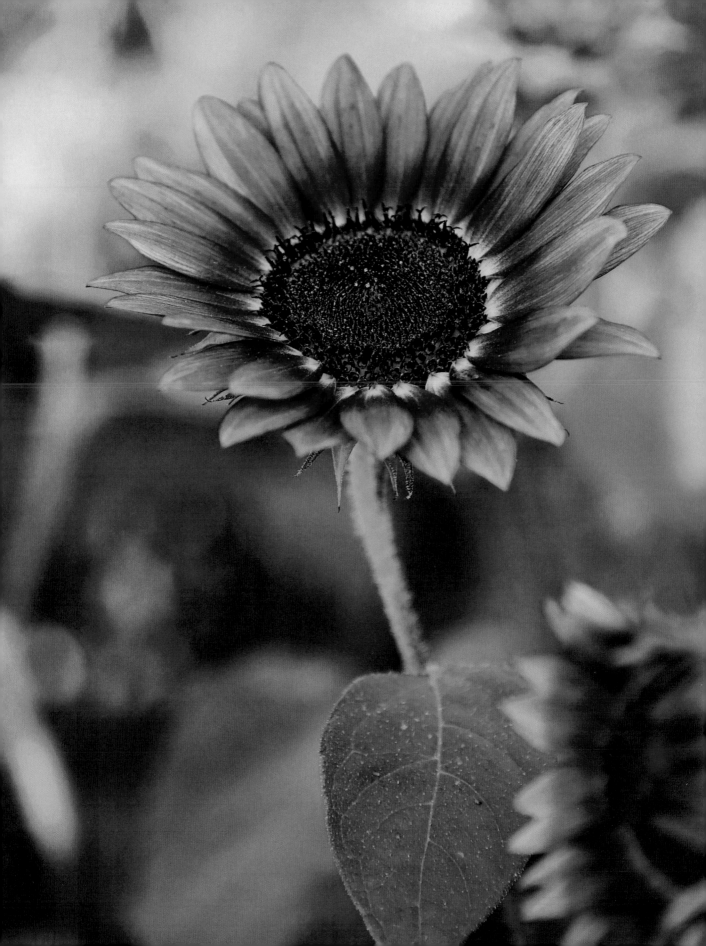

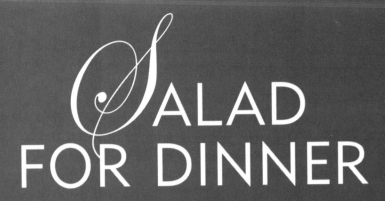

SALAD FOR DINNER

Salads need not be relegated to appetizer or side status! A gorgeous, crunchy salad bursting with color and flavor (and veggies and protein and cheese and all sorts of other fun stuff) is sometimes all you need at suppertime. (Plus, look at it this way: You'll feel less guilty about dessert!) Go ahead and crunch your way to bliss with these main dish beauties.

GINGER STEAK SALAD

MAKES 2 OR 3 SERVINGS

I love steak salads in pretty much any form, and this Asian-inspired beauty is a favorite of mine. You can grill the steak fresh or—one of my favorite tricks—use leftover grilled steak right out of the fridge. The flavors are fab, the textures terrific, and the colors . . . pretty.

I couldn't think of an adjective that conveyed "pretty" but began with the letter "C." Sorry.

So I think I'll just make the salad.

DRESSING/MARINADE

¼ cup low-sodium soy sauce

¼ cup olive oil

2 tablespoons sherry or white wine vinegar

2 tablespoons fresh lime juice

1 tablespoon brown sugar

4 garlic cloves, minced

2 tablespoons finely minced fresh ginger

½ jalapeño, seeded and finely diced

SALAD

One 8-ounce rib-eye, strip, or sirloin steak

2 tablespoons olive oil

5 cups salad greens (baby lettuce, endive, radicchio—whatever you like!)

4 green onions, sliced

1 cup assorted cherry tomatoes, halved

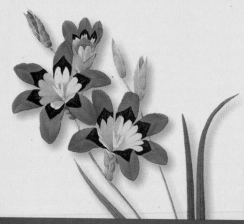

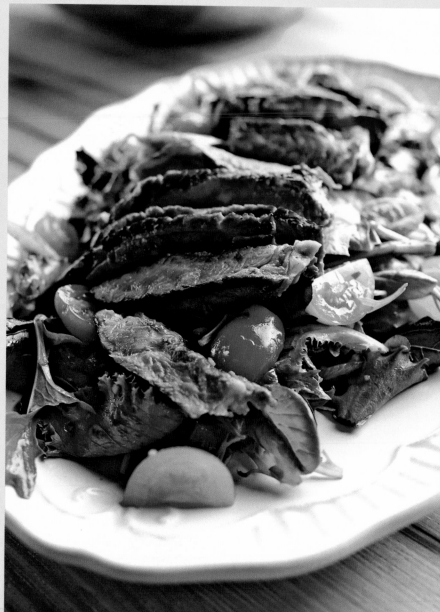

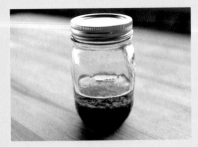

1. Make the dressing: Combine the soy sauce, olive oil, sherry, lime juice, brown sugar, garlic, ginger, and jalapeño in a small jar.

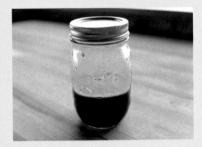

2. Shake it for a good 30 to 40 seconds, until it's all combined. Give it a taste and add more of whatever you'd like! (Some folks like it a little sweeter, some like it more spicy, and so on.)

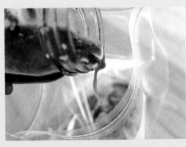

3. Place the steak in a plastic bag and pour in half the dressing/marinade. Seal the bag, forcing out the air, and let the steak marinate in the fridge for an hour, or up to 6 hours if you have the time! Store the remaining dressing in the fridge.

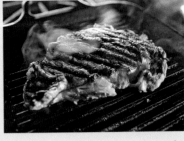

4. After the steak has marinated, heat the olive oil in a grill pan or skillet over medium-high heat. Cook the steak for 1½ to 2 minutes per side, or until medium-rare. (The thickness of your steak will determine the cooking time.)

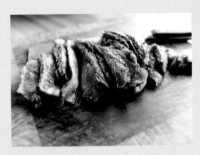

5. Remove the steak from the pan and allow it to rest for 5 minutes, then slice it into strips.

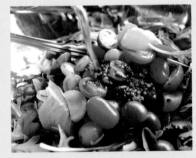

6. In a large bowl, combine the greens, green onions, and tomatoes. Pour in the rest of the dressing, toss to combine, and transfer the salad to a large serving platter.

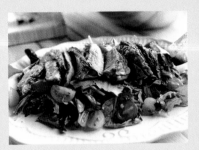

7. Arrange the strips of steak all over the top.

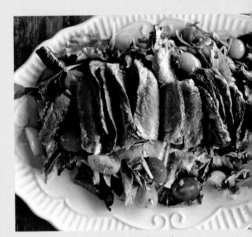

Mmmm. Steak salad. Definitely one of my favorite things!

M MAKE AHEAD

Grill the steak up to 12 hours in advance and store in the fridge. Slice it just before serving, and serve the steak cold.

Make the dressing/marinade up to 3 days in advance and store it in the fridge. Give it a good shake before using!

V VARIATION

Top the salad with grilled shrimp or chicken instead of steak.

S SERVE WITH

The Bread (page 336)

Chow Mein (page 174)

Sweet Potato Fries (page 308)

SESAME CHICKEN SALAD

MAKES 6 SERVINGS

I ordered a salad similar to this one while Paige and I were in Kansas for a soccer tournament one cold fall weekend. We had gone back to the hotel room after her first morning game and planned to take advantage of being in civilization by getting all spiffed up and going out for lunch at an area restaurant, then doing a little shopping.

Instead, once we got back to the room, we took off our shoes, splayed out on the bed, and decided to order room service. I mean, we don't get the opportunity to go out to eat in restaurants together on a daily basis . . . but we *sure* don't get the opportunity to order room service. So we picked the more indulgent of the two luxuries—room service—and enjoyed every darn bite.

Here's my take on the room service salad I ordered: The flavors are yummy, but the colors are just gorgeous, too. One of the purtiest salads this side of the Mississippi!

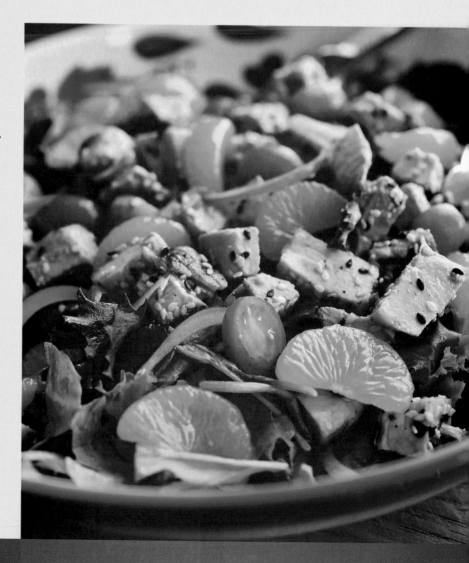

DRESSING

⅔ cup olive oil

¼ cup low-sodium soy sauce

¼ cup rice vinegar or white vinegar

2 garlic cloves, minced

2 tablespoons minced fresh ginger

1 teaspoon toasted sesame oil

2 tablespoons brown sugar, more to taste

¼ teaspoon red pepper flakes

SALAD

Olive oil, for drizzling

2 boneless, skinless chicken breasts

Kosher salt and black pepper to taste

1 tablespoon white sesame seeds

1 tablespoon black sesame seeds

8 cups mixed greens

½ red onion, very thinly sliced

1 cup red grape or cherry tomatoes, halved

One 11-ounce can mandarin oranges, drained

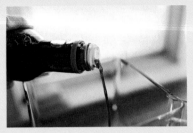

1. To make the dressing, combine the olive oil, soy sauce, vinegar, garlic, ginger, sesame oil, brown sugar, and red pepper flakes in a blender.

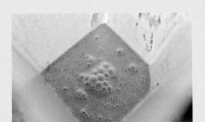

2. Blend until completely emulsified. Taste the dressing and adjust to your liking!

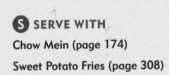

3. Heat a grill pan or skillet over medium heat and drizzle with olive oil. Sprinkle both sides of the chicken with salt and pepper and cook until done in the middle, about 5 minutes per side.

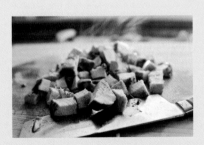

4. Cut the chicken into cubes.

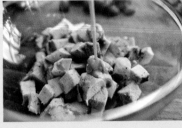

5. Throw the chicken into a bowl and pour in about one-third of the dressing, tossing to coat the chicken.

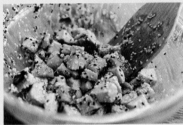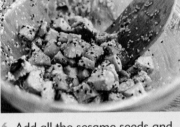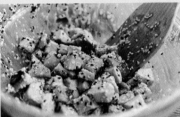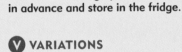

6. Add all the sesame seeds and toss the chicken to coat.

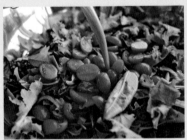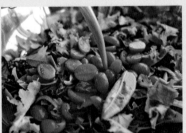

7. Place the greens, onion, and tomatoes in a large bowl. Pour on half the remaining dressing, reserving the rest if you'd like more later. Toss to coat.

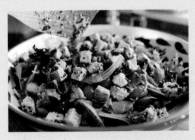

8. Top the salad with the sesame chicken . . .

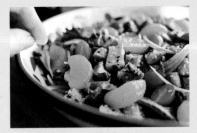

9. Then arrange the mandarin oranges all over the top.

You'll love this salad!

Ⓜ MAKE AHEAD

Make the dressing up to 24 hours in advance and store in the fridge.

Ⓥ VARIATIONS

Swap in thawed Ready-to-Go Grilled Chicken (page 110) to save time.

Use grilled shrimp or sliced grilled steak instead of chicken.

Add halved, seeded, and sliced cucumber to the salad with the tomatoes.

Use shaved kale (as prepared on page 41) instead of mixed greens.

Ⓢ SERVE WITH

Chow Mein (page 174)

Sweet Potato Fries (page 308)

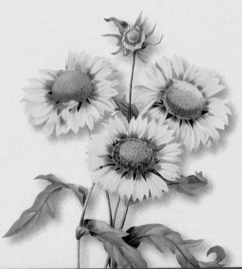

KALE CITRUS SALAD

MAKES 4 SERVINGS

A couple of years ago, I needed to go to Los Angeles for a couple of days, so I took along my two lifelong friends Connell and Becky, since the three of us don't get to see one another much. We had such a fun time: stayed in a swanky (for us, anyway!) hotel, ate, walked around Hollywood, ate, shopped, ate, reminisced, ate, laughed, ate, ate, ate, and ate.

We had more than one delicious meal on our girls' trip, but ironically, the dish that left the greatest impression on me was a salad like this one, which we had in the restaurant of our hotel! I wound up re-creating it within a day of returning to the ranch because it was truly the most enjoyable salad I'd ever had in my life.

If you are a lover of all things kale, this salad will knock your socks off. And if you don't have much experience with kale . . . well, consider this the perfect introduction.

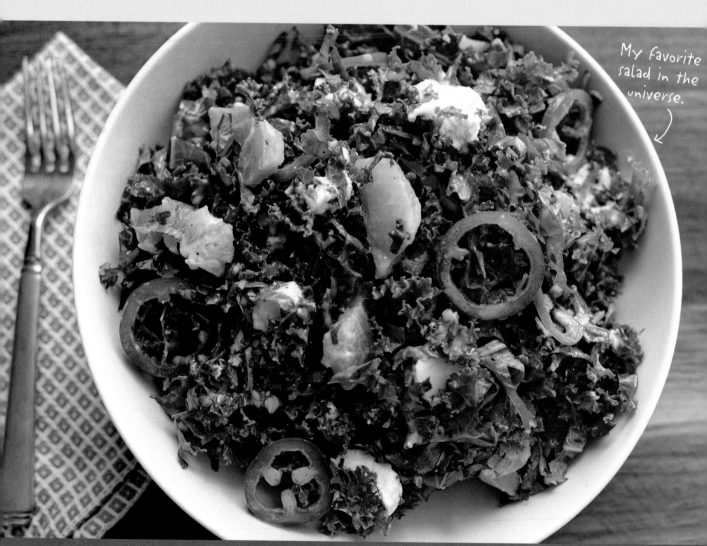

My favorite salad in the universe.

SALAD

1 bunch kale

1 jalapeño

3 tangerines or clementines

4 ounces goat cheese

CREAMY CITRUS DRESSING

¼ cup orange juice

1 garlic clove

2 tablespoons olive oil

1 teaspoon sugar

Pinch of kosher salt

Pinch of black pepper

1 heaping tablespoon sour cream or Greek yogurt

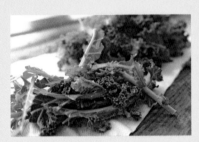

1. Start by prepping the kale: Rinse it well, then pull the leaves off the stalks. (The stalks can be discarded.)

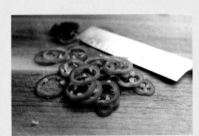

4. Next, cut the ends off the jalapeño and use a sharp knife to cut very thin slices. Use a spoon to clear as many seeds out of the centers as you can so that you mostly just have green circles.

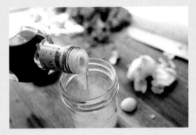

7. Add the olive oil . . .

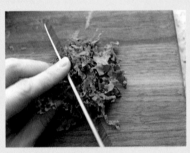

2. Working in bunches, roll up the kale leaves into a tight roll and use a sharp knife to slice it very thin.

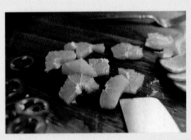

5. Peel the tangerines or clementines, then slice them and cut them into chunks.

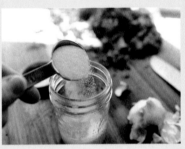

8. Along with the sugar, salt, and pepper. Put the lid on the jar and shake it vigorously for about 30 seconds. And congratulations! You've just gotten your exercise for the day.

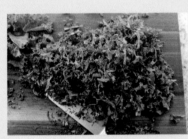

3. Keep going until you have a big pile of gorgeous shaved kale!

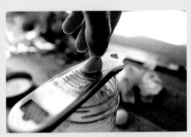

6. To make the dressing, pour the orange juice into a small jar and grate or press in the garlic.

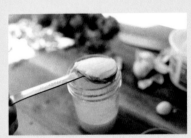

9. Finally, add the sour cream or Greek yogurt, whichever you prefer . . .

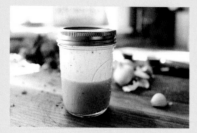

10. And shake it again until it's all incorporated. This dressing is *GOOD* with a capital G. Actually, a capital G, O, O, and D. Creamy, bright, and sassy. Great on lots of different salads!

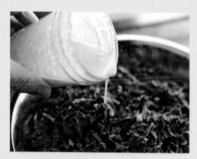

11. Put the kale in a large bowl . . .

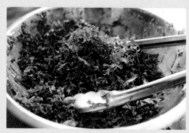

12. And pour on half the dressing. Toss the kale and let it sit for a few minutes. (That, by the way, is the great thing about kale: It holds up and almost gets better if it sits in the dressing for a bit.)

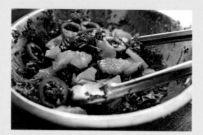

13. After it has sat for a bit, add the jalapeños and citrus and toss to combine . . .

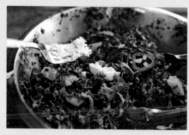

14. Just before serving, crumble in the goat cheese and very lightly toss it in. (The kale will stick to the goat cheese, and each bite of it is just about the loveliest thing on earth.)

Ⓜ MAKE AHEAD

Prep the kale, peel and chop the clementines, slice the jalapeños, and make the dressing up to 24 hours ahead of time and store them in separate containers in the fridge. Makes assembling the salad easy!

Ⓥ VARIATIONS

Substitute feta cheese for the goat cheese.

Substitute strawberries for the citrus.

Sprinkle sunflower seeds or chopped pecans over the finished salad.

Add grilled chicken or shrimp.

Ⓢ SERVE WITH

Crusty dinner rolls

Cheese Biscuits (page 332)

Sweet Potato Fries (page 308)

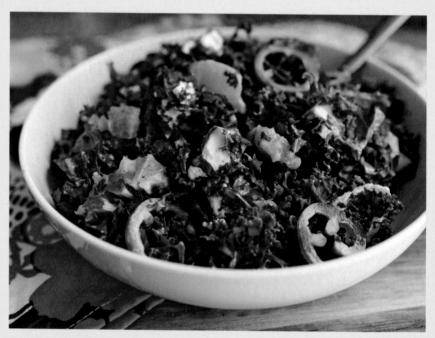

Ohhhh, baby. Do I love this salad. I know you'll love it, too!

GRILLED CHICKEN AND STRAWBERRY SALAD WRAP

MAKES 8 SERVINGS

Would it be a cliché to say "yum" in a cookbook? If so, I'm in big, big trouble.

And furthermore: *Yum*.

I made this deliciously simple salad one Sunday after church, and since I was ravenously ravenous, I decided to introduce some carbs into the picture and turn the salad into a wrap. It was so utterly delightful: fresh, crunchy, with a nice combination of protein and fruit and greens . . . oh, and goat cheese.

Oh, and a few other things, too.

2 boneless, skinless chicken breasts

½ cup balsamic vinaigrette (bottled, or make your own as on page 65), more as needed

Olive oil, for drizzling

6 cups mixed salad greens

12 medium strawberries, hulled and quartered

4 ounces goat cheese

8 whole wheat tortillas (optional)

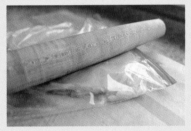

1. Place the chicken breasts in a large plastic bag. Seal the bag and use a rolling pin to pound the breasts to a uniform ½ inch thick.

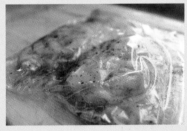

3. Then seal the bag and let the breasts marinate in the fridge for 1 hour.

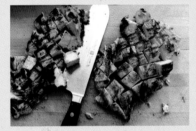

5. Let the chicken cool slightly, then dice it into bite-size pieces.

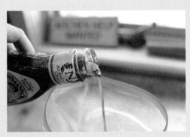

2. Pour in ¼ cup of the balsamic vinaigrette . . .

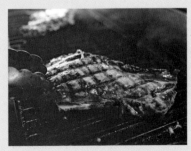

4. Heat a grill pan or skillet over medium heat and drizzle with olive oil. Cook the chicken until done in the middle, 3 to 4 minutes per side.

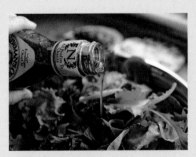

6. To assemble the salad, place the greens in a large bowl and pour the remaining ¼ cup (or more, if you'd like!) vinaigrette over the top. Toss to coat.

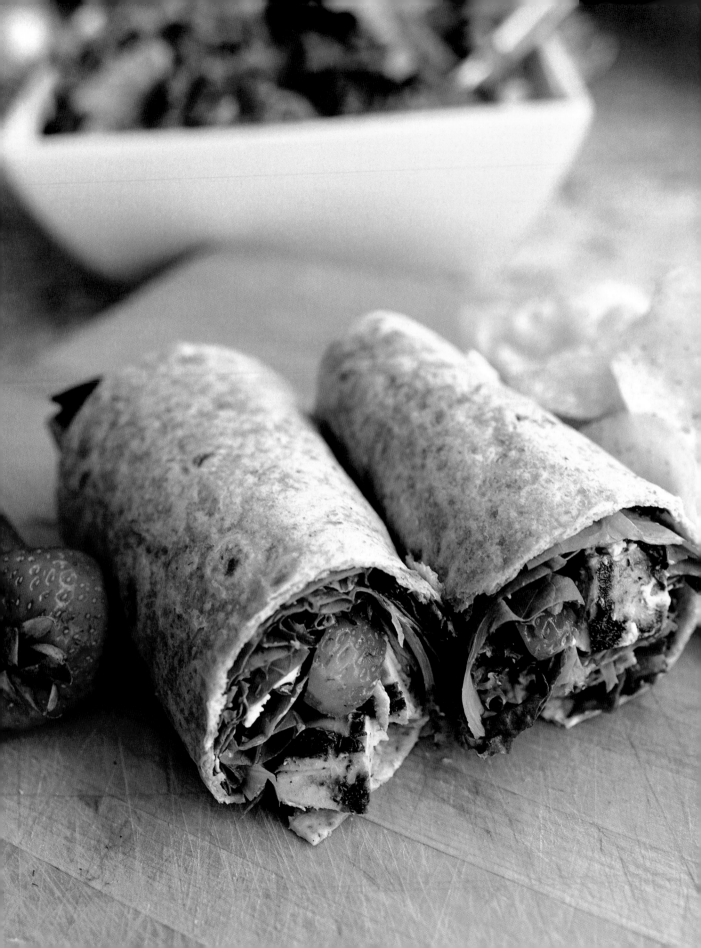

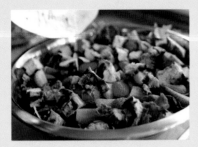

7. Add the strawberries and the chicken.

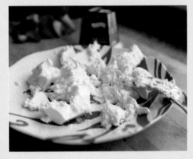

8. Use a fork to break up the goat cheese into large chunks . . .

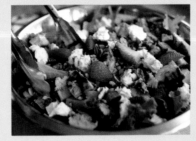

9. Then add the goat cheese to the salad and toss all the ingredients together. Serve it as is on big dinner plates . . .

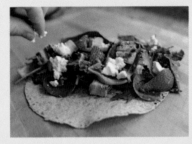

10. Or pile some of the salad onto a whole wheat tortilla . . .

11. Then roll it up and slice it in half. Such a tasty, fresh meal!

Ⓜ MAKE AHEAD

Marinate and grill the chicken up to 2 days in advance and store in the fridge. Dice before serving.

Ⓥ VARIATIONS

Use shaved kale (as prepared on page 41) instead of salad greens.

Add cubed fresh mozzarella cheese to the salad.

Add blueberries along with the strawberries.

Omit the chicken for a vegetarian salad.

Ⓢ SERVE WITH

The Bread (page 336)

Refrigerator Rolls (page 334)

Roasted Asparagus (page 280)

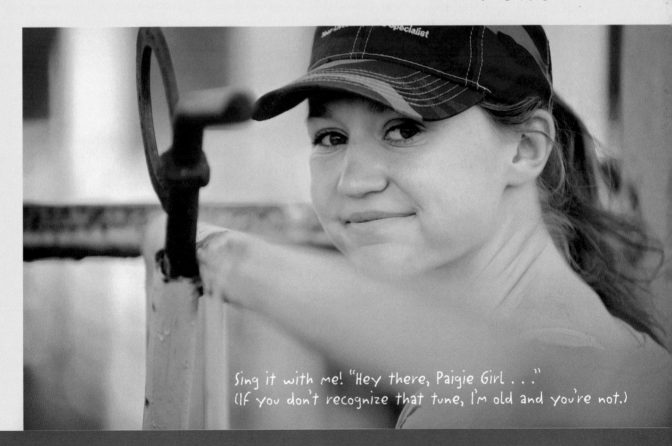

Sing it with me! "Hey there, Paigie Girl . . ."
(If you don't recognize that tune, I'm old and you're not.)

PANZANELLA

MAKES 8 SERVINGS

In a very tasty nutshell, panzanella is tomato-bread salad. I imagine it was originally created as a way to use up old, staling bread, as that is panzanella's key component. And I can't remember the first time I ever tried it, but panzanella has been one of my favorite delights for years and years. There's just something special about it, and it makes for a simply lovely dinner.

1 loaf very crusty Italian bread, preferably day-old, cut into 1-inch cubes

¼ cup olive oil, plus more for drizzling

1 tablespoon red wine vinegar

Kosher salt and black pepper to taste

6 tomatoes (different colors are nice), cut into wedges

1 English cucumber, halved, seeded, and thinly sliced

Block of Parmesan cheese, for shaving

25 basil leaves, more to taste, cut into chiffonade

½ red onion, very thinly sliced

1. Preheat the oven to 275°F.

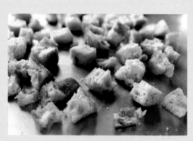

2. Arrange the bread cubes on a rimmed baking sheet, drizzle them lightly with olive oil, and bake for 20 to 25 minutes, or until crisped slightly. Set aside to cool.

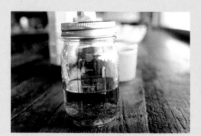

3. Next, make the super-simple dressing: Place the olive oil, vinegar, and salt and pepper in a jar . . .

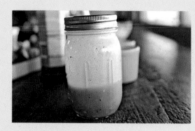

4. And shake it for 30 to 45 seconds, until it's totally combined.

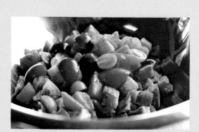

5. Place the bread cubes in a large bowl and throw in the tomatoes.

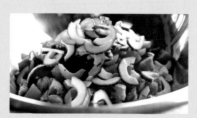

6. Add the cucumber . . .

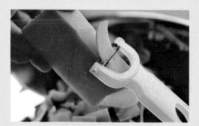

7. Then shave in a good amount of Parmesan . . .

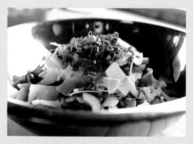

8. And add the basil.

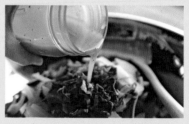

9. Drizzle the dressing all over the top . . .

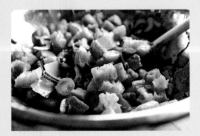

10. And toss until everything is combined.

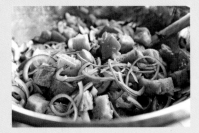

11. Finally, toss in the red onion! And if you have time, cover the bowl and let it sit at room temperature for an hour before serving.

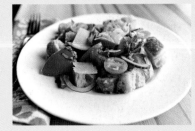

12. I'm not sure I've ever been able to wait that long, though. I love it so much!

Ⓜ MAKE AHEAD

You may cut the bread into cubes, lay them on baking sheets, and allow them to stale naturally at room temperature for 48 hours. Omit the crisping process in the oven.

The salad can be assembled up to 2 hours before serving.

Ⓥ VARIATIONS

Add cooled Beautiful Roasted Vegetables (page 290) to the bowl with the bread and tomatoes.

Add cubed fresh mozzarella cheese.

Add shaved kale (as prepared on page 41) along with the tomatoes.

Ⓢ SERVE WITH

Ready-to-Go Grilled Chicken (page 110)

Potato Soup (page 74)

Pan-Fried Pork Chops (page 156)

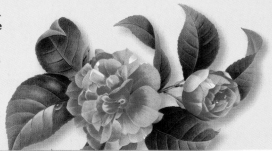

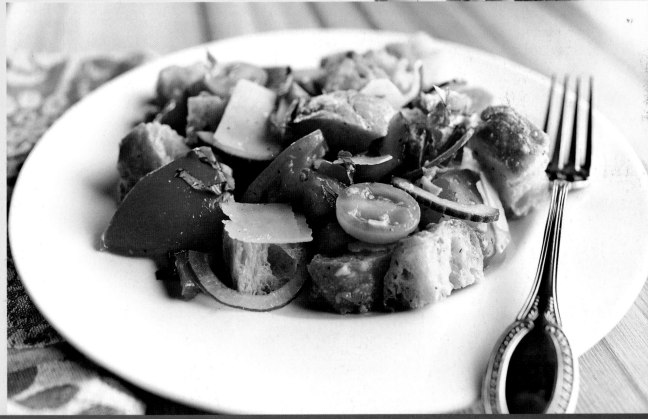

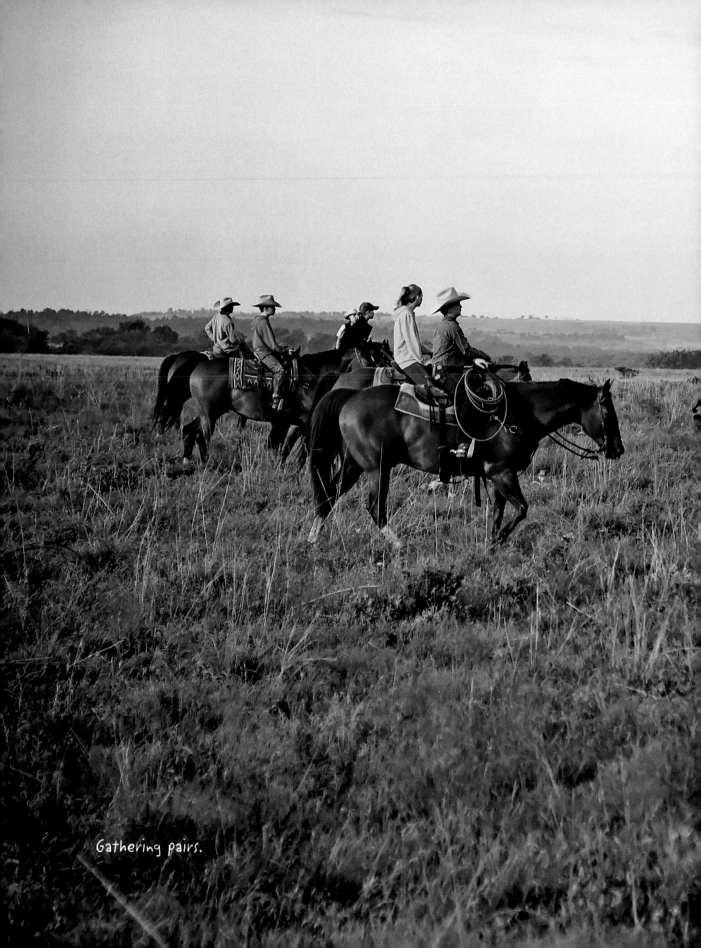

Gathering pairs.

COBB SALAD

MAKES 8 TO 12 SERVINGS

I love a good Cobb salad. My mom used to order them at restaurants when I was younger, and I knew I had truly become a grown-up when I started ordering them, too. (And when I could no longer eat Ding Dongs with impunity . . . but that's another story for another time.) I love Cobb salads because there are so many different things going on, and it's really hard to get bored: crisp greens, grilled chicken, eggs, bacon, avocado, tomato. And to tie it all together, creamy blue cheese dressing. A perfectly satisfying supper, whether for your family or for company.

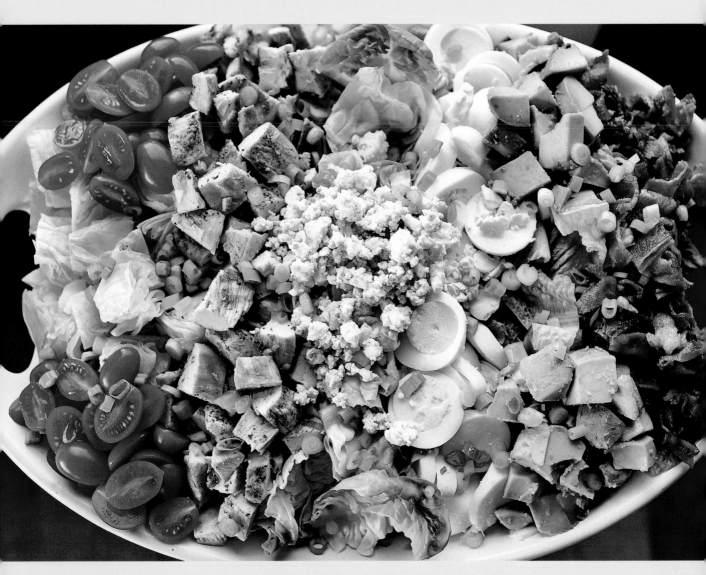

BLUE CHEESE DRESSING

1 cup mayonnaise

½ cup sour cream

½ cup buttermilk (or mix ½ cup milk with 1 tablespoon white vinegar and let it sit for 3 minutes to make homemade buttermilk)

4 ounces blue cheese, crumbled (about ½ cup)

2 tablespoons chopped chives

3 dashes of Worcestershire sauce

Pinch of kosher salt

½ teaspoon black pepper

SALAD

2 boneless, skinless chicken breasts, sliced in half down the middle (you'll be left with 4 very thin breast-shaped chicken pieces)

Olive oil, for drizzling

Kosher salt and black pepper to taste

2 romaine lettuce heads, chopped

1 iceberg lettuce head, cut into chunks

2 Bibb lettuce heads, cored and leaves separated

6 hard-boiled eggs (see Note), peeled and sliced

2 avocados, pitted, peeled, and diced

1 pound thin bacon, fried until crisp and chopped

2 cups red grape tomatoes, halved

⅓ cup crumbled blue cheese

Black pepper to taste

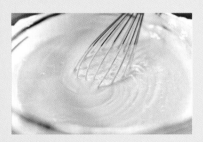

1. To make the dressing, in a medium bowl, mix together the mayonnaise, sour cream, and buttermilk until smooth.

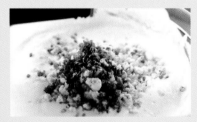

2. Add the blue cheese, chives, Worcestershire, salt, and pepper . . .

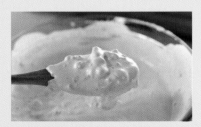

3. And stir it all together. Yum!

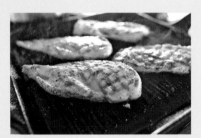

4. Heat a grill pan or skillet over medium-high heat and drizzle with olive oil. Sprinkle the chicken with salt and pepper and cook until done in the middle, about 3 minutes per side (it's nice and thin, so doesn't take too long).

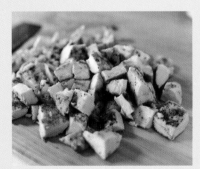

5. Let the chicken cool, then dice it up and set it aside.

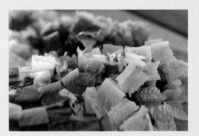

6. To assemble the salad, arrange the three lettuces on a large platter in separate piles.

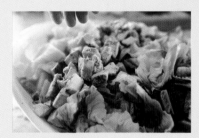

7. Lay on the chicken . . .

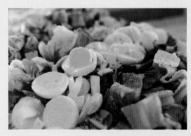

8. And the hard-boiled eggs . . .

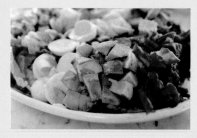

9. Then add a pile of avocado, a pile of chopped bacon . . .

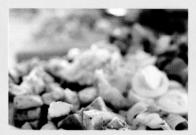

10. And a pile of tomatoes.

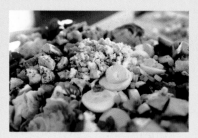

11. Place a pile of blue cheese in the center, then sprinkle some black pepper all over the salad.

12. Serve with a dish of blue cheese dressing and a hearty salad appetite.

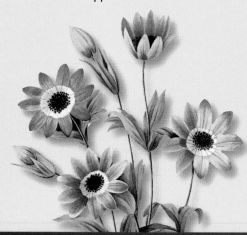

N NOTE

To make perfect hard-boiled eggs, place eggs in a saucepan and cover with 3 inches of cold water. Bring the water to a rolling boil, then turn off the heat. Allow the eggs to sit in the water for 12 minutes, then drain off the hot water and replace it with 6 cups of ice. Allow the eggs to cool down in the ice (it will melt!), then peel and use them as needed (or store them in the fridge for up to 1 week).

M MAKE AHEAD

Prep the lettuces and store in the fridge.

Grill and dice the chicken and store in the fridge.

Fry and chop the bacon, and store in the fridge. Heat it in the microwave for 20 seconds just before adding to the salad.

Slice the eggs and tomato and store in the fridge.

Make the dressing up to 3 days in advance and store in the fridge.

V VARIATIONS

Use thawed Ready-to-Go Grilled Chicken (page 110) to save time.

Substitute grilled shrimp for the chicken.

Use crumbled feta instead of blue cheese.

Add grilled corn to the salad.

Add a couple of spoonfuls of salsa to the dressing to give it a zesty kick.

S SERVE WITH

Crusty Italian bread

Cheese Biscuits (page 332)

The Bread (page 336)

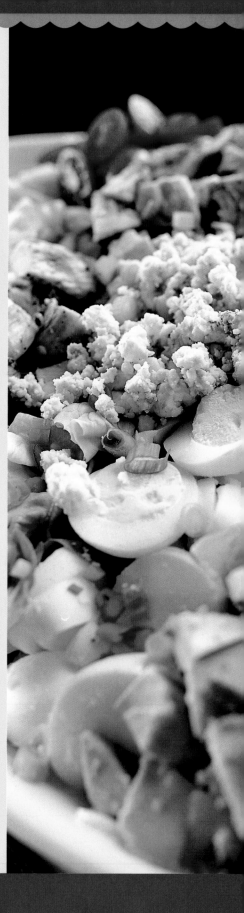

CHICKEN TACO SALAD

MAKES 8 SERVINGS

You can pretty much put any taco ingredient in a taco salad, but instead of stuffing it all inside taco shells, you crumble the taco shells and sprinkle them on top! It's as pretty as it is satisfying, and when you're all done eating, your appetite won't even notice that you just had a salad for dinner.

I love playing mind games with my stomach!

That made absolutely zero sense.

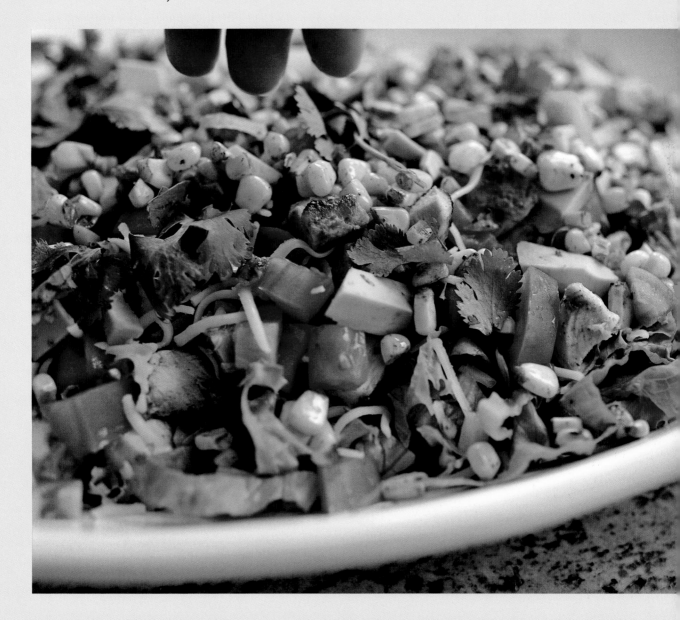

CHICKEN

2 boneless, skinless chicken breasts

2 tablespoons taco seasoning (store-bought, or your own mix)

¼ cup vegetable oil

DRESSING

¾ cup ranch dressing (bottled or homemade)

¼ cup salsa (as spicy as you'd like!)

3 tablespoons chopped cilantro

SALAD

2 ears fresh corn, husks and silk removed

1 large head green-leaf lettuce, thinly shredded

3 Roma tomatoes, diced

½ cup grated pepper Jack cheese

2 avocados, peeled, pitted, and diced

½ cup cilantro leaves

Tortilla chips of your choice, slightly crushed

3 green onions, sliced

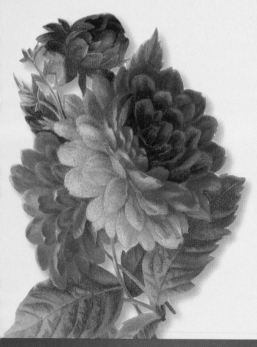

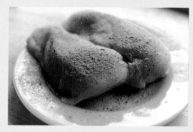

1. Season the chicken generously on both sides with the taco seasoning . . .

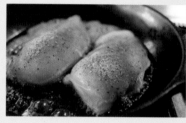

2. Then heat the vegetable oil in a large skillet over medium-high heat and cook the chicken on both sides until it's done in the middle, about 8 to 12 minutes total, depending on thickness.

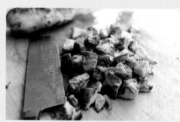

3. Remove the chicken from the pan, let it rest for 10 minutes, and then dice it up.

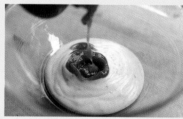

4. Meanwhile, make the dressing: Combine the ranch dressing and salsa in a bowl . . .

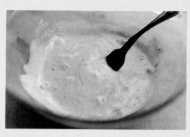

5. Stir it together . . .

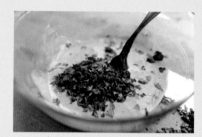

6. Then add the cilantro and stir until it's all combined.

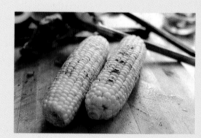

7. To make the salad, grill the corn in a grill pan or a skillet until there's a little color on the outside.

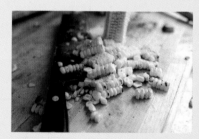

8. Then, using a sharp knife, slice off the kernels.

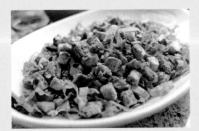

9. Now assemble the gorgeous salad! Pile the shredded lettuce on a platter, then sprinkle the chicken all over the top.

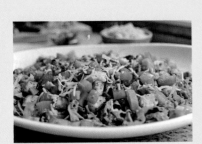

10. Add a layer of tomatoes . . .

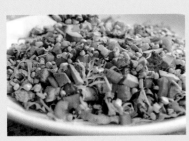

11. A sprinkling of cheese . . .

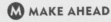

12. The diced avocado and grilled corn . . .

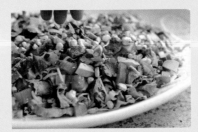

13. A generous sprinkling of cilantro leaves . . .

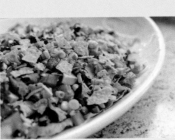
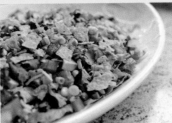

14. And a nice crunchy layer of crushed chips.

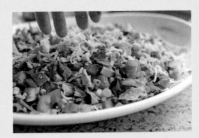

15. Finally, some green onion . . .

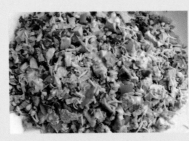

16. And some drizzled dressing (alliteration alert!).

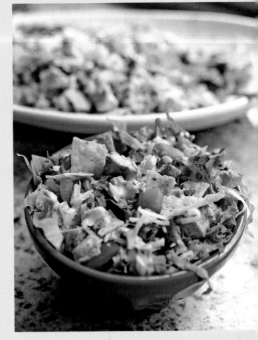

17. Serve in individual bowls with a little extra dressing on the side.

Mighty zesty and flavorful—enjoy!

M MAKE AHEAD

Swap in Ready-to-Go Grilled Chicken (page 110) instead of cooking it in the skillet.

Make the dressing up to 2 days in advance and store it in the fridge, but do not stir in the cilantro until just before serving.

Grill the corn up to 2 days in advance. Store cobs in the fridge, then slice off the kernels just before serving.

V VARIATIONS

Substitute cooked ground beef with taco seasoning for the chicken.

Heat up a can of seasoned pinto or black beans and spoon them over the salad with the chicken.

Use thawed frozen corn instead of grilled.

ROASTED BUTTERNUT SQUASH SALAD

MAKES 6 SERVINGS

I had a roasted butternut squash dish at the Purple Pig in Chicago a while back, and it was so beautiful in its simplicity, I knew I had to make it as soon as I returned to the ranch and unpacked my clothes, which of course was fourteen years after I returned to the ranch.

I hate unpacking. Have I ever told you that before?

Anyway, at the restaurant, the squash was served in a little crock as a side dish. At home, I decided to sprinkle it on top of salad greens . . . and it has become one of my favorite salads ever!

3 tablespoons pine nuts	Kosher salt and black pepper to taste	1 tablespoon balsamic vinegar
1 medium butternut squash		¼ cup olive oil
4 tablespoons (½ stick) butter	¼ cup freshly grated Parmesan cheese, more to taste	6 cups mixed salad greens

1. Preheat the oven to 375°F.

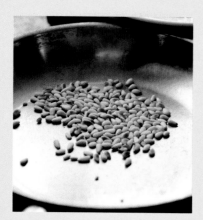

2. Place the pine nuts in a small skillet over low heat and slowly toast them, stirring, until they're golden brown and fragrant, about 2 minutes. Set them aside off the heat.

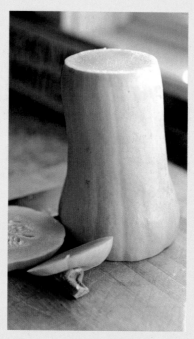

3. To prepare the butternut squash, lop off the top and bottom . . .

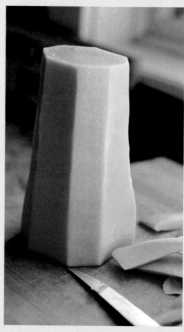

4. Then use a sharp knife or a vegetable peeler to remove the hard skin.

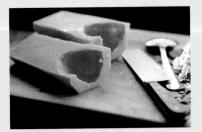

5. Cut the squash in half lengthwise and remove the seeds with a spoon . . .

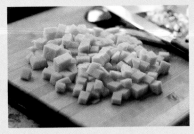

7. And slice the sticks into cubes.

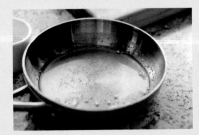

9. And skim off as much of the foam as you can.

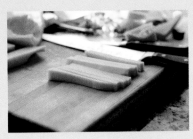

6. Then slice the squash into sticks . . .

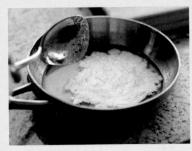

8. Meanwhile, melt the butter in a small skillet or saucepan over low heat . . .

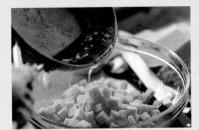

10. Place the squash in a bowl and pour in the melted butter . . .

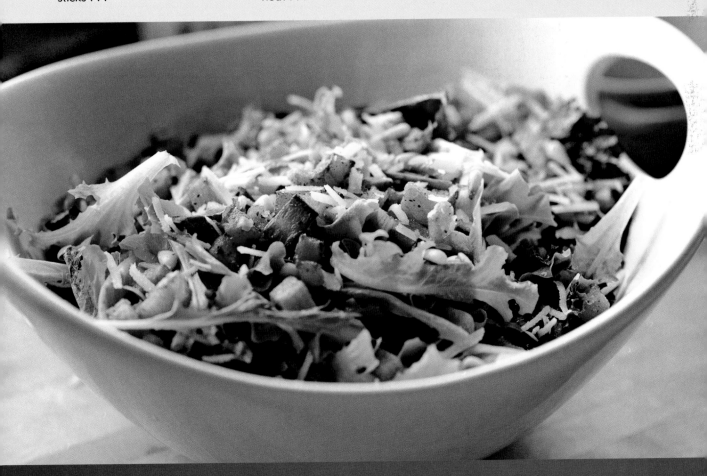

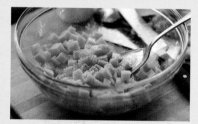

11. Then sprinkle with salt and pepper.

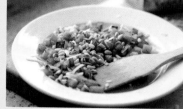
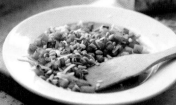

15. Then pour the squash into a bowl and toss in the pine nuts.

V VARIATIONS

Use baby spinach instead of salad greens.

Use thinly sliced kale (as prepared on page 41).

S SERVE WITH

The Bread (page 336)

Cheese Biscuits (page 332)

12. Spread the squash out on a rimmed baking sheet . . .

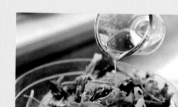

16. Mix the balsamic with the olive oil and sprinkle in a little salt and pepper. Put the salad greens in a bowl and toss with half the dressing. Serve the extra dressing on the side.

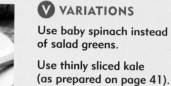

Loading hay bales.

13. And roast it for 20 to 25 minutes, shaking the pan once or twice during baking. Crank up the heat to 400°F and roast for 15 minutes or so, until the squash is sizzling and golden brown around the edges. Set the pan aside to cool for 5 minutes.

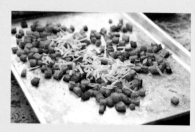

14. Add the Parmesan and toss it quickly so the cheese doesn't melt . . .

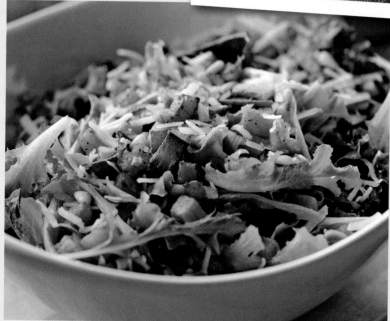

17. Add the squash mixture and lightly toss it in.

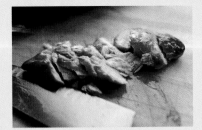

7. Slice the chicken . . .

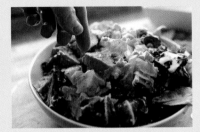

8. And place the chicken pieces over each of the salads.

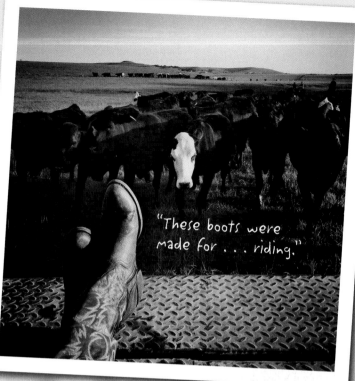

"These boots were made for . . . riding."

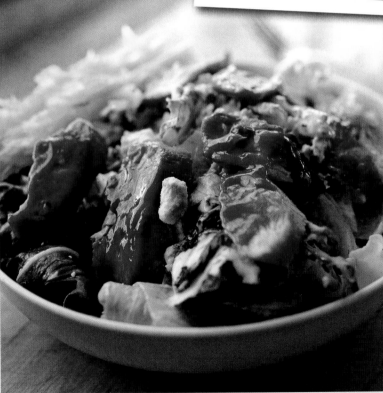

9. Sprinkle on extra blue cheese crumbles and serve with celery sticks.

M MAKE AHEAD

Make the dressing up to 3 days in advance and store in the fridge.

Swap in Ready-to-Go Grilled Chicken (page 110) instead of cooking it in the skillet.

V VARIATIONS

Use ranch dressing instead of blue cheese for a different flavor!

Slice the celery and mix it in with the salad greens.

Swap in deli rotisserie chicken meat; just coat it in warm sauce.

S SERVE WITH

The Bread (page 336)

Cheese Biscuits (page 332)

Refrigerator Rolls (page 334)

MEDITERRANEAN ORZO SALAD

MAKES 12 SERVINGS

A delicious main course salad or a colorful, pretty main side dish for so many things.
You know what Confucius always said: "There's just something about that orzo. . . ."

¼ cup extra-virgin olive oil

Juice of 1 lemon

1 garlic clove, minced

1 teaspoon kosher salt, more to taste

¾ teaspoon black pepper, more to taste

12 ounces orzo pasta, cooked, drained, and cooled

1 cup red grape or cherry tomatoes, halved

1 cup yellow grape or cherry tomatoes, halved

1 cup pitted Kalamata olives, halved

1 cup crumbled feta cheese

1 cup cooked chickpeas (I use canned)

½ red onion, diced

Minced parsley, for garnish

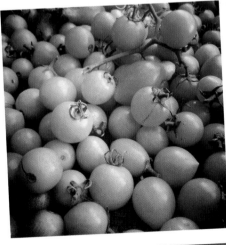

'Maters from my garden.

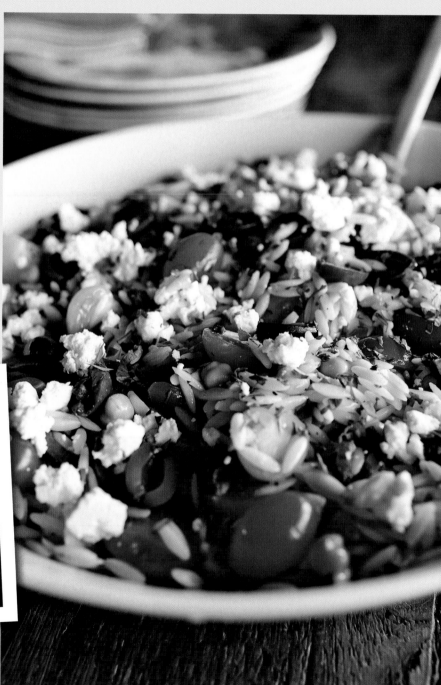

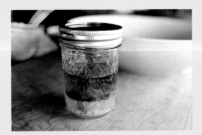

1. Combine the olive oil, lemon juice, garlic, salt, and pepper in a jar . . .

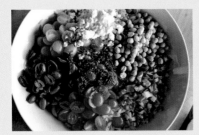

2. And shake it for approximately 38.5736222 seconds to combine. Give or take a year.

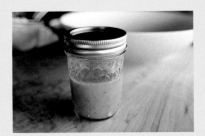

3. Place the orzo in a large bowl with all the rest of the ingredients . . .

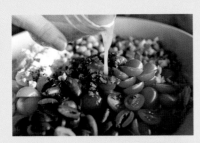

4. And pour over two-thirds of the dressing.

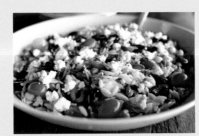

5. Toss it all around until the dressing coats everything. Give it a taste and add more dressing, more salt and pepper, and/or more of any other ingredient you like!

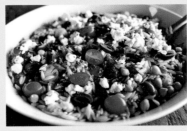

6. Sprinkle on some minced parsley to make it extra yummy.

M MAKE AHEAD

The salad can be assembled up to 12 hours before serving and kept in the fridge. Hold back half the feta to stir in right before serving.

V VARIATIONS

Add Parmesan shavings to the salad.

Add diced Ready-to-Go Grilled Chicken (page 110) to the salad.

Add peeled, sliced cucumber to the salad.

S SERVE WITH

Grilled Chicken (page 110)

Chicken with Mustard Cream Sauce (page 146)

Pork Chops with Wine and Roasted Garlic (page 246)

Italian Meatloaf (page 212)

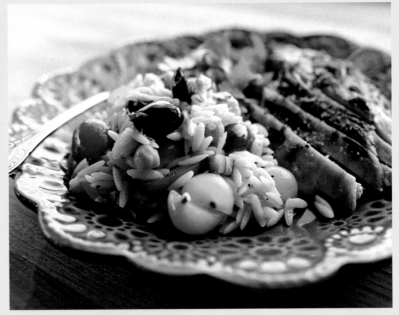

7. Serve with grilled chicken, fish, a green salad, or whatever you'd like!

QUINOA CAPRESE

MAKES 12 GENEROUS SERVINGS

I have fallen in love with quinoa over the past couple of years, which is approximately four billion years after the rest of America fell in love with it, but I live on an isolated ranch in Oklahoma and trends generally take a little longer to get here. I don't make quinoa in my own kitchen very often, but I get to eat it in delis if I happen to be in New York City, or when I stop at a nice market in the big city every now and again.

I won't illustrate all the benefits of this ancient grain. I'll just say that if you haven't tried it, you should! Even though it looks a little weird, with its spiraled germ and all, it is absolutely wonderful, whether as the basis for a salad like this one *or* mixed with butter, brown sugar, and cream for a warm breakfast treat.

And it's very, very, very, very good for you. (Unless you mix it with butter, brown sugar, and cream. Ha.)

2 cups uncooked red quinoa

½ teaspoon kosher salt, more as needed

½ cup olive oil

2 tablespoons balsamic vinegar

½ teaspoon black pepper, more to taste

1 cup red grape tomatoes, halved lengthwise

1 cup yellow cherry tomatoes, halved lengthwise

8 ounces fresh mozzarella, cubed

24 basil leaves, cut into chiffonade

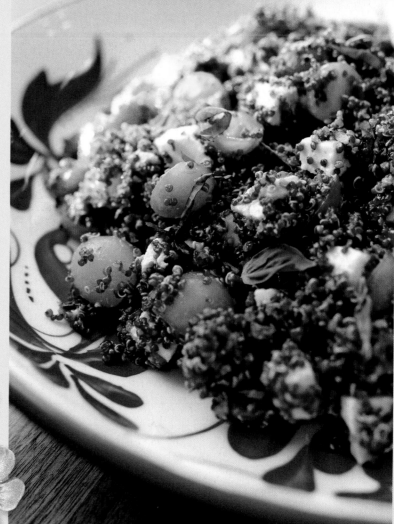

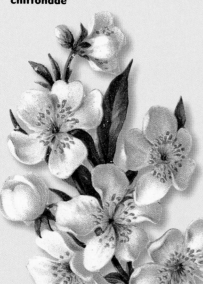

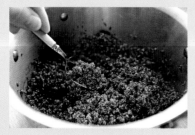

1. Bring 4 cups water to a boil. Add the quinoa and a dash of salt and simmer, covered, until the spiral germs pop out, about 15 minutes.

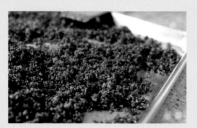

2. Spread the quinoa into an even layer on a baking sheet and set it aside to cool.

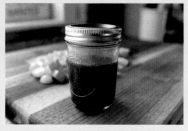

3. Whip up a simple vinaigrette by combining the olive oil, balsamic, salt, and pepper and shaking or whisking to combine.

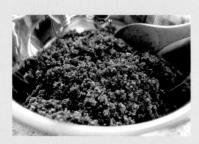

4. When the quinoa has cooled to room temperature, throw it into a big bowl . . .

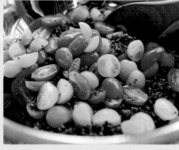

5. Then add the tomatoes . . .

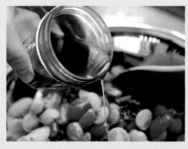

6. And pour on two-thirds of the dressing. (Save the rest in case the salad needs more at the end.)

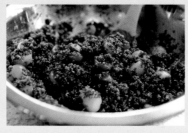

7. Toss everything around to distribute the dressing . . .

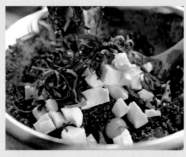

8. Then add the mozzarella and basil . . .

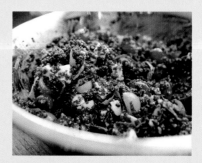

9. And toss everything to combine. Give the salad a taste and add more dressing and/or more salt and pepper, if needed . . .

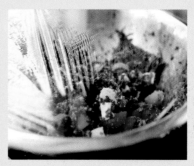

10. Then cover the bowl and refrigerate the salad for a couple of hours before serving.

V VARIATIONS

Add cubed Ready-to-Go Grilled Chicken (page 110) to the salad.

Add sliced grilled steak to the top of each serving of salad.

Add seeded and sliced cucumber to the salad.

Stir in Beautiful Roasted Vegetables (page 290) instead of tomatoes.

S SERVE WITH

Kale Citrus Salad (page 40)

Ready-to-Go Grilled Chicken (page 110), steak, or fish

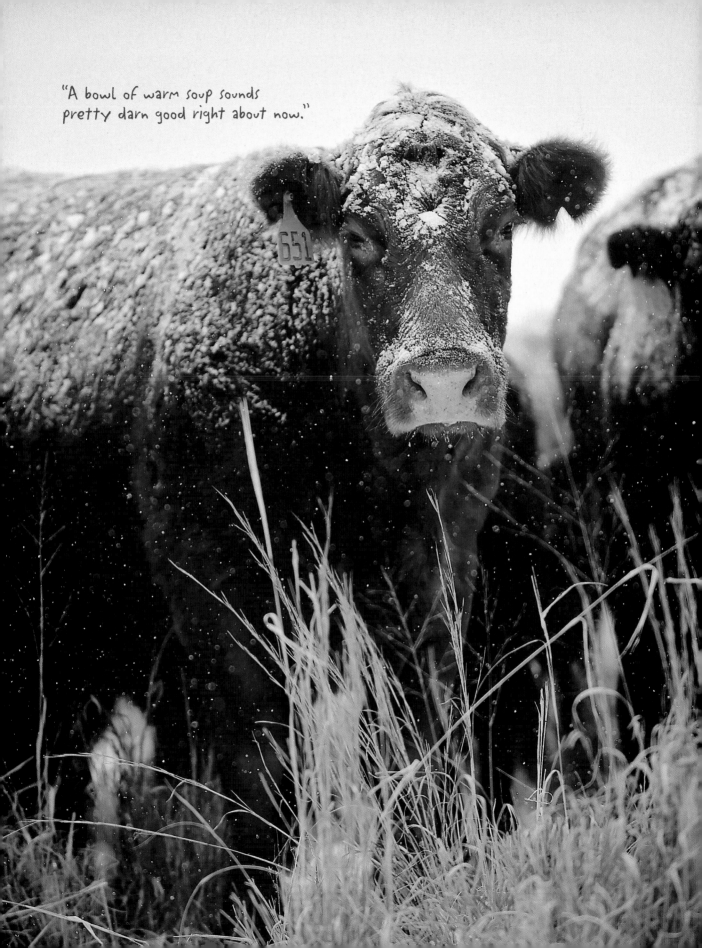

"A bowl of warm soup sounds pretty darn good right about now."

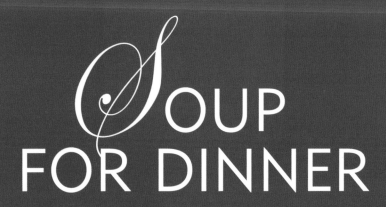

SOUP FOR DINNER

A pot of soup simmering on the stove reminds us of yesterday, makes us happy about today, and gives us hope for tomorrow. I've served my children every category of recipe under the sun, and I still say that nothing makes them feel more at home than when I hand them a big bowl of soup. It also helps somewhat that I'm doing this in our home. But still. Here are some of my family's most treasured soup recipes. Enjoy every slurp!

TOMATO SOUP WITH PARMESAN CROUTONS

MAKES 12 SERVINGS

On a freezing, frigid winter day, few things sound better to me, both physically and psychologically, than a bowl of warm tomato soup. It's one of those things that instantly takes me back to childhood, when my mom would bring me soup on a tray with a glass of Sprite as I watched *The Brady Bunch* and tried to figure out how I could get my hair as straight as Marcia's and where I could find a boyfriend as cute as Peter.

Peter was always my favorite Brady brother. (No offense, Greg and Bobby! You both were groovy, too!)

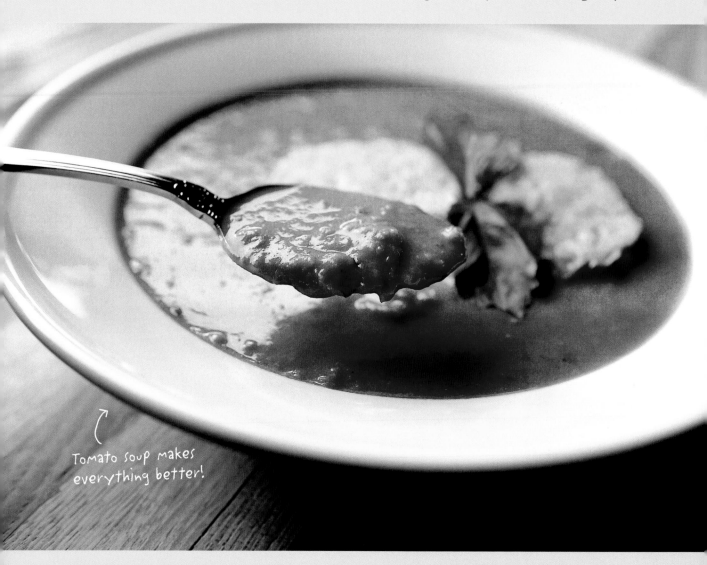

Tomato soup makes everything better!

SOUP

1 tablespoon butter

1 tablespoon olive oil

1 garlic clove, grated

1 medium onion, finely diced

3 large carrots, finely diced

2 tablespoons tomato paste

4 cups vegetable or chicken broth

Three 28-ounce cans whole tomatoes

½ cup heavy cream

2 tablespoons chopped parsley

2 tablespoons chopped basil, plus leaves for garnish

Kosher salt and black pepper to taste

PARMESAN CROUTONS

½ baguette, cut into ½-inch slices

¼ cup olive oil

½ cup grated Parmesan cheese

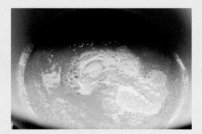

1. In a big ol' pot, melt the butter in the olive oil over medium-high heat . . .

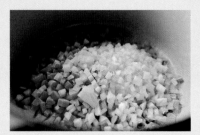

2. Then add the garlic, onion, and carrots.

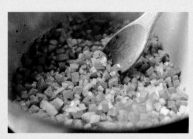

3. Stir the veggies around and cook 'em for 5 minutes or so, until they start to soften.

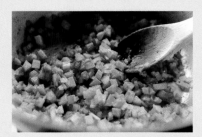

4. Add the tomato paste and stir it into the veggies, letting it cook and release its flavor for a couple o' minutes.

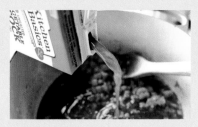

5. Next, add 1 cup water along with the broth!

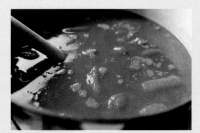

6. Add the tomatoes. Stir the mixture around, bring it to a boil, then reduce the heat to low, cover the pot, and let it simmer for 15 to 20 minutes.

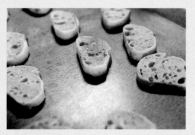

7. While the soup is simmering, make the croutons! Place the baguette slices on a rimmed baking sheet and drizzle them with the olive oil.

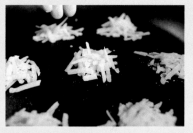

8. In a large nonstick skillet, mound the Parmesan cheese in individual piles . . .

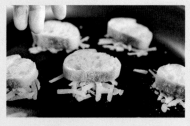

9. Lay a baguette slice on each Parmesan pile, then turn the heat to medium.

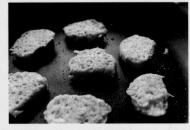

10. When the cheese is nice and melted and starting to bubble, carefully flip the croutons over to toast a bit on the other side.

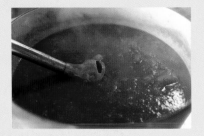

11. And guess what? The soup is almost done! You can serve it as is, but there will be some mighty big chunks of tomatoes and carrots in there, so I like to stick in an immersion blender and puree it about halfway. (You can also transfer it in small batches to a blender if you prefer. But always be careful when blending hot soup!)

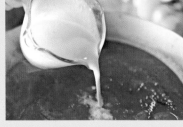

12. To soften the tomato flavor a bit, add the cream . . .

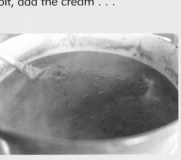

13. Then stir the soup and let it cook for a few minutes more.

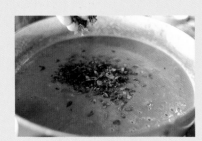

14. Finally, sprinkle in some chopped parsley and basil, along with some salt and pepper to taste.

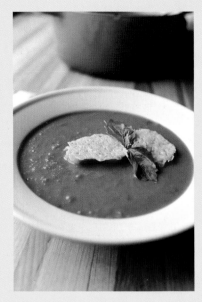

15. Serve it in a bowl with a couple of the croutons and a little more basil.

Ⓜ MAKE AHEAD

The soup will keep in the fridge for up to 3 days.

Ⓥ VARIATIONS

Add 8 roasted garlic cloves to the soup.

Puree the soup fully for more of a tomato bisque.

Ladle the soup into small crocks, top with grated mozzarella cheese, and melt the cheese under the broiler before serving.

Top with sliced or diced Ready-to-Go Grilled Chicken (page 110).

Use the croutons for any of the other soups in this chapter!

Ⓢ SERVE WITH

The Bread (page 336)

Refrigerator Rolls (page 334)

Cheese Biscuits (page 332)

Any crusty Italian or French loaf

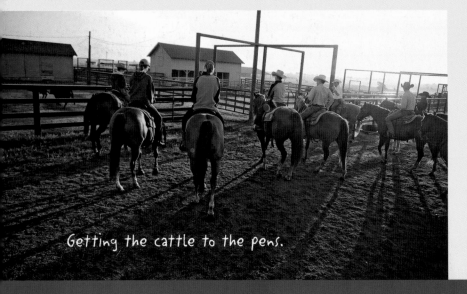

Getting the cattle to the pens.

HAMBURGER SOUP

MAKES 12 SERVINGS

I made this glorious hamburger soup one Sunday in winter for three very important reasons: One, it was so ding dang cold outside, all I could think about was soup. Two, church was canceled (Church? Canceled? I don't understand.) and I didn't have anything else to do. Three, I was hungry, man.

I love hamburger soup so much because it's meaty and hearty and flavorful and satisfying. *Mmmmmm!* It just feels good to eat it, and as a bonus, it always reminds me of my grandmother Ga-Ga.

And that always means it's going to be delicious.

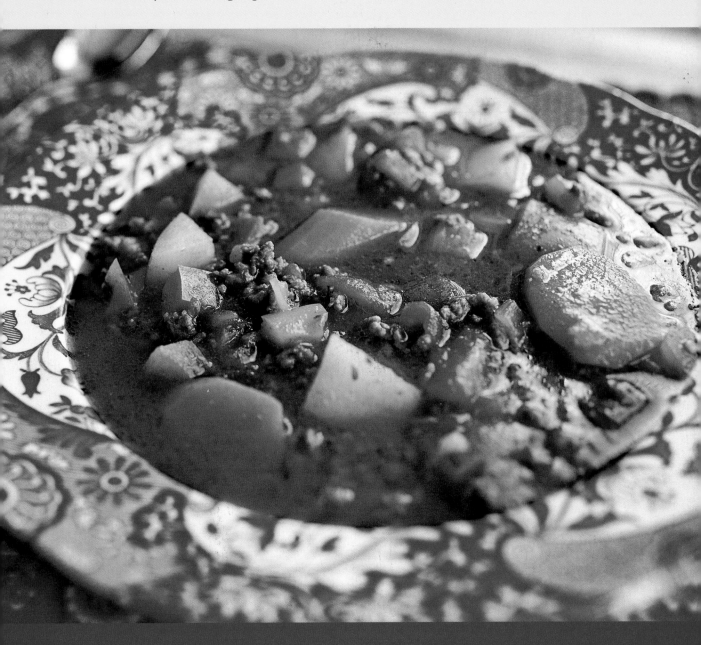

2½ pounds ground chuck or other ground beef

1 large yellow onion, diced

2 celery stalks, diced

3 garlic cloves, minced

One 14.5-ounce can whole tomatoes

1 yellow bell pepper, seeded and diced

1 red bell pepper, seeded and diced

1 green bell pepper, seeded and diced

4 carrots, peeled and sliced on the diagonal

5 large red potatoes, scrubbed and cut into 1-inch chunks

3 cups beef broth, more as needed

3 tablespoons tomato paste

½ teaspoon kosher salt, more to taste

½ teaspoon black pepper

2 teaspoons dried parsley

½ teaspoon ground oregano

¼ teaspoon cayenne pepper

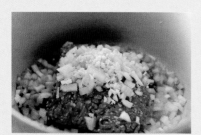

1. In a large pot, combine the meat, onion, celery, and garlic.

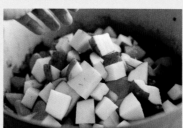

4. Then throw in the potatoes!

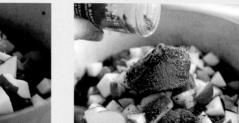

7. And the salt, black pepper, parsley, oregano, and cayenne.

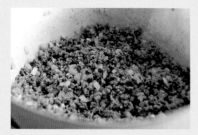

2. Cook the mixture over medium-high heat until the meat is totally browned, then drain off and discard as much fat as you can.

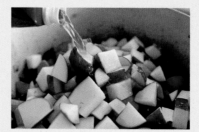

5. Next, add the beef broth . . .

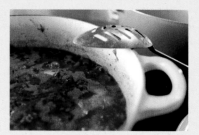

8. Stir everything together, then bring the mixture to a boil.

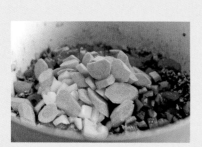

3. Add the tomatoes and their juices, bell peppers, and carrots . . .

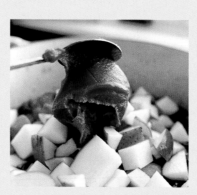

6. The tomato paste . . .

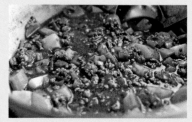

9. Reduce the heat, cover the pot, and simmer the soup for 15 to 20 minutes, or until the potatoes are tender but not overly mushy. If the soup is too thick for your taste, just splash in a cup or two of beef broth until it's the consistency you like.

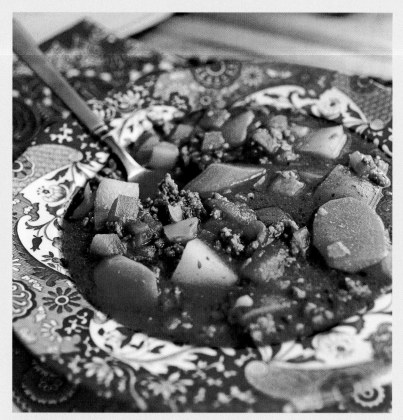

M MAKE AHEAD

For some reason, this soup always seems to taste better the next day! Feel free to make this ahead of time and store it in the fridge for up to 3 days. If soup is overly thick when reheated, add a little extra beef broth or water to thin it to your liking.

V VARIATIONS

Add any veggies you'd like to the soup: diced zucchini, corn kernels, cut green beans, or mushrooms.

Use ground turkey instead of ground beef.

Add peeled, diced parsnips or peeled, diced butternut squash to the soup.

S SERVE WITH

The Bread (page 336)

Refrigerator Rolls (page 334)

Cheese Biscuits (page 332)

10. Dish it up and serve it piping hot!

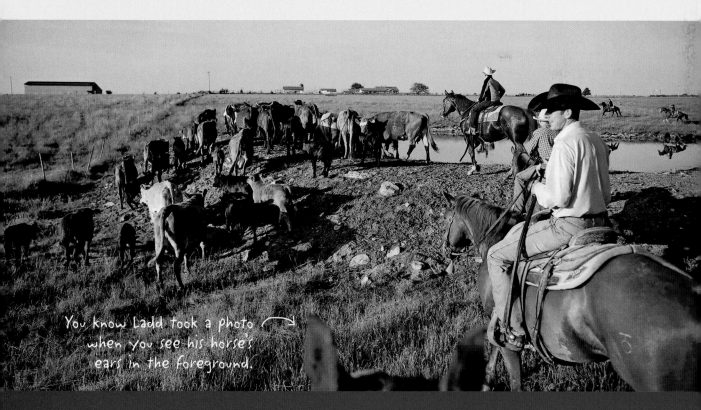

You know Ladd took a photo when you see his horse's ears in the foreground.

POTATO SOUP

MAKES 12 SERVINGS

I have a confession to make. Are you ready? Here goes.

Ahem. Clearing my throat. Singing a couple of scales to warm up.

I'M PICKY ABOUT POTATO SOUP.

I don't want it to be too creamy, with no variance in texture.

I don't want it to be too lumpy. Potato soup has to have a pureed, smooth potato component.

It has to be full of flavor or I'll die a thousand deaths.

And most of all . . . it has to make me close my eyes, sigh, and feel like everything is going to be okay.

But other than those things, I'm not the least bit picky about potato soup! Let me show you how I make it.

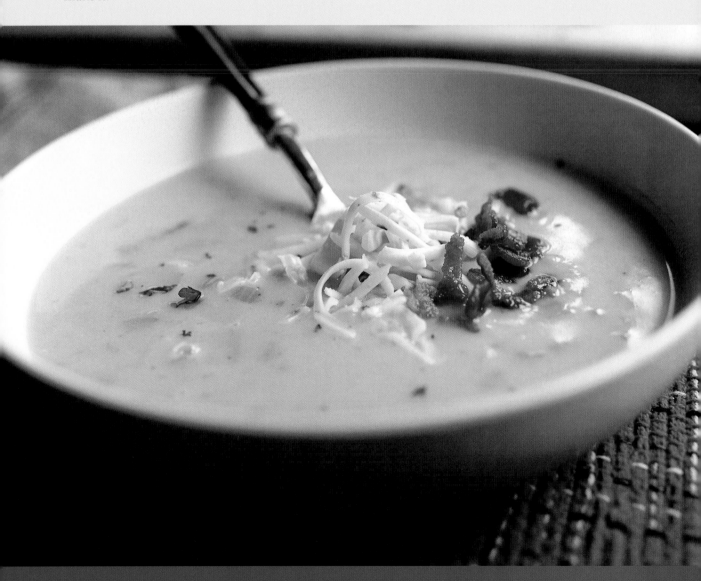

6 thin slices bacon, cut into 1-inch pieces

1 medium yellow onion, diced

3 carrots, scrubbed and diced

3 celery stalks, diced

6 small russet potatoes, peeled and diced

½ teaspoon kosher salt, more to taste

Black pepper to taste

½ teaspoon Cajun spice or other spicy seasoned salt

8 cups low-sodium chicken or vegetable broth

3 tablespoons all-purpose flour

1 cup milk

½ cup heavy cream

1 teaspoon minced parsley, plus more for serving

1 cup grated cheese (Cheddar, Monterey Jack, or whatever you like)

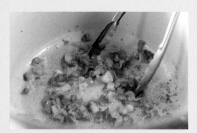

1. Cook the bacon in a large pot over medium heat until the bacon is crisp and the fat is rendered.

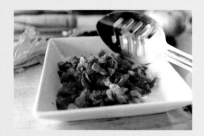

2. Remove the bacon from the pot and set it aside. Pour most of the grease from the pot, but don't clean the pot. That's where the flavor is, baby!

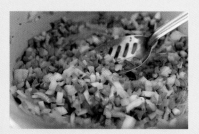

3. Return the pot to medium-high heat and add the onion, carrots, and celery. Stir and cook for 2 minutes, or until the onion has softened a bit . . .

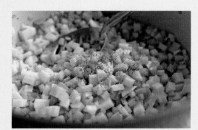

4. Then add the potatoes, salt, pepper, and Cajun spice and cook for 5 minutes more.

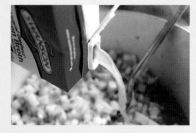

5. Add the broth and bring the mixture to a gentle boil.

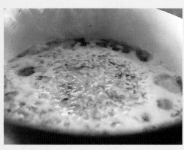

6. Cook for 10 minutes, or until the potatoes are starting to get tender.

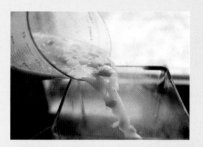

7. In a small bowl, whisk together the flour and the milk, then pour the mixture into the soup, stir to combine, and let the soup cook and thicken for 5 minutes.

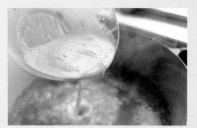

8. Working in batches, remove half the soup from the pot and pour it into a blender.

Important note: Do not fill the blender more than half full of hot soup! Use caution when blending hot soup. If possible, allow the soup to cool before blending. Alternatively, you may use an immersion blender to partially puree the soup directly in the pot.

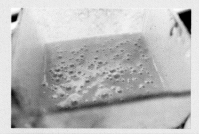

9. Puree the soup until completely smooth . . .

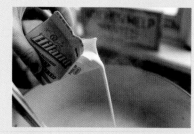

11. Add the heavy cream . . .

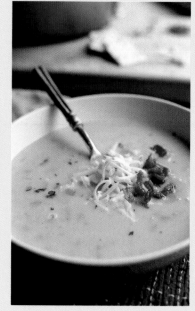

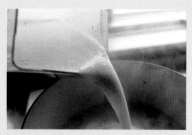

10. Then pour the pureed soup back into the pot with the rest of the soup.

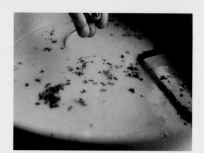

12. And the parsley. Stir and heat through.

13. Serve with a little extra parsley on top, as well as some of the bacon and grated cheese.

You will love every last drop!

V VARIATIONS

Puree all the soup in batches for a perfectly smooth cream-of-potato soup.

Don't puree any of the soup for a more chunky soup.

Add 2 sliced leeks with the veggies when you start the soup, puree the soup perfectly smooth, and serve it cold. Vichyssoise!

Stir in 1½ to 2 cups grated cheese for a cheesy potato soup.

Add 2 tablespoons prepared pesto for an herby edge!

S SERVE WITH

The Bread (page 336)

Refrigerator Rolls (page 334)

Cheese Biscuits (page 332)

Any crusty Italian or French loaf

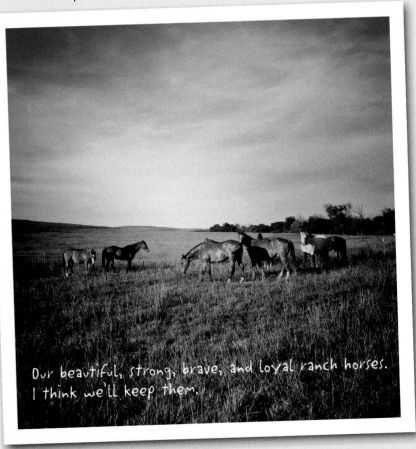

Our beautiful, strong, brave, and loyal ranch horses. I think we'll keep them.

BLACK BEAN SOUP

MAKES 8 SERVINGS

I'm a very inquisitive person. As such, I have a question. Please advise.

What is the difference between black beans and black bean soup?

Seriously. Think about it.

I don't really expect an answer. I'm just putting it out there.

Here's how I made the beans. I mean bean soup. I mean beans. I mean bean soup.

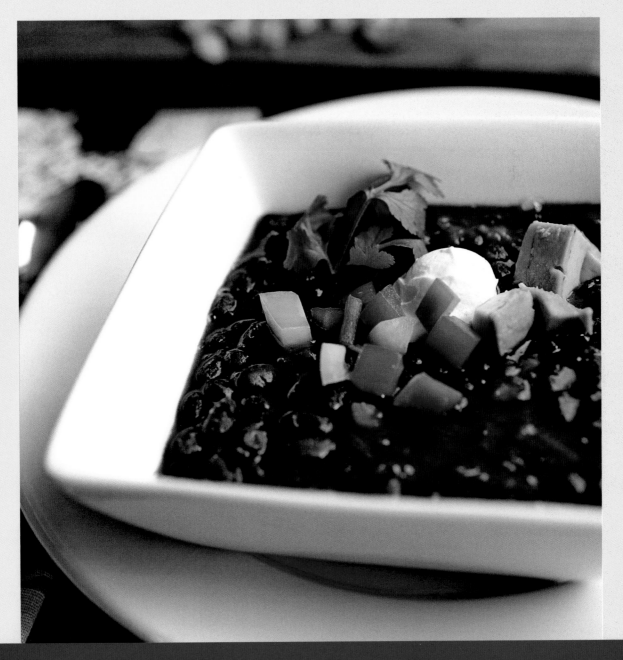

1 pound dried black beans

4 cups low-sodium chicken broth

3 garlic cloves, minced

1 medium onion, diced

1 red bell pepper, seeded and diced

1 green bell pepper, seeded and diced

1 yellow bell pepper, seeded and diced

1 teaspoon kosher salt, more to taste

1½ teaspoons chili powder, more to taste

1½ teaspoons ground cumin, more to taste

FIXINS

Diced bell pepper

Sour cream

Diced avocado

Cilantro leaves

Corn tortilla strips

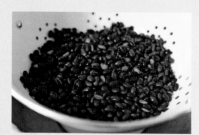

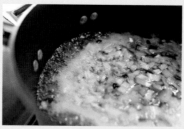

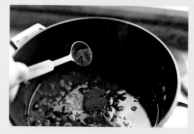

1. Place the beans in a bowl or pot, cover with cold water, and let them soak overnight. (Or, for the quick-soak method, boil the beans for 2 minutes, then turn off the heat and let the beans soak for 1 hour.) Drain the beans and rinse them with cold water when you're ready to proceed.

4. Bring the mixture to a boil over high heat . . .

7. Add the salt, chili powder, and cumin . . .

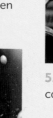

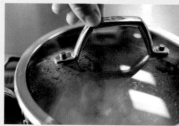

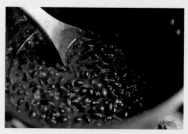

2. In a medium pot, combine the beans, broth, and 2 cups water . . .

5. Then reduce the heat to low, cover the pot . . .

8. Then cover and simmer for 30 minutes to 1 hour more, until the soup is as thick as you want it (anywhere from very thick to a thinner soup is fine!). Taste and adjust the seasonings as needed.

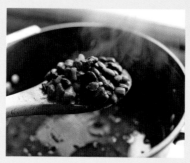

6. And simmer for 1½ hours. The beans will be slightly tender but not soft.

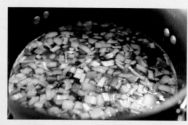

3. And stir in the garlic, onion, and bell peppers.

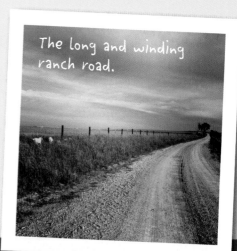

The long and winding ranch road.

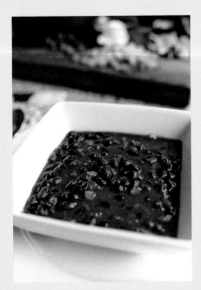

9. Serve it plain and beautiful . . .

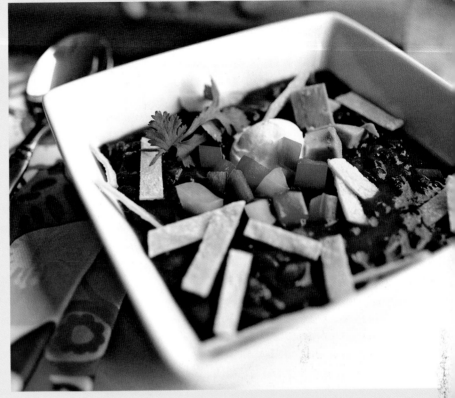

Is to sprinkle on soft corn tortilla strips. A sincerely satisfying and stunning soup!

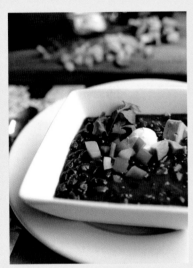

Or add a delicious topping of extra diced bell pepper, avocado, sour cream, and cilantro!

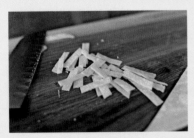

Another thing I like to do . . .

Ⓜ MAKE AHEAD

The soup can be made up to 24 hours in advance and stored in the fridge. Add a little broth while reheating if the soup is too thick.

Ⓢ SERVE WITH

Chips and guacamole

Pico de gallo (see page 23)

Cornbread

Ⓥ VARIATIONS

Add chunks of baked ham to the soup for a heartier meal.

Add ¼ cup lime juice toward the end of cooking for great flavor.

Use a potato masher to mash part of the beans for a different texture.

Add 1 or 2 seeded, diced jalapeños for a spicier bean soup.

Top with grated Monterey Jack cheese.

Add 12 roasted garlic cloves to the soup toward the end of the cooking time.

Cook until thick, then use the beans in burritos, on nachos, or in tacos.

SPINACH SOUP

MAKES 8 SERVINGS

When I was a little girl, I took piano lessons from Mrs. Boucher, and at the end of every year, she would have what she called "spinach soup parties" for her students. New students would recoil at the thought of celebrating their first year of piano by eating green soup, but once they realized that "spinach soup" was actually code for "ice cream sundaes," they chuckled and helped perpetuate the joke for years to follow.

It can't compete with sundaes, of course, but spinach soup is actually wildly delicious! And with a chunk of buttered bread and a glass of wine, it makes a tasty (and verdant!) dinner.

2 tablespoons olive oil

1 bunch spinach (10 to 12 ounces)

2 garlic cloves, minced

4 tablespoons (½ stick) butter

½ medium onion, chopped

¼ cup all-purpose flour

3 cups whole milk

½ cup half-and-half

1½ teaspoons kosher salt, more to taste

¾ teaspoon black pepper

Dash of cayenne pepper

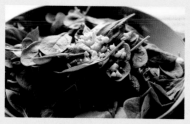

1. In a large skillet, heat the olive oil over medium heat. Add the spinach and garlic . . .

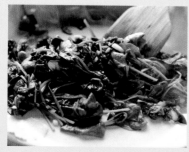

2. And cook for 2 to 3 minutes, stirring continuously, until the spinach is wilted.

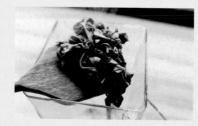

3. Remove the cooked spinach and add to a blender or food processor . . .

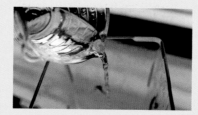

4. And pour in ¼ cup hot water.

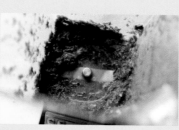

5. Pulse the spinach until it's totally pureed, then set it aside.

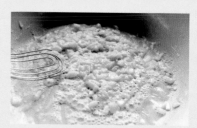

6. Melt the butter in a large pot over medium heat. Add the onion and cook until it begins to soften, 3 to 4 minutes. Sprinkle in the flour and stir it to combine. Cook the roux over medium heat for about 2 minutes, whisking continuously, until it's light golden brown . . .

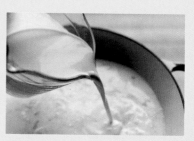

7. Then add the milk and half-and-half . . .

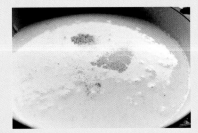

8. Along with the salt, black pepper, and cayenne. Stir and cook the mixture until it starts to thicken, 3 to 4 minutes . . .

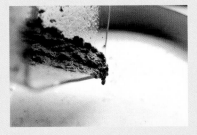

9. Then pour in the spinach puree.

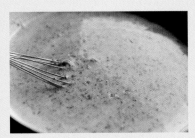

10. Stir to combine, taste and adjust the seasonings (add more salt if it needs it!), and let the soup heat through.

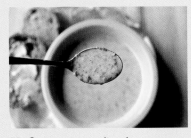

11. Serve it immediately.

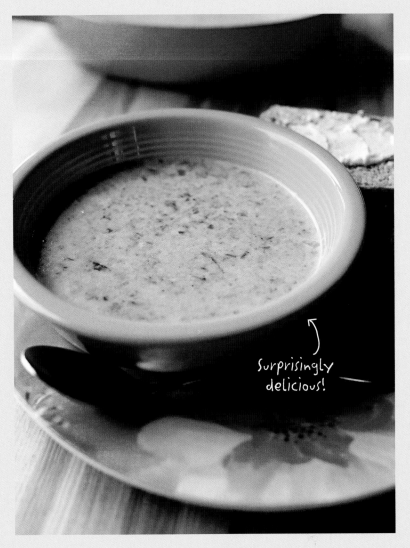

Surprisingly delicious!

V VARIATIONS

Cook a mix of greens (spinach, kale, collard greens) for a super-healthy soup.

Add a couple of grilled shrimp to the top of each bowl of soup.

Add strips of roasted red pepper to the top of each bowl of soup.

Sprinkle crumbled bacon over each bowl of soup.

Swirl a little sour cream, crème fraîche, or Greek yogurt into each bowl of soup.

S SERVE WITH

The Bread (page 336)

Refrigerator Rolls (page 334)

Cheese Biscuits (page 332)

Any crusty Italian or French loaf

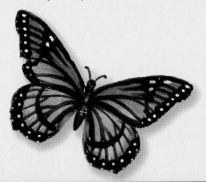

MINESTRONE

MAKES 8 SERVINGS

Minestrone is nothing more than an Italian soup with a whole bunch of ingredients. There is no Italian magistrate who has created a ruling on just what ingredients must be used to constitute minestrone, but it looks something like this:

Broth. Veggies. Beans. Pasta. Tomatoes. And whatever else you feel like throwing in.

And if those are the criteria, this one passes with flying colors!

2 zucchini, halved, cut into thick strips, and cubed

2 summer squash, halved, cut into thick strips, and cubed

8 ounces white mushrooms, stemmed and quartered

4 tablespoons (¼ cup) olive oil

Kosher salt to taste

2 carrots, scrubbed (not peeled) and chopped

1 medium onion, diced

3 celery stalks, sliced (leaves included)

8 cups low-sodium chicken broth

Black pepper to taste

Two 15-ounce cans cannellini beans, drained and rinsed

2 cups fresh or frozen green beans, cut into 1-inch pieces

One 14.5-ounce can diced tomatoes

1½ cups miniature pasta shells, cooked to al dente and drained

3 tablespoons minced parsley

Parmesan cheese shavings, for serving

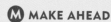 MAKE AHEAD

Roast the veggies up to 24 hours ahead of time and store in the fridge.

Prep the other vegetables (except for the potatoes) ahead of time and store them in the fridge until cooking time.

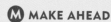 VARIATIONS

Add 2 tablespoons tomato paste with the broth for a tangy, tomato-y broth.

Add ¼ cup red or white wine with the broth for a nice "grown-up" flavor.

Roast any diced vegetable you'd like: carrots, parsnips, eggplant, turnips, and so on.

Add red pepper flakes for a little spice.

Use cooked elbow macaroni instead of shells.

Omit the pasta altogether if you prefer.

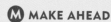 SERVE WITH

The Bread (page 336)

Refrigerator Rolls (page 334)

Cheese Biscuits (page 332)

Any crusty Italian or French loaf

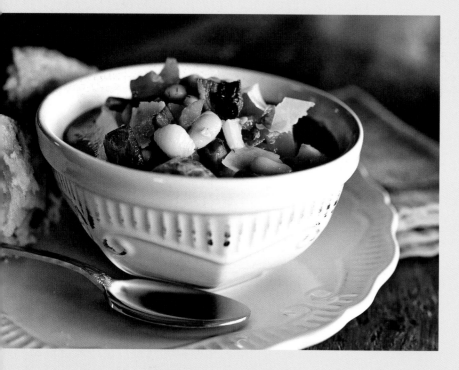

1. Preheat the oven to 500°F.

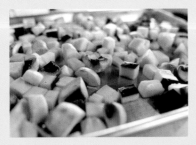

2. Mix the zucchini, squash, and mushrooms in a large bowl with 2 tablespoons of the olive oil and a little salt. Arrange on two rimmed baking sheets to avoid overcrowding . . .

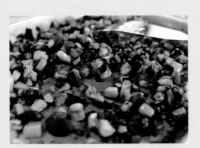

3. And roast for 10 to 12 minutes, shaking the pan once or twice during roasting, until brown bits begin to show. Remove the veggies from the oven and set aside.

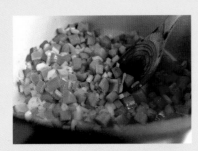

4. In a large pot, heat the remaining 2 tablespoons olive oil over medium heat and add the carrots, onion, and celery. Cook the mixture for 3 to 4 minutes, or until the onion is softened . . .

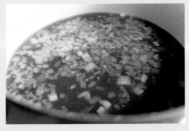

5. Then add the broth and salt and pepper to taste and bring it to a boil. Reduce the heat to low and simmer the mixture for 10 minutes.

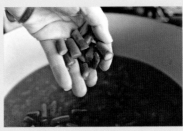

6. Add the cannellini beans, green beans, and tomatoes with their juices . . .

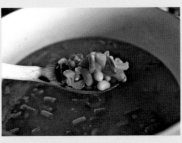

7. And simmer on low for 5 minutes.

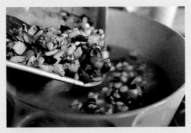

8. Finally, stir in the roasted veggies . . .

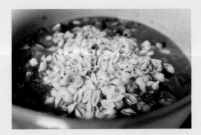

9. The pasta . . .

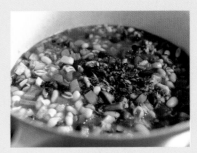

10. And the parsley. Stir and simmer for 5 minutes more, or until the soup is piping hot. Taste and adjust the seasonings, adding more salt and pepper, if needed.

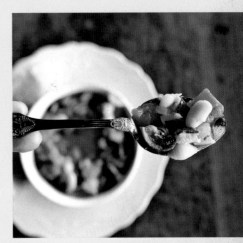

11. Serve the minestrone in a bowl with thick shavings of Parmesan. Delicious!

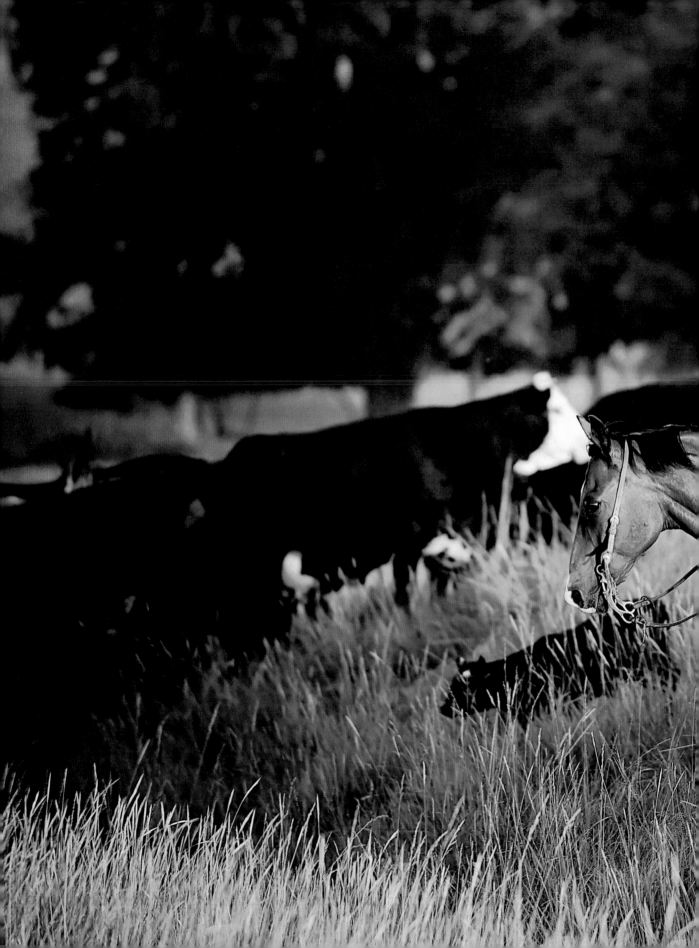

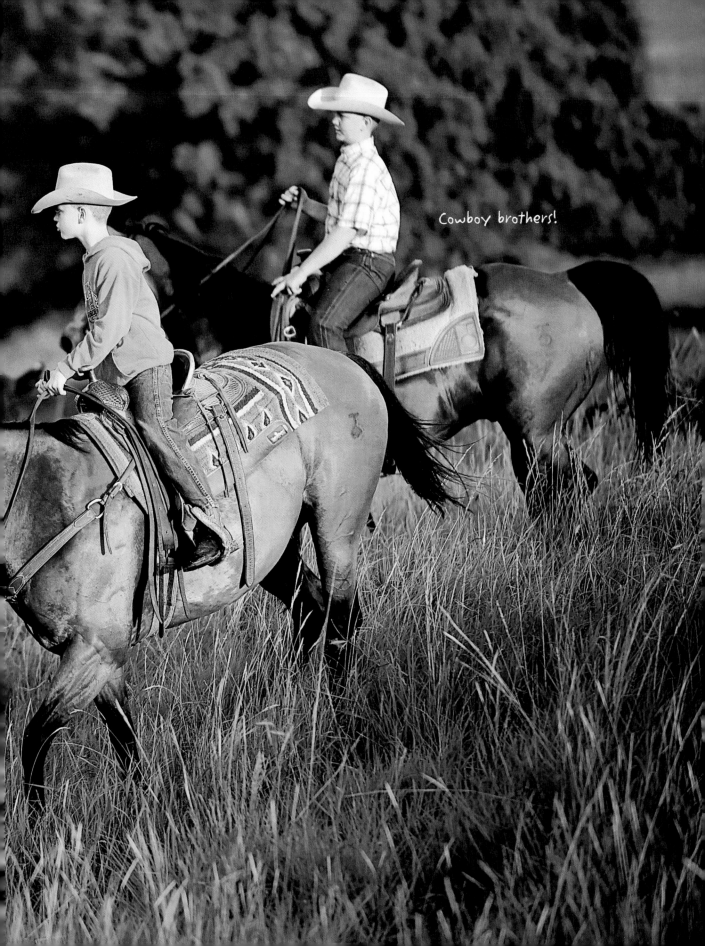

Cowboy brothers!

SAUSAGE, POTATO, AND KALE SOUP

MAKES 12 SERVINGS

This is a make-at-home version of Olive Garden's Zuppa Toscana. Now, if you actually live in civilization and have an Olive Garden near your house, you may choose not to make this at home. You may choose instead to get in your car, drive to Olive Garden, get out of your car, go inside, order Zuppa Toscana, and enjoy every bite. Then have someone else do the dishes. Restaurants are good like that.

If, however, you are like me and don't have an Olive Garden anywhere near your dwelling, making a batch at home is the next best thing.

(On a related note, my kids pretty much think Olive Garden is the best restaurant on the face of the planet. I figure this will save our family a lot of money on that whole eating-our-way-through-Italy vacation we no longer need to take.)

1½ pounds Italian sausage

1 large onion, diced

3 cups whole milk

2 cups half-and-half

¼ cup cream

1 quart (4 cups) low-sodium chicken broth

½ teaspoon dried oregano

½ teaspoon red pepper flakes

Kosher salt and black pepper, to taste

8 to 10 medium red potatoes, boiled until almost tender

1 or 2 bunches kale, stalks removed, torn into bite-size pieces

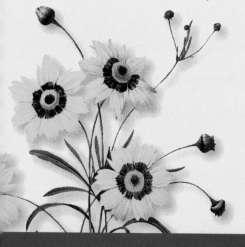

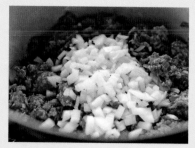

1. In a large pot over medium-high heat, sauté the Italian sausage with the onion . . .

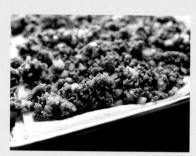

2. Until the sausage is totally cooked, 5 to 7 minutes. Drain off the excess fat, then pour the sausage mixture onto a rimmed baking sheet lined with paper towels in order to remove as much fat as possible. Set aside.

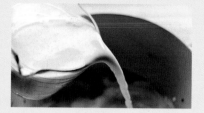

3. Wipe the pot clean, then return it to the stove over medium heat. Pour in the milk, half-and-half, and cream . . .

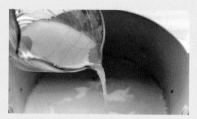

4. And the broth.

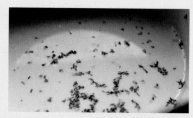

5. Add the oregano, red pepper flakes, and salt and pepper . . .

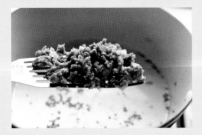

6. Then add the sausage back in . . .

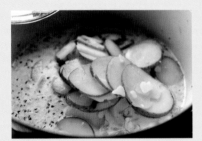

7. And bring it to a gentle boil, stirring.

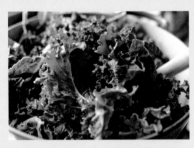

8. Slice the potatoes and add them in . . .

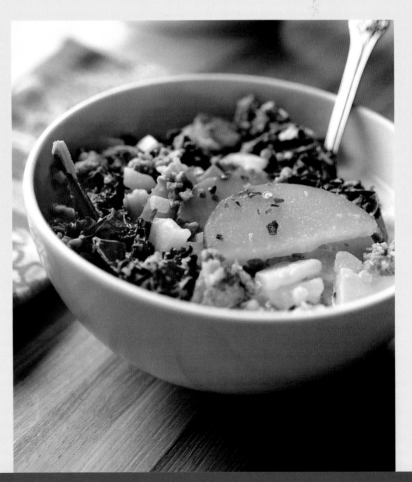

9. Along with all the kale! Stir the soup gently until the kale wilts and shrinks a bit, just 1 to 2 minutes.

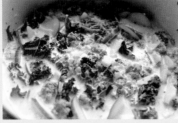

10. Reduce the heat to low, cover the pot, and let the soup simmer for 10 minutes.

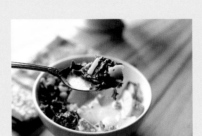

11. Serve it to hungry humans!

V VARIATIONS

Add 2 tablespoons prepared pesto to the soup for nice flavor.

Substitute dry white wine for ½ cup of the broth.

Use hot Italian sausage instead of regular.

Omit the sausage for a meat-free soup.

Add chopped collard or mustard greens along with the kale.

Stir 1 cup grated Parmesan cheese into the soup just before serving.

S SERVE WITH

The Bread (page 336)

Refrigerator Rolls (page 334)

Cheese Biscuits (page 332)

Any crusty Italian or French loaf

BUTTERNUT SQUASH SOUP

MAKES 12 SERVINGS

I love butternut squash however I can get it, but pureed butternut squash soup is at the top of my list. It's creamy and smooth and so unbelievably decadent. (Splashes of cream and maple syrup only make it more fabulous.)

I want to dive in right now!

2 medium butternut squash, peeled, seeded, and cut into cubes, as shown on page 57

¼ cup plus 2 tablespoons olive oil

1 medium onion, diced

4 cups vegetable or chicken broth

½ cup heavy cream, plus more for serving (optional)

¼ cup maple syrup

½ teaspoon kosher salt, more to taste

Sour cream, for serving (optional)

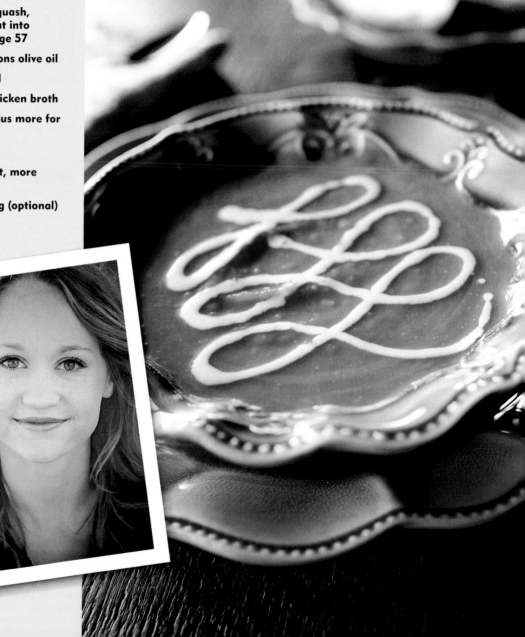

She's even prettier on the inside. ♥

1. Preheat the oven to 350°F.

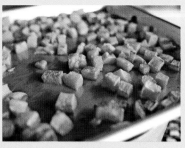

2. Spread the squash on two rimmed baking sheets and drizzle it with ¼ cup of the olive oil. Roast until it's soft and light brown, 30 to 40 minutes, shaking the pan halfway through. Set the squash aside.

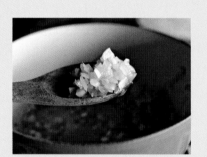

3. In a large pot, cook the onion in the remaining 2 tablespoons olive oil over medium heat until soft and lightly caramelized, 7 to 8 minutes.

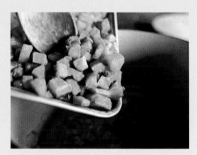

4. Add the roasted squash . . .

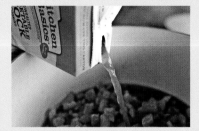

5. And the broth . . .

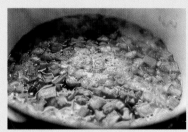

6. And heat the mixture until bubbling.

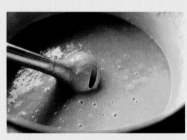

7. Use an immersion blender to puree the soup in the pot until totally smooth. You can also transfer the mixture in batches to a regular blender; just don't fill it more than halfway full since the soup is hot! Transfer the pureed soup back to the pot when it's done.

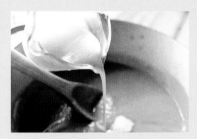

8. Finally, add the cream . . .

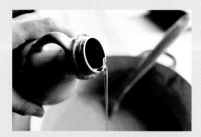

9. The maple syrup . . .

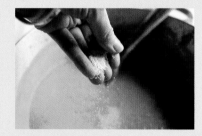

10. And the salt.

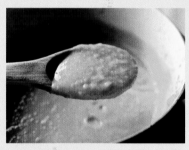

11. Then stir it around and let it simmer for 5 minutes more. Give it a taste and add more salt to your liking.

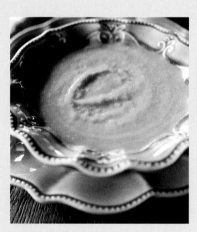

12. Serve the soup plain . . .

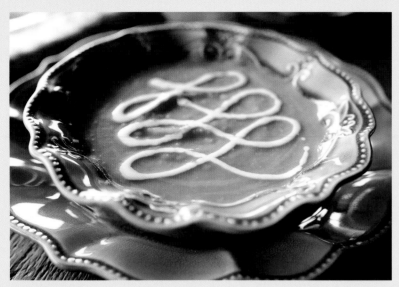

Or mix together equal parts cream and sour cream and drizzle little designs on the surface.

Ⓜ MAKE AHEAD

The squash can be roasted up to 48 hours ahead of time and kept in the fridge. Just proceed with the soup as instructed.

Ⓥ VARIATIONS

Use a combination of root vegetables (parsnips, turnips, carrots) along with the butternut squash.

Roast a garlic head along with the squash, then squeeze the cloves into the pot with the squash to give the soup a roasted garlic flavor.

Puree the soup only halfway for a chunkier soup.

Add chopped herbs of your choice for an herby soup.

Ⓢ SERVE WITH

Ready-to-Go Grilled Chicken (page 110)

Kale Citrus Salad (page 40)

The Bread (page 336)

Refrigerator Rolls (page 334)

Cheese Biscuits (page 332)

Any crusty Italian or French loaf

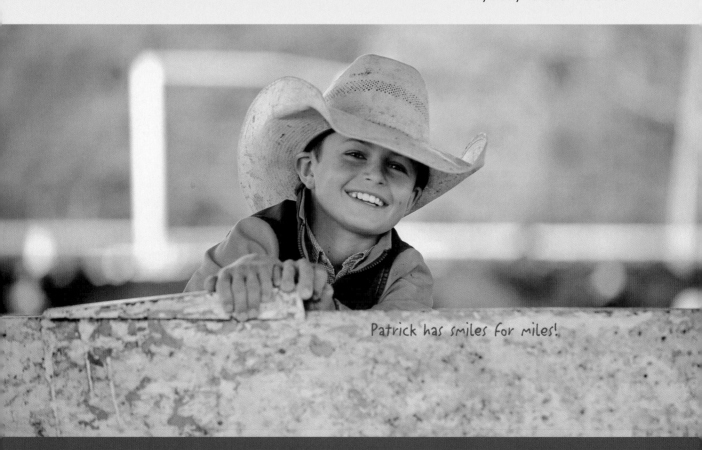

Patrick has smiles for miles!

CHEESY CAULIFLOWER SOUP

MAKES 12 SERVINGS

This is a variation of my mom's famous cauliflower soup, which was pretty much perfect to begin with, but of course I'm not happy in life until I take every last one of my mom's recipes and add cheese and bacon to them.

It's the kind of daughter I am.

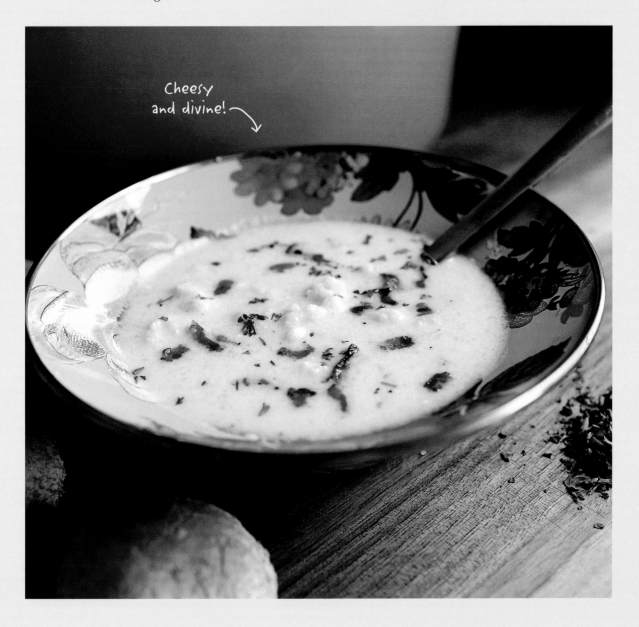

Cheesy and divine!

4 thin slices bacon, cut into small pieces

1 large onion, finely diced

1 cauliflower head, cut into small florets

½ teaspoon Cajun spice, more to taste

½ teaspoon black pepper, more to taste

8 cups low-sodium chicken broth

4 tablespoons (½ stick) butter

¼ cup flour

2 cups whole milk

1 cup half-and-half

¼ cup sour cream

3 cups grated Monterey Jack cheese, more to taste

2 tablespoons minced parsley

Kosher salt to taste (optional)

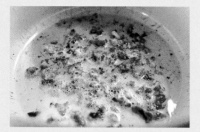

1. In a large pot, fry the bacon pieces over medium-high heat until crisp.

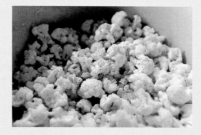

4. Add the cauliflower, sprinkle with the Cajun spice and pepper . . .

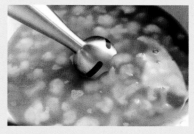

7. Next, use an immersion blender . . .

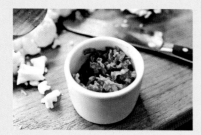

2. Remove the bits from the pan and drain on a paper towel. Pour off the grease and return the pot to the stove, leaving the bacon bits to the side for now.

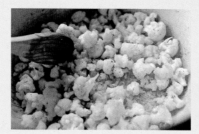

5. And cook for 3 to 4 minutes more, or until the cauliflower starts turning golden brown.

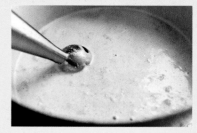

8. To puree the soup slightly, or all the way, if you prefer. (Or use a regular blender and puree the soup in batches; don't fill it more than halfway when the soup is hot!)

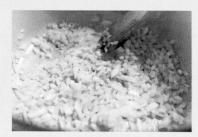

3. Add the onion to the pot and cook over medium-high heat, stirring continuously, for 3 to 4 minutes, or until translucent.

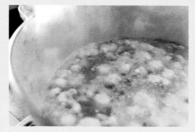

6. Pour in the broth, stir, and reduce the heat to a simmer. Cook for 15 minutes.

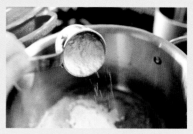

9. In a separate saucepan or skillet, melt the butter over medium heat. Sprinkle in the flour . . .

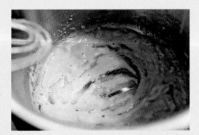

10. And whisk to form a roux. Cook the roux for about 2 minutes . . .

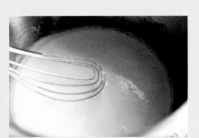

11. Then pour in the milk. Cook, whisking continuously, until the mixture becomes thick, about 4 minutes. Remove from the heat and stir in the half-and-half.

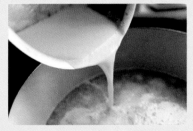

12. Pour the white sauce into the partially pureed soup.

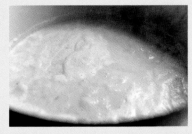

13. Turn the heat to medium-high and bring the soup back to a boil for 3 to 5 minutes to thicken it.

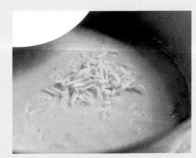

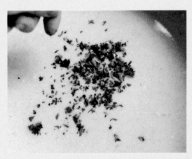

14. Reduce the heat to low and add the sour cream and cheese. Stir until fully melted.

15. Finally, stir in the parsley. Taste and adjust the seasonings, adding salt if desired.

Ⓜ MAKE AHEAD

Make the soup up to 24 hours in advance, but wait to stir in the cheese until just before serving, while you are reheating it.

Ⓥ VARIATIONS

Replace the cauliflower with broccoli for a cheesy broccoli soup.

Use half cauliflower and half broccoli.

Add diced carrots, celery, parsnips, or other vegetables to the pot with the cauliflower.

Use Cheddar, pepper Jack, Swiss, or any cheese you'd like.

Add several dashes of hot sauce to give the soup some kick!

Ⓢ SERVE WITH

The Bread (page 336)

Refrigerator Rolls (page 334)

Cheese Biscuits (page 332)

Any crusty Italian or French loaf

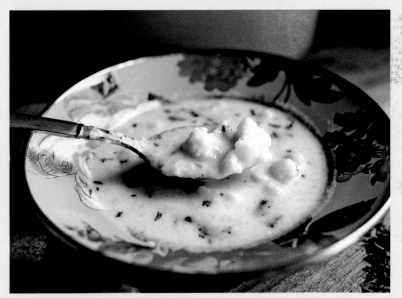

16. And serve it piping hot in a bowl!

CHICKEN SOUP

MAKES 8 SERVINGS

Chicken soup . . . ah, what is there to say? It's perfect for a rainy day. It's also perfect for a sunny day. It's also perfect for a partly cloudy day. It's also perfect for a snowy day. It's also perfect for a drizzly day.

It's also perfect . . . for every day!

Good chicken soup takes a little time, but it's worth every single second.

1 whole fryer chicken, cut into 8 pieces

1 large onion, chopped

3 celery stalks, cut into thin slices

3 carrots, diced

3 parsnips, peeled and diced

1 bay leaf

4 cups unsalted (or low-sodium) chicken broth

½ teaspoon kosher salt, more to taste

¼ teaspoon black pepper

½ teaspoon ground thyme

½ teaspoon ground oregano

8 ounces cooked egg noodles, or ½ cup cooked white rice (optional)

Chopped parsley, for garnish

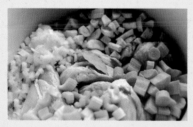

1. Throw the chicken, onion, celery, carrots, parsnips, and bay leaf into a large pot.

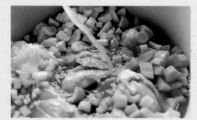

2. Pour in the broth . . .

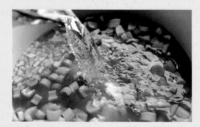

3. And 4 cups water.

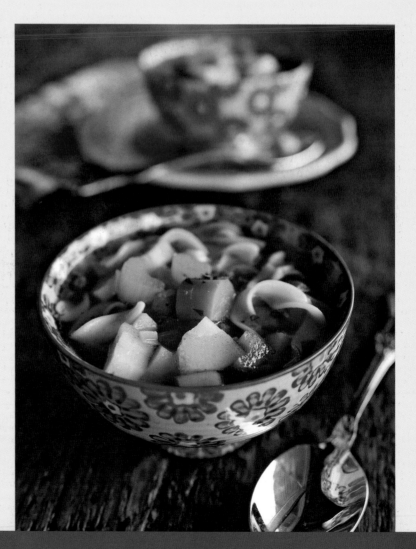

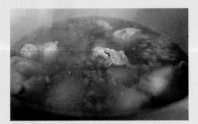

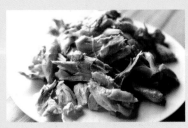

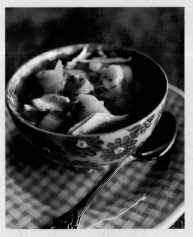

4. Bring the mixture to a boil over high heat, then reduce the heat to low. Cover the pot and simmer the soup for 1½ to 2 hours, or until the chicken is very tender.

8. Until it's all off the bones (discard the bones and skin). Transfer the chicken to a large plastic bag or container and refrigerate it alongside the soup.

11. Sprinkle the top of each serving with chopped parsley.

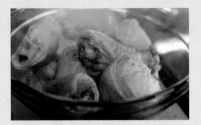

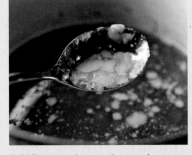

V VARIATIONS

If you prefer, omit the refrigeration step and serve the soup when it is finished cooking. It will have a little more fat in the broth, but it will still be delicious.

Add a splash of heavy cream to the finished soup for a little richness.

5. Remove the chicken from the pot and set it aside to cool slightly.

9. When you're ready to reheat the soup, use a spoon to remove as much as the hardened fat from the surface as you can. Discard the fat.

S SERVE WITH

The Bread (page 336)
Refrigerator Rolls (page 334)
Cheese Biscuits (page 332)
Any crusty Italian or French loaf
Saltine or oyster crackers

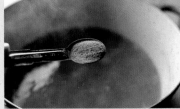

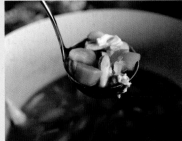

6. Add the salt, pepper, thyme, and oregano and simmer the soup for 15 minutes. Let the soup cool to room temperature, then refrigerate (either in the pot or in a separate container) for several hours or overnight.

10. Return the soup to the stove, add the chicken, and heat the soup until hot and simmering. Taste and adjust the seasonings as you go. If you like, stir in cooked egg noodles or cooked rice, or whatever makes your skirt fly up!

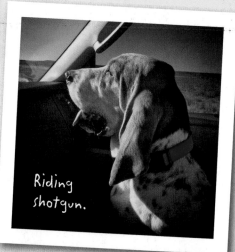

Riding shotgun.

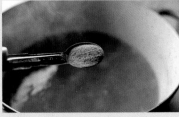

7. Use two forks to shred the chicken . . .

VEGGIE CHILI

MAKES 12 SERVINGS

Good veggie chili is soooo good that you won't even notice there's no meat in it! This is chock-full of all the good things in life: veggies, beans, and a lot of spice. One of my favorite meatless marvels on the planet.

2 tablespoons olive oil

1 large onion, diced

3 garlic cloves, minced

1 red bell pepper, seeded and diced

1 yellow bell pepper, seeded and diced

1 green bell pepper, seeded and diced

1 jalapeño, seeded and finely diced

2 carrots, diced

2 celery stalks, diced

½ teaspoon kosher salt

1 teaspoon ground oregano

1 tablespoon ground cumin

2 tablespoons chili powder, more to taste

3 cups low-sodium vegetable broth

One 12-ounce can tomato sauce

One 10-ounce can diced tomatoes and chiles (such as Ro-Tel)

One 14-ounce can kidney beans, drained and rinsed

One 14-ounce can pinto beans, drained and rinsed

One 14-ounce can black beans, drained and rinsed

One 14-ounce can chickpeas, drained and rinsed

1 large or 2 medium zucchini, chopped

¼ cup masa harina (corn flour) or regular cornmeal

Crumbled Cotija cheese, for serving (optional)

Cilantro leaves, for serving (optional)

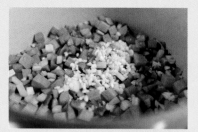

1. In a large pot over medium-high heat, heat the olive oil. Add the onion, garlic, bell peppers, jalapeño, carrots, and celery and cook, stirring occasionally, until the vegetables start to turn deep golden brown, 5 to 7 minutes.

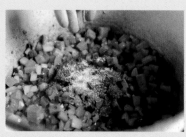

2. Add the salt, oregano, cumin, and chili powder . . .

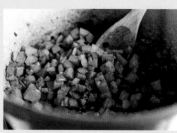

3. And cook for 2 minutes more. Pour in the broth, the tomato sauce . . .

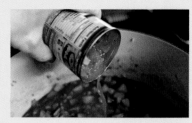

4. And the diced tomatoes and chiles.

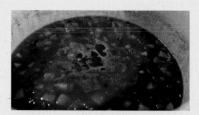

5. Let the mixture come to a boil, then reduce the heat to low, cover the pot, and simmer, stirring occasionally, for 30 minutes.

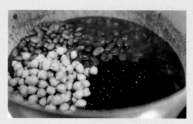

6. Add the beans and chickpeas . . .

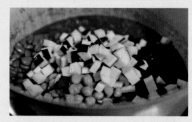

7. And the zucchini . . .

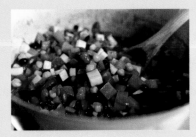

8. And stir to combine. Cover and simmer for 30 minutes more.

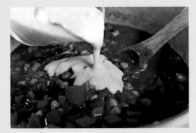

9. Mix the masa harina with ½ cup warm water and pour it into the chili.

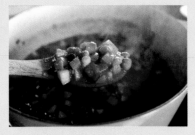

10. Simmer the chili for 15 minutes more, or until it's thick and rich and perfect! Taste and adjust the seasonings, adding more of whatever it needs.

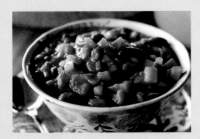

11. Serve it plain and unadorned . . .

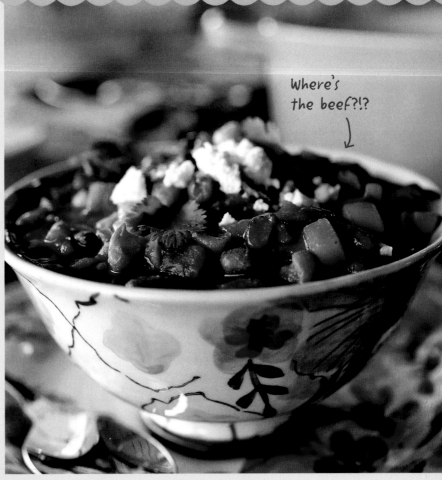

Where's the beef?!?

12. Or with crumbled Cotija and cilantro leaves.

Ⓥ VARIATIONS

Add 2 tablespoons tomato paste for a richer tomato flavor.

Substitute a bottle of Mexican beer for 1 cup of the broth.

Add chopped mushrooms, diced butternut squash, diced parsnips, or any vegetable you'd like.

Top with a big spoonful of pico de gallo (see page 23) or chopped fresh tomatoes.

Top with a dollop of sour cream.

Top with grated sharp Cheddar.

Put on top of a plate of cheese nachos.

Put inside crisp taco shells with cheese, lettuce, and tomatoes.

Ⓜ MAKE AHEAD

The chili will keep in the fridge for up to 3 days. Just add a little broth as you're reheating if it's too thick.

Ⓢ SERVE WITH

Corn or flour tortillas

Corn chips or tortilla chips, for dipping

Baked potatoes

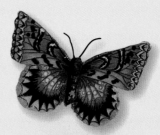

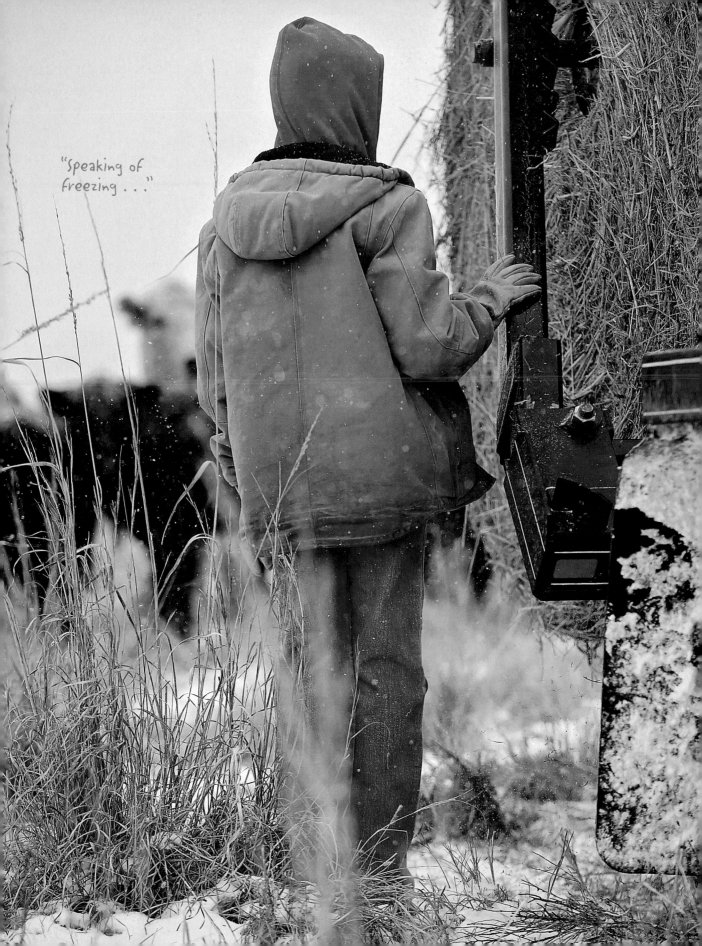

"Speaking of freezing . . ."

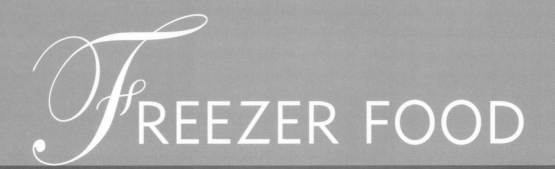

FREEZER FOOD

When we've had a particularly crazy day on the ranch—the cow ate Bryce's schoolwork, the horse ate my sunflowers, the dog ate Paige's boot, and other typical challenges—I can't tell you the comfort that a freezer full of dinner options brings me!

FREEZER FOOD

Because I'm always trying to rise above my impulses, I'm going to attempt to articulate how essential freezer food is in my life without using exaggeratory language. It will be somewhat difficult, but here goes: IF FREEZER FOOD DIDN'T EXIST, I WOULD JUST DIE.

I'd say that went well!

But really. *Freezer food.* I love the stuff. To say it's a lifesaver is an understatement. Here are the whys, whats, and hows!

THE BENEFITS OF FREEZER FOOD

1. You don't have to think about dinner. That's already been done another day, another time.

2. It's efficient! You can spend a Saturday stocking up on freezer dishes, and, in the process, free yourself from a bunch of daily headaches trying to figure out supper the following week.

3. It's flexible. Depending on the size of your family, you can make big batches of freezer food and divide them up in whatever size freezer containers you wish. Use small individual foil loaf pans all the way up to 2-gallon freezer bags. Customize the size!

4. It's a safety net. If your kids decide to throw an impromptu slumber party, your husband decides to bring five of his coworkers home for dinner, or you have to dash out the door and leave your family in charge of their own dinner, there are plenty of options behind the freezer doors.

5. It facilitates generosity. You have a friend just returning from a long trip, a neighbor who has just lost a loved one, or a mom just home from the hospital with her new baby. Delivering a frozen casserole or meal kit with the instructions attached is one of the best ways to say, *I'm thinking about you.*

FREEZER SUPPLIES

1. Zipper bags. All shapes and sizes. Store raw meat, cooked meat, soups, sauces, raw vegetables . . . anything goes!

2. Pint and quart food storage containers. You might also call these Chinese food containers, but I call them little miracles. They can be reused, which I love, and they stack beautifully.

3. Foil pans. These come in all shapes and sizes—round, square, rectangular, octagonal (just kidding)— and they're great to use because they keep you from having to tie up your glass and ceramic pans for freezing. I reuse these a lot; they hold up well!

4. Aluminum foil. Heavy-duty foil is perfect for making custom-shaped freezer parcels; just rip off the size you want and form it into whatever shape you need. But here's my favorite way to use foil for the freezer: Before assembling a casserole in the pan, line a glass or ceramic pan with foil, letting the foil hang over the edges of the pan at least 4 inches on all sides, tucking them flat under the pan. Spray the foil with cooking spray, then assemble the casserole as you normally would. Cover the pan with additional foil and freeze until the casserole is completely frozen solid. Then remove the pan from the freezer and use the foil overhangs to carefully lift the frozen casserole out of the pan. Fold the foil overhangs over the top of the casserole, then wrap the casserole in additional foil (or place it into an oversize plastic zipper bag) and freeze until you need it. To bake it, simply remove it from the freezer, take off all the wrap, and place the frozen casserole into the same size glass or ceramic pan for baking and serving. Brilliant!

5. Permanent markers. For labeling—not just what's inside, but also the date it was frozen and reheating instructions to take away the guesswork.

PACKIN' FOR SUCCESS

Four words: **Air is the enemy.** That's one of the most important things to know. Air causes freezer burn and other disasters, so when you pack things for the freezer, force out the excess air and place the wrapping right against the surface of the food—anything to eliminate (or at least diminish!) the airspace.

Two words: **Flash freezing!** It's one of my favorite freezer tricks. When you flash freeze, you place uncovered food straight into the freezer to do a quick freeze of the surface in order to make it easier (and less messy) to pack and store. Things like grilled chicken breasts, raw or cooked meatballs, rounds of cookie dough, hamburger patties—they all benefit from flash freezing! Just pop them straight into the freezer for a good 30 minutes, until the surface is frozen and they're slightly firm, then remove them and quickly pop them into their permanent (well, semi-permanent) storage container.

Five words: **Make wise use of space.** If you have a freezer the size of a small horse barn, this isn't as much of a concern, but if you're more limited on freezer space, you'll want to pack things to maximize the space you have. Store things flat in zipper bags, whether it's grilled meat or hamburger soup, and stack them neatly as high as you can go. You would be astounded by how many flat freezer bags you can fit in a standard freezer! Just label the bags as clearly as you can and keep the most recently frozen items toward the back or at the bottom, so you're using up things in the right order.

MY FAVORITE THINGS TO FREEZE

Unbaked casseroles
Grilled chicken breasts
Raw, formed hamburger patties

Meatballs, cooked or raw
Browned hamburger, sausage, and ground turkey

Soups and sauces
Nonacidic raw vegetables such as corn, green beans, and carrots

READY-TO-GO FREEZER MEATBALLS

MAKES 125 MEATBALLS

You want to be happy and content in life? Have at least five bags of these meatballs in your freezer at all times. All you have to do is whip up the sauce of your choosing, throw in the meatballs straight out of the freezer, and cook the sauce long enough for them to thaw and heat up. They're tasty and versatile, and you'll get hooked on how easy it is to turn them into a delicious dinner.

They're the answer to all your dinnertime prayers.

5 pounds ground beef

1½ cups plain breadcrumbs

1 teaspoon kosher salt

1 teaspoon black pepper

4 large eggs

2 heaping tablespoons grainy mustard

½ cup whole milk

¼ cup heavy cream

¼ cup chopped parsley

½ teaspoon red pepper flakes

Olive oil, for frying

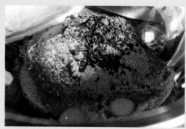

1. Combine all the ingredients (except the olive oil) in a large bowl.

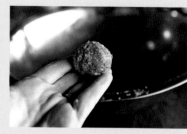

3. Scoop out 1-tablespoon portions of the meat mixture and roll them into neat balls.

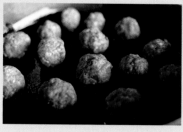

5. To brown the meatballs, heat ¼ cup olive oil in a large skillet over medium-high heat. Working in batches, add some meatballs to the skillet . . .

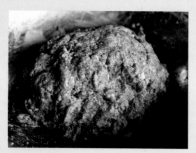

2. Knead it all together well with your hands until it's well combined.

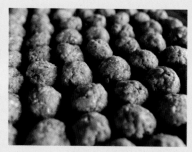

4. Place them on parchment-paper-lined rimmed baking sheets as you go, then put the sheets in the freezer for about 10 minutes to firm them up before frying.

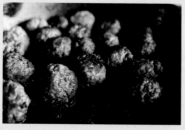

6. And cook them on all sides until they have great color on the surface and are fully cooked inside, about 5 to 6 minutes.

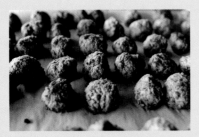

7. Drain the meatballs on paper towels when they're done, then line them up on clean parchment-paper-lined baking sheets.

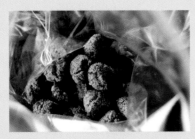

8. Place them in the freezer, uncovered, for 30 to 45 minutes, or until they're frozen and firm on the surface.

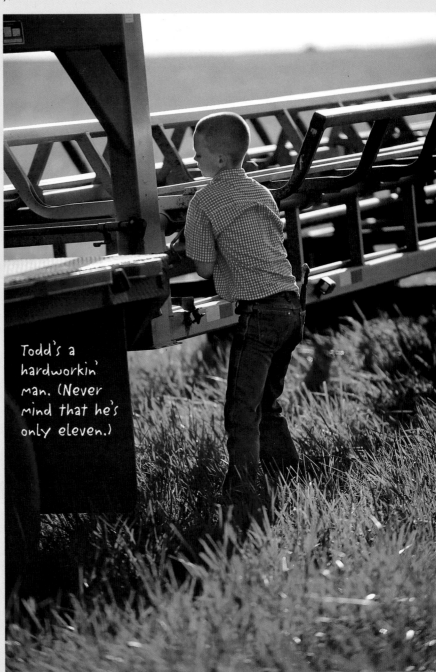

9. Then just pop them into 5 to 7 separate freezer bags (roughly 25 per bag) . . .

10. And freeze them immediately. They'll be there when you need them!

FREEZER INSTRUCTIONS

Freeze the meatballs for up to 6 months. To use them in sauces or soups, simply add them to the hot sauce or soup and allow it to simmer long enough for the meatballs to thaw and heat up.

—OR—

Allow the meatballs to thaw in the fridge for 24 hours, then use them as you'd like.

Todd's a hardworkin' man. (Never mind that he's only eleven.)

SWEET-AND-SOUR MEATBALLS

MAKES 4 TO 6 SERVINGS

This sweet, tangy, slightly spicy dinner is one of the best ways to use my beloved Freezer Meatballs. It's marvelous.

2¼ cups pineapple juice

½ cup packed brown sugar

½ cup rice vinegar or white vinegar

¼ cup ketchup

1 tablespoon low-sodium soy sauce

1 tablespoon cornstarch

One 25-count bag frozen Ready-to-Go Freezer Meatballs (page 102)

1 tablespoon sriracha or other hot sauce, more to taste

1 cup drained canned or fresh pineapple chunks

4 tablespoons sliced green onions

1½ cups long-grain or basmati rice, cooked (about 4½ cups), for serving

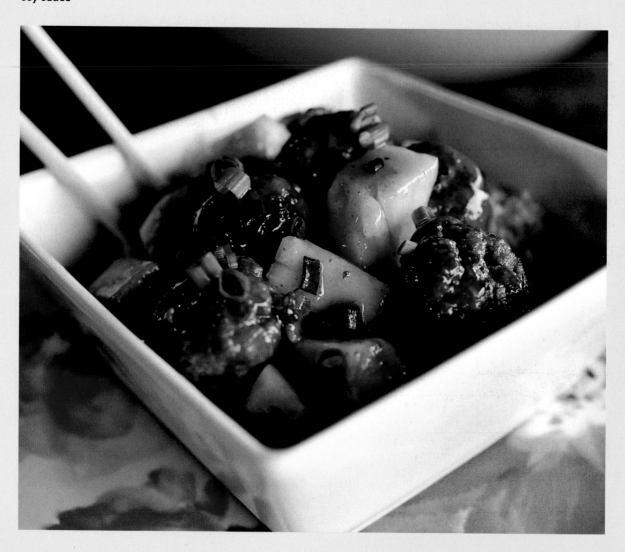

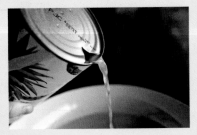

1. In a large skillet (with a lid), combine 2 cups of the pineapple juice . . .

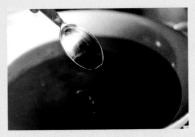

2. With the brown sugar, vinegar, ketchup, and soy sauce.

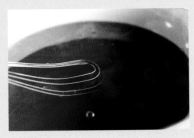

3. Stir the mixture around and bring it to a gentle boil over medium-high heat.

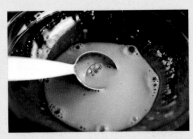

4. To thicken the sauce, make a slurry by mixing the cornstarch with the remaining ¼ cup pineapple juice until smooth . . .

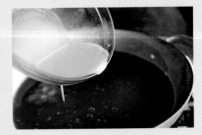

5. Then add it to the sauce, whisking to combine.

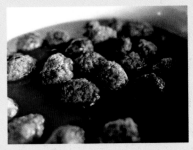

6. Add the frozen meatballs . . .

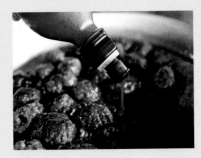

7. Then the sriracha . . .

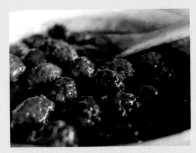

8. And toss to combine. Cover the skillet and cook for 8 to 10 minutes, until the sauce has thickened and the meatballs are heated through.

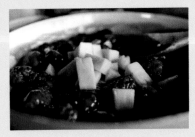

9. Stir in the pineapple . . .

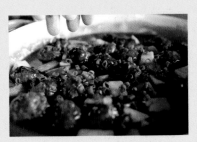

10. Then sprinkle in 2 table-spoons of the green onions.

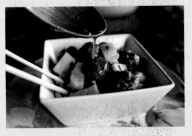

11. Serve the meatballs and sauce over the rice and sprinkle on the rest of the green onions at the end!

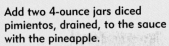 **VARIATIONS**

Add two 4-ounce jars diced pimientos, drained, to the sauce with the pineapple.

Add coarsely chopped red or green bell pepper to the sauce with the meatballs.

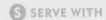 **SERVE WITH**

Pineapple Fried Rice (page 261)

Chow Mein (page 174)

SWEDISH MEATBALLS

MAKES 4 TO 6 SERVINGS

Savory . . . creamy . . . with the slightly unexpected hint of allspice. Mmmm, too good for words! If you've never had Swedish Meatballs before, these will totally rope you in.

2¼ cups beef broth

1 tablespoon Worcestershire sauce

¼ cup grainy brown mustard

Pinch of ground allspice

1 tablespoon cornstarch

¼ cup heavy cream

One 25-count bag frozen Ready-to-Go Freezer Meatballs (page 102)

12 ounces egg noodles, cooked according to the package directions

2 tablespoons butter

2 tablespoons minced parsley, plus more for serving

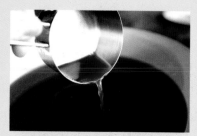

1. In a large skillet, combine 2 cups of the broth . . .

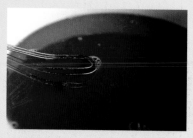

4. And allspice. Whisk the mixture together and bring it to a gentle boil over medium-high heat.

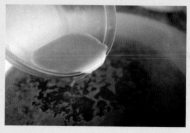

6. When the sauce is beginning to boil, pour in the slurry, whisking to combine.

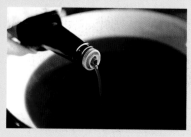

2. The Worcestershire . . .

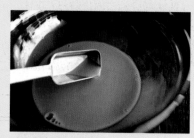

5. Make a slurry by mixing the cornstarch with the remaining ¼ cup broth until it's smooth.

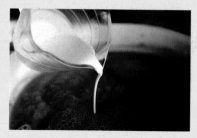

7. When the sauce starts to thicken, slowly add the cream, whisking continuously.

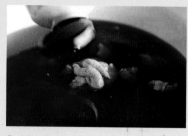

3. Mustard . . .

Ⓥ VARIATION

Use ½ cup room-temperature Greek yogurt or sour cream instead of heavy cream.

Ⓢ SERVE WITH

Polenta (page 322)

Rice Pilaf (page 320)

Stovetop Mashed Potatoes (page 310)

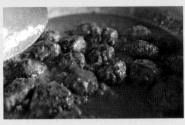

8. Add the meatballs, stir to coat, then cover the pan, reduce the heat to low, and simmer for 8 to 10 minutes, until the sauce has thickened and the meatballs are heated through.

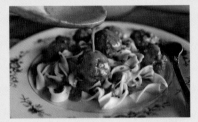

9. To serve, toss the cooked noodles with the butter and parsley. Spoon the meatballs and sauce over the noodles . . .

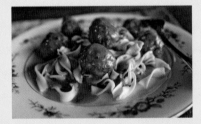

10. And sprinkle with more parsley.

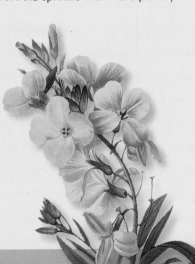

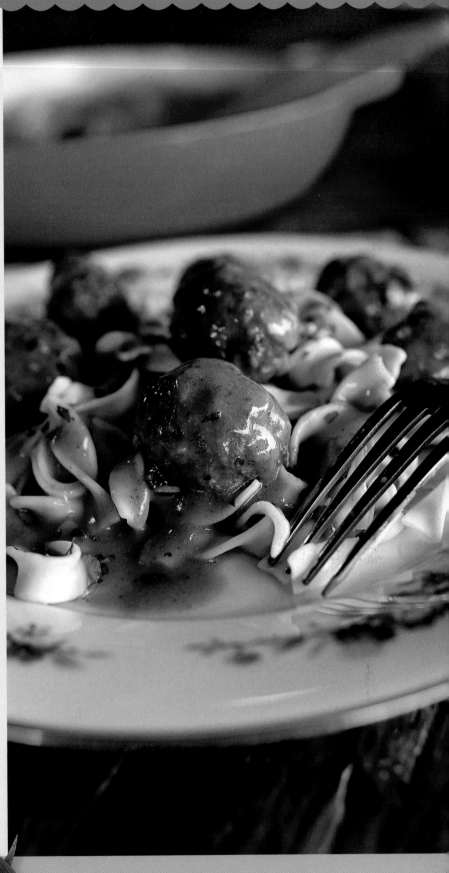

BBQ MEATBALLS

MAKES 4 TO 6 SERVINGS

If you've got a bag of meatballs in your freezer and a bottle of barbecue sauce in your pantry, you're well on your way to one of the easiest dinners in the Milky Way galaxy.

2 cups barbecue sauce

2 tablespoons white vinegar

1 teaspoon hot sauce, such as Tabasco

1 teaspoon Worcestershire sauce

1 tablespoon brown sugar

One 25-count bag frozen Ready-to-Go Freezer Meatballs (page 102)

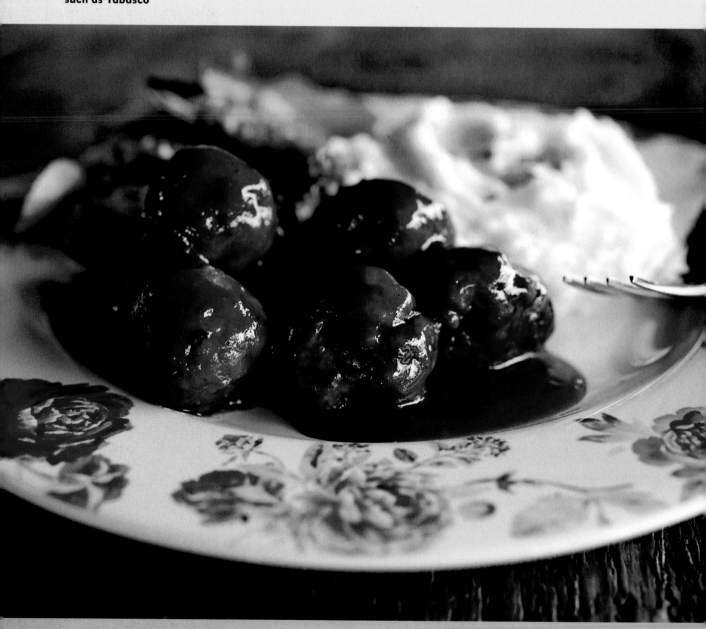

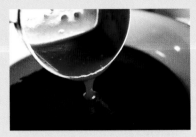

1. In a large skillet, bring the barbecue sauce to a gentle boil over medium-high heat.

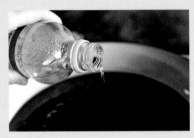

2. Add the vinegar . . .

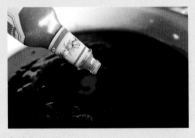

3. Hot sauce . . .

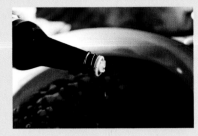

4. Worcestershire . . .

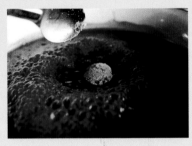

5. And brown sugar. Stir the mixture all around and let it bubble up . . .

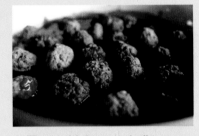

6. Then add the meatballs . . .

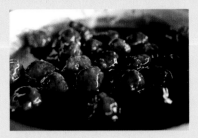

7. And toss them to coat. Cover the pan, reduce the heat to low, and simmer for 8 to 10 minutes, or until the meatballs are heated through.

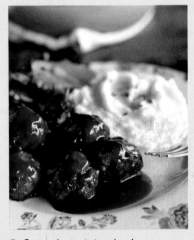

8. Serve 'em piping hot!

V VARIATIONS

Just use your favorite barbecue sauce as is, without "doctoring" it, to make the meatballs even more quickly!

Add ½ teaspoon red pepper flakes for a spicier dish.

Serve the meatballs on a toasted sub roll with thinly sliced red onion on top!

S SERVE WITH

Stovetop Mashed Potatoes (page 310)

Buttered Parsley Noodles (page 324)

Polenta (page 322)

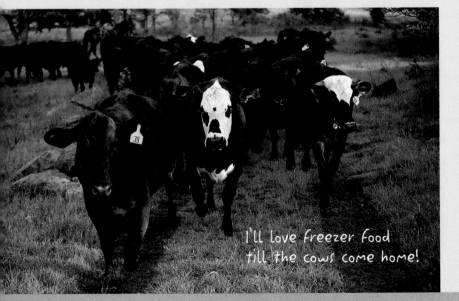

I'll love freezer food till the cows come home!

READY-TO-GO GRILLED CHICKEN

MAKES 12 GRILLED CHICKEN BREASTS OR 24 THIN CUTLETS

On the list of the Most Versatile Foods of All Time, basic grilled chicken breasts have to rank pretty high. They're perfect on salads, inside quesadillas and sandwiches, or stirred into pasta dishes, and once you get used to having them ready to go in your freezer, you won't ever want to go back to the way it was before.

Here's my basic marinade, but feel free to add anything you want to make it your own.

12 boneless, skinless chicken breasts

2 cups olive oil

Juice of 12 lemons (about 2 cups)

3 heaping tablespoons Dijon mustard

½ cup honey

1 tablespoon dried thyme

1 tablespoon ground oregano

1 tablespoon kosher salt

1 teaspoon black pepper

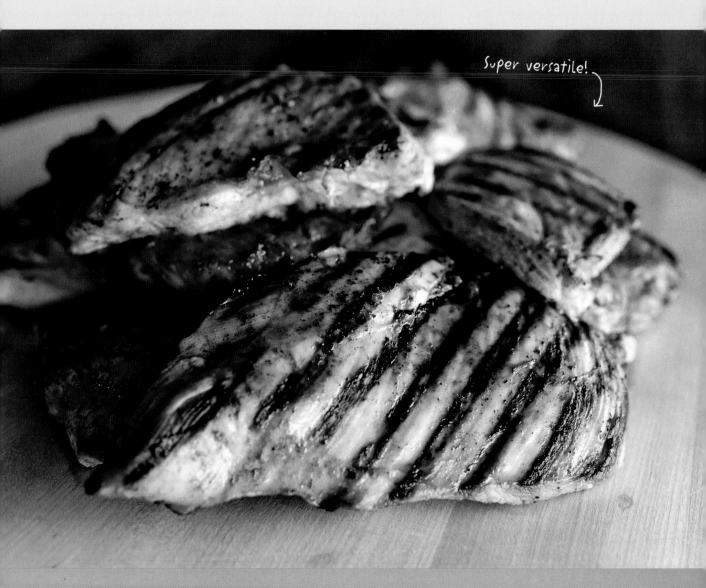

Super versatile!

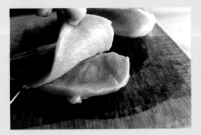

1. Leave the breasts as they are, or if you want 24 thinner cutlets, slice the chicken breasts in half horizontally.

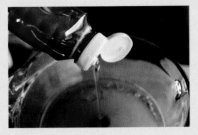

2. In a bowl, combine the olive oil, lemon juice, Dijon, and honey . . .

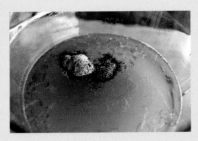

3. Then add the thyme, oregano, salt, and pepper . . .

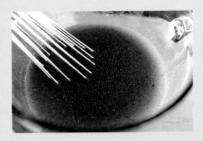

4. And whisk to combine.

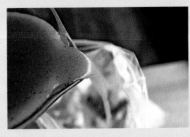

5. Place the chicken breasts or cutlets in one or two large plastic bags and cover them with the marinade . . .

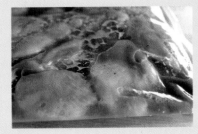

6. Then seal the bags and let them marinate in the fridge for 8 to 12 hours.

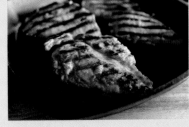

7. Grill the chicken on an outdoor grill (or indoor grill pan) on both sides for 7 to 10 minutes total, depending on thickness, until golden brown and completely cooked through.

V VARIATIONS

Add 1 tablespoon chili powder to the marinade for a spicier chicken.

Freeze the raw chicken in the marinade to have ready-to-go chicken to thaw and put on the grill.

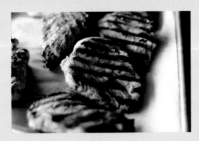

8. To prepare them for freezing, let them cool, then place them on a parchment-paper-lined baking sheet and place them directly in the freezer for 30 to 45 minutes to "set" the surface.

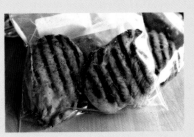

9. From there, transfer them into small or large freezer bags and store in the fridge. (Force as much air out of the bags as possible before freezing.)

REHEATING INSTRUCTIONS

Thaw frozen chicken packets in the fridge for 24 to 48 hours. Serve cold in salads, or warm in a skillet, microwave, or oven for various recipes.

S SERVE

On Chicken Caesar Salad (page 112)

On Chicken Taco Salad (page 53)

In Cobb Salad (page 50)

On sandwiches, nachos, in tacos . . . the list goes on!

CHICKEN CAESAR SALAD

MAKES 8 SERVINGS

Mmmmm, Caesar salad. There's just nothing like it in the world, is there? The tangy sharpness of the dressing, the crispness of the romaine, the reference to the ancient Roman statesman Julius Caesar. It's a food lover's—and homeschooling mother's—dream.

And never mind on the Julius Caesar reference. Caesar salad is actually named after its creator, Caesar Cardini, an Italian immigrant who opened restaurants in the United States.

But it doesn't matter for whom the salad was named (Speaking of homeschooling mothers, notice my correct use of the preposition in the preceding clause? Do I get an A?)—this will always be one of my lifelong favorites and, on a slightly different note, my most oft-ordered hotel room service dish!

There you go. You now know everything there is to know about me. So let's go ahead and make Caesar salad together!

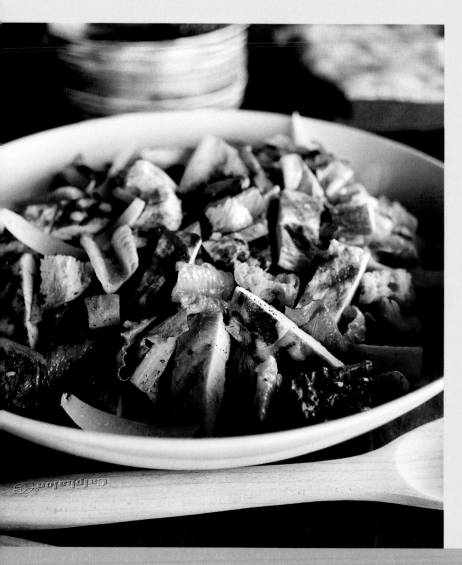

DRESSING

4 anchovy fillets

2 garlic cloves

3 tablespoons Dijon mustard

1 tablespoon balsamic or red wine vinegar

Juice of ½ lemon

3 or 4 dashes Worcestershire sauce

¼ teaspoon kosher salt, more to taste

Black pepper to taste

¼ cup freshly grated Parmesan cheese

½ cup olive oil

CROUTONS

¼ cup olive oil

3 garlic cloves, minced

½ loaf crusty Italian or French bread, cut into 1-inch cubes

Kosher salt to taste

SALAD

2 Ready-to-Go Grilled Chicken breasts (page 110), chilled

3 romaine lettuce hearts

Fresh Parmesan shavings

Black pepper to taste

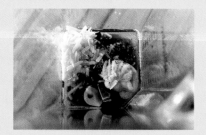

1. To make the dressing, combine all the dressing ingredients except the olive oil in a blender or food processor.

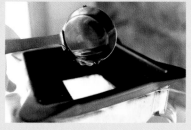

2. With the machine on low, drizzle in the olive oil in a small stream until it's all incorporated.

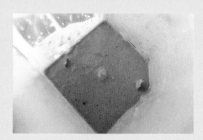

3. Scrape down the sides, blend it again for a few seconds, then give the dressing a taste and add more of whatever ingredient it needs. Make it all yours!

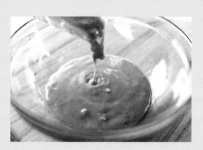

4. Transfer the dressing to a bowl.

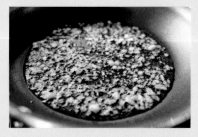

5. When it's getting close to salad time, make the croutons: Preheat the oven to 200°F. In a skillet, gently heat the olive oil with the garlic over medium heat . . .

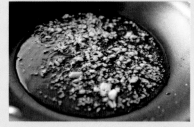

6. Until the garlic is lightly golden, about 3 minutes (don't let it burn!).

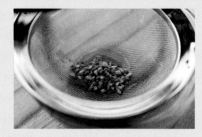

7. Strain out the garlic so you're left with perfect, pure garlic oil. Yum!

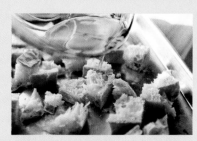

8. Spread the bread cubes on a rimmed baking sheet, drizzle on the garlic oil, sprinkle them with salt, and toss them to coat.

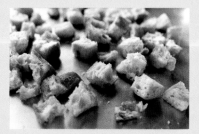

9. Bake the croutons for 1 hour, shaking the pan a couple of times. After 1 hour, crank up the oven to 400°F and bake the croutons for 5 minutes more. Set the pan aside to cool.

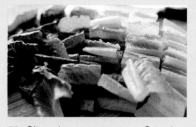

10. To assemble the salad, slice the grilled chicken into strips or chunks, whatever makes your skirt fly up.

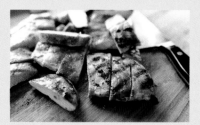

11. Slice the romaine into 2-inch pieces and throw them into a large bowl.

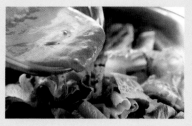

12. Pour on two-thirds of the dressing . . .

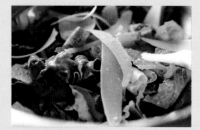

13. Add a good amount of fresh Parmesan shavings . . .

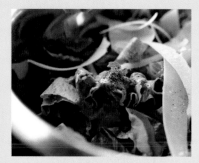

14. And sprinkle on some pepper.

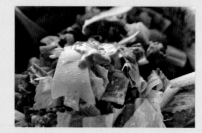

15. Toss to combine and give the salad a taste, then add more dressing and/or Parmesan to taste.

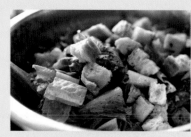

16. Finally, toss in the croutons . . .

Ⓜ MAKE AHEAD

Make the dressing up to 5 days ahead of time and store in the fridge.

Make the croutons up to 2 days ahead of time and store in a plastic bag at room temperature.

Ⓥ VARIATIONS

Make the croutons from cornbread instead of Italian/French bread.

Use grilled shrimp instead of chicken.

Top the salad with Beautiful Roasted Vegetables (page 290) instead of chicken for a colorful, tasty salad.

Drop the chicken altogether and serve as a regular Caesar salad with any number of main courses.

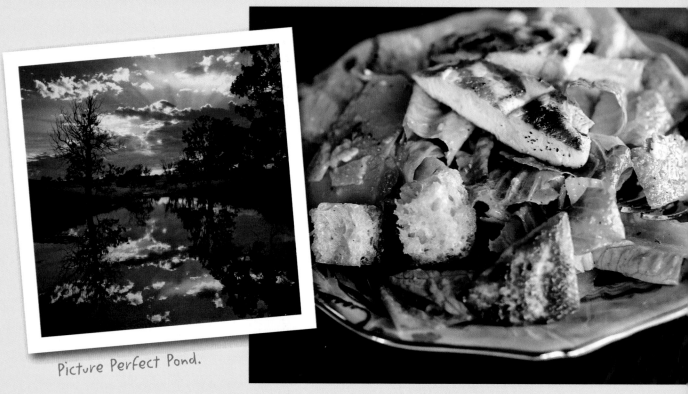

Picture Perfect Pond.

17. And serve it to Caesar salad–loving humans!

READY-TO-GO CHILI PACKETS

MAKES TWELVE 2-CUP FREEZER PACKETS

This is the Simple, Perfect Chili recipe I've made for years and years (I make it so much, in fact, that it's in my first cookbook, albeit in half this quantity), and I've found that keeping a ready-to-use stash in my freezer at all times really does contribute to my all-around contentment and satisfaction in life. Chili is just one of those things that opens up a world of possibilities, from chili dogs to nachos, and since it's a great thing to make in bulk, you can knock out a huge batch all at once.

Fill your freezer with chili packets! It'll make ya happy, I promise.

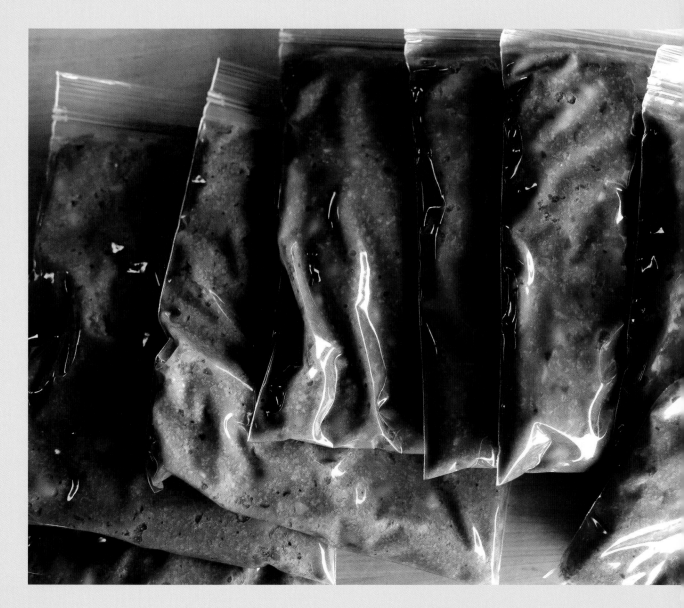

4 pounds ground beef

6 garlic cloves, minced

Two 8-ounce cans tomato sauce

One 6-ounce can tomato paste

¼ cup chili powder, more to taste

2 teaspoons ground cumin

2 teaspoons ground oregano

2 teaspoons kosher salt

½ teaspoon cayenne pepper, more to taste

Two 15-ounce cans kidney beans, drained and rinsed

Two 15-ounce cans pinto beans, drained and rinsed

½ cup masa harina (corn flour) or regular cornmeal

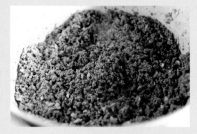

1. In a large, heavy pot, brown the ground beef with the garlic until it's totally cooked. Drain off most of the excess fat, leaving a little behind for moisture and flavor.

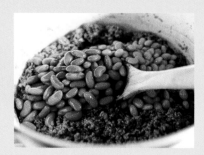

4. After an hour, stir in all the beans.

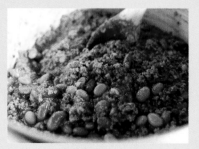

7. Let the chili simmer for another 10 minutes to thicken, then turn off the heat and let it cool.

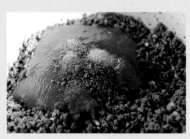

2. Add the tomato sauce, tomato paste, chili powder, cumin, oregano, salt, and cayenne.

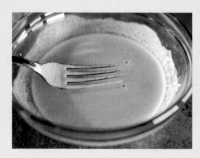

5. In a small bowl, combine the masa harina with ½ cup water and stir together with a fork until it's smooth.

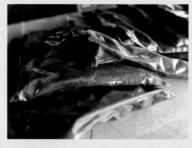

8. Fill large or small freezer bags (or other freezer containers) according to your preference . . .

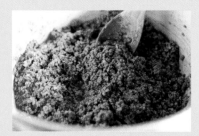

3. Stir together well, cover the pot, and reduce the heat to low. Simmer for 1 hour, stirring occasionally. If the liquid level seems low, add up to 1 cup water to keep it from burning.

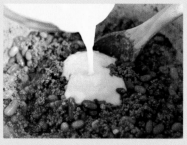

6. Pour the masa mixture into the chili. Stir together well, then taste the chili and adjust the seasonings.

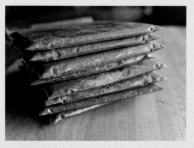

9. And freeze them flat for easy stacking.

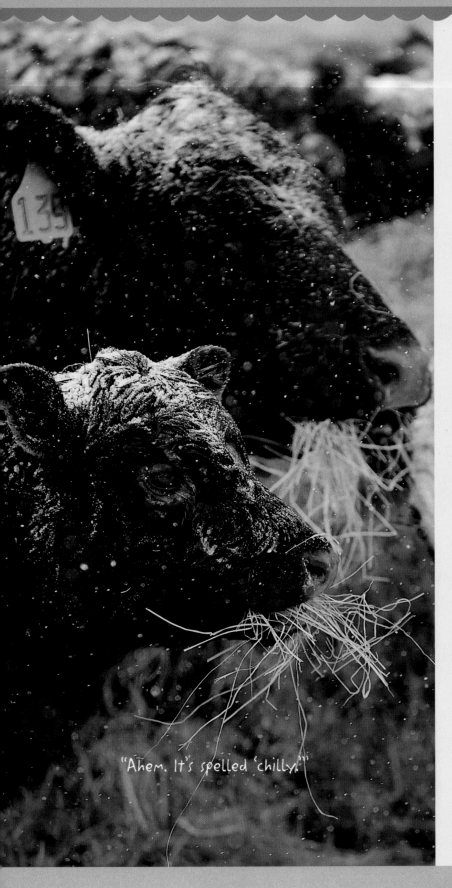

"Ahem. It's spelled 'chilly.'"

REHEATING INSTRUCTIONS

Let individual bags of chili thaw in the fridge for 24 hours, then reheat in a saucepan, adding ¼ cup water if necessary for consistency.

—OR—

Lay a bag of frozen chili on a microwave-safe plate and defrost it in the microwave according to your microwave's instructions. Transfer to a bowl (for the microwave) or a saucepan for reheating.

—OR—

Place a bag of frozen chili in a microwave-safe bowl and reheat according to your microwave's instructions.

Ⓥ VARIATIONS

Omit the beans for a simpler, meat-only chili.

Add diced bell pepper (any color) to the chili.

Substitute ground turkey for part of the ground beef.

Ⓢ SERVE

On top of cheeseburger patties

In Chili Dogs (page 118)

On tortilla chips, topped with cheese

In a bowl with sour cream, grated cheese, and chopped onion

In taco shells as a taco filling

CHILI DOGS

MAKES 2 BIG, BEAUTIFUL CHILI DOGS

Chili dogs are so crazy-good, and so crazy . . . well, crazy. But make no apologies! Eat that chili dog with abandon and pride! (Just don't do it more than once or twice a year.)

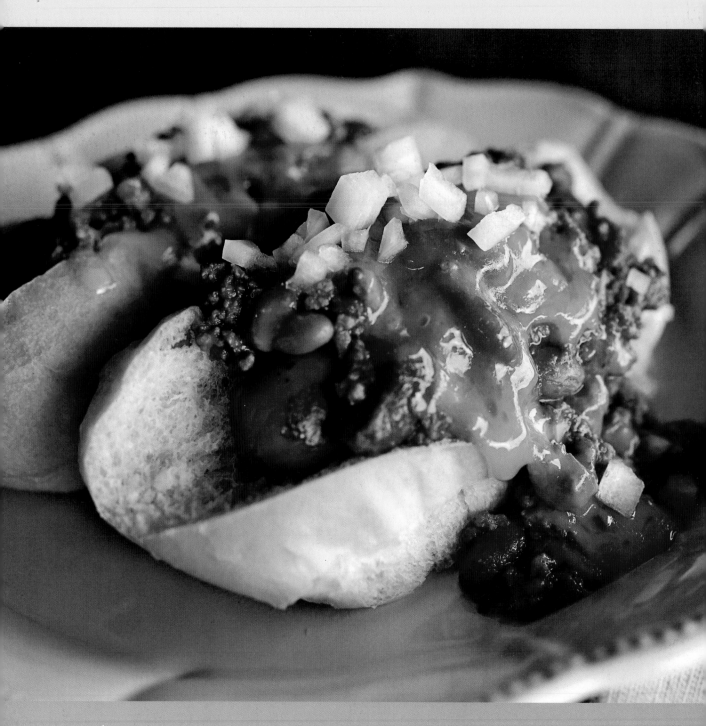

2 good-quality hot dog buns
2 good-quality beef franks

2 cups (1 packet) Ready-to-Go Chili Packet (page 115), thawed and reheated

½ cup grated Cheddar cheese
2 tablespoons finely diced onion

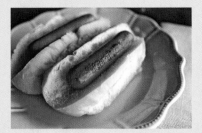

1. Lightly toast the buns under the broiler and brown the franks in a small skillet over medium heat. Place the franks on the buns . . .

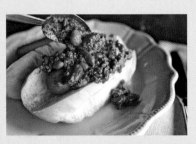

2. And spoon on a bunch of chili.

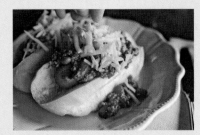

3. Add the cheese all over the top . . .

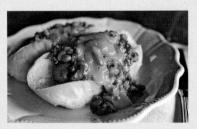

4. Then heat in the microwave to melt the cheese, 25 to 35 seconds. (Or, if you're using an oven-safe plate, place it under a low broiler until the cheese melts, about 1 minute.)

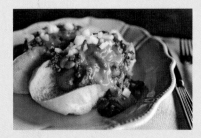

5. Sprinkle with the onion . . .

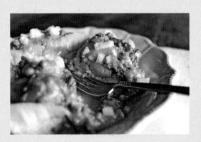

6. And dive in.

A fork and knife are recommended!

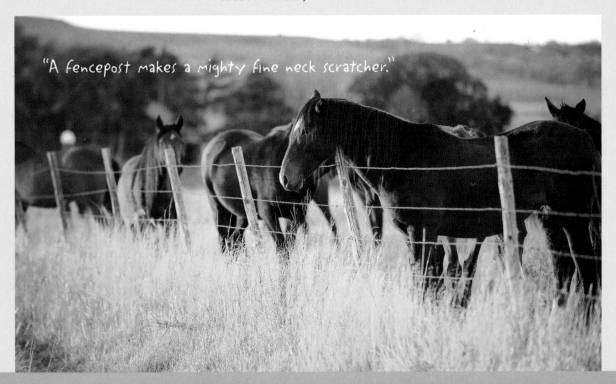

"A fencepost makes a mighty fine neck scratcher."

READY-TO-GO TACO CHICKEN

MAKES ABOUT 6 CUPS

This flavorful shredded chicken is just the thing for tacos, nachos, quesadillas, tostadas, taco salad, taco pizza . . . the list is endless! It's nice and saucy, so it packs extra flavor wherever you use it. Double it, triple it . . . make as much of it as you think you'll need. Then just freeze it in smaller bags so you can pull out the portion you need. With this taco meat, all things are possible!

6 boneless, skinless chicken breasts

¼ cup taco seasoning

2 tablespoons chili powder

Kosher salt (optional)

¼ cup vegetable oil

Two 8-ounce cans tomato sauce

Several dashes of hot sauce, such as Cholula or Tabasco

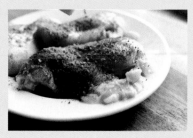

1. Coat both sides of the chicken with the taco seasoning and the chili powder. Rub it into the meat so the chicken is totally coated. Add salt if the taco seasoning you use does not contain salt.

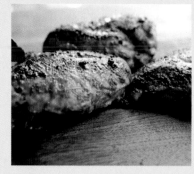

3. Set the chicken aside to cool slightly.

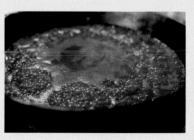

5. Bring the sauce to a gentle boil over medium-high heat, then reduce the heat to low and simmer for a few minutes while you shred the chicken.

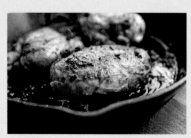

2. Heat a large skillet over medium heat and add the oil. Working in batches, cook the chicken breasts on both sides until they're deep golden on the outside and done in the middle, about 4 minutes per side.

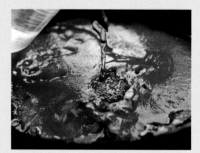

4. In the same skillet, combine the tomato sauce and 1 cup hot water, stirring and scraping the bottom of the skillet to loosen all the flavorful bits.

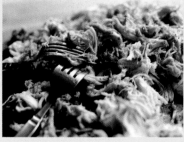

6. Use two forks to completely shred the chicken . . .

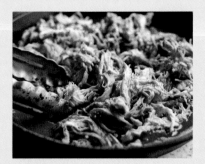

7. Then transfer it to the sauce . . .

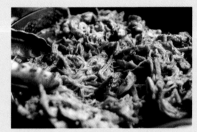

8. And stir the chicken to coat it with the sauce. Simmer on low for 5 minutes more, then turn off the heat.

S SERVE

In Chicken Nachos (page 122)

In Chicken Taco Salad, instead of the cubed chicken (page 53)

In tacos

In quesadillas

On taco pizza

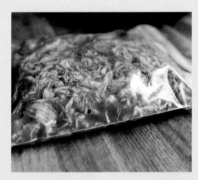

FREEZER INSTRUCTIONS

Allow the mixture to cool almost to room temperature, then pack the taco chicken in plastic freezer bags (or other freezer containers) according to the sizes you need. Freeze for up to 6 months.

To reheat, place the bag(s) in the refrigerator and allow them to thaw for 24 to 36 hours, then reheat in a saucepan or in a microwave-safe dish in the microwave. For a quick thaw, place the bag in the microwave and heat in 1- to 2-minute intervals, flipping/squishing the bag after each, until the meat is thawed.

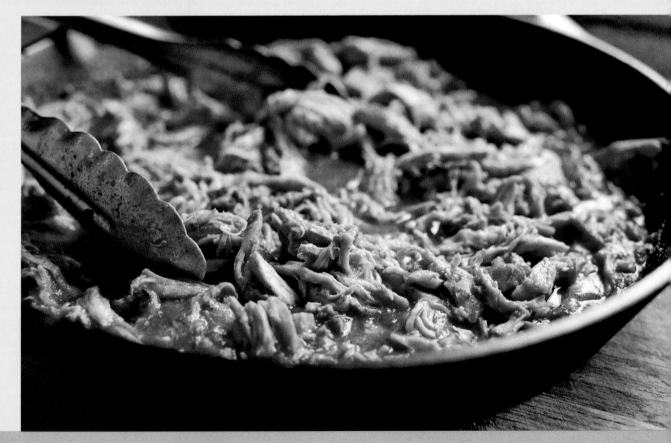

CHICKEN NACHOS

MAKES 4 SERVINGS

Have you heard the news? Nachos make a perfectly legitimate dinner! This is especially true if you pile on delicious meat and serve them with a big salad on the side. Or turn the nachos into a complete meal themselves by piling on tomatoes, lettuce, and other fixins.

The guys in my house love this simple version. (The girls in my house do, too!)

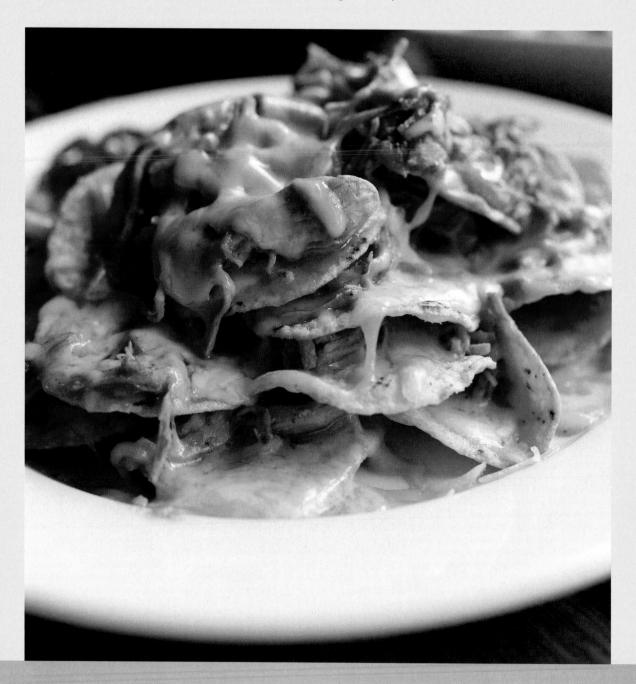

4 to 6 ounces good-quality tortilla chips

½ pound Cheddar-Jack cheese, grated (about 1½ cups)

2 cups Ready-to-Go Taco Chicken (page 120), thawed and heated

1. Preheat the oven to 325°F. (If you're using the microwave, skip this step.)

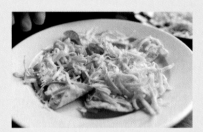

2. On an oven-safe/microwave-safe plate, arrange some of the chips in a single layer, overlapping them slightly. Sprinkle on a good layer of cheese . . .

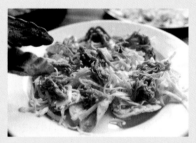

3. Then add a layer of the chicken . . .

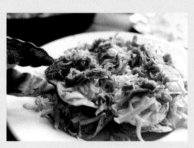

4. Then another round of chips, cheese, and chicken.

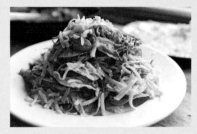

5. And keep going until you feel you've successfully built Mount St. Nacho!

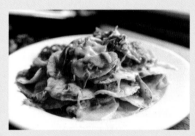

6. Place the plate in the oven and heat the nachos for 4 to 5 minutes, until the cheese is totally melted. (Alternatively, microwave the nachos for about 2 minutes, until the cheese is melted.)

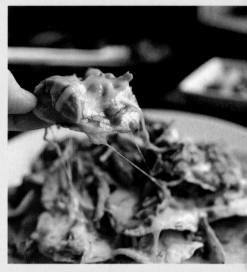

7. Then dive right in and devour 'em!

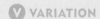 **VARIATION**

Add any of the following fixins: pinto beans, pico de gallo (see page 23), chopped tomatoes, guacamole, sliced avocado, sour cream, jalapeño slices, shredded lettuce.

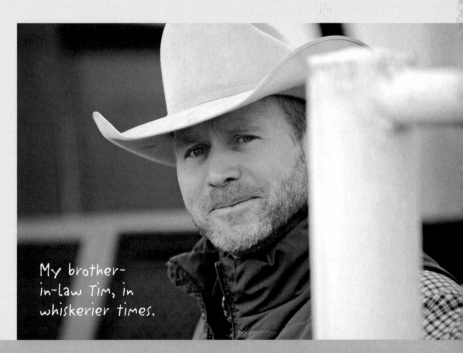

My brother-in-law Tim, in whiskerier times.

READY-TO-GO BEEF TACO FILLING

MAKES TWELVE 2-CUP FREEZER PACKETS

Beef taco meat isn't really wildly different from beef chili, except taco meat generally doesn't contain beans and the seasonings take a slightly different approach. But the truth is, you can use them interchangeably: Add beans to this meat to turn it into chili, or use Ready-to-Go Chili Packets (page 115) in your tacos.

In case you like to keep things separate and compartmentalized, though, here's my favorite taco meat recipe! So great to have on hand.

4 pounds ground beef

Two 10-ounce cans Mexican red sauce or red enchilada sauce

2 tablespoons chili powder

1 teaspoon cayenne pepper

1 tablespoon ground cumin

2 teaspoons garlic salt

2 teaspoons kosher salt

1 tablespoon black pepper

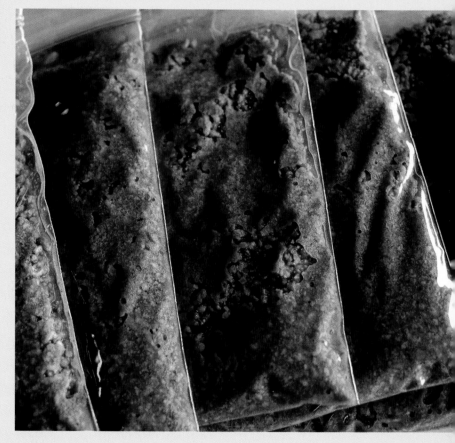

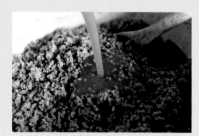

1. In a large pot, brown the beef over medium-high heat. Drain off the excess fat, leaving behind a little bit for moisture and flavor. Add the red sauce . . .

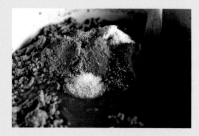

2. Along with the chili powder, cayenne, cumin, garlic salt, kosher salt, and black pepper.

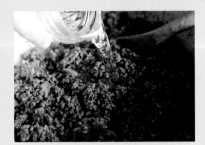

3. Pour in 1½ cups water . . .

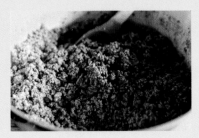

4. Then stir it around, reduce the heat, cover the pot, and simmer for 30 minutes, stirring occasionally.

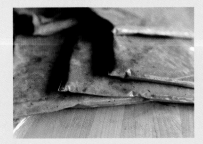

5. Let the meat cool, then package it in quart-size freezer bags (or other freezer containers) and freeze them flat for easy stacking.

S SERVE

On Salad Tacos (page 126)

On nachos, covered in grated Cheddar cheese

Inside burritos, with refried beans and cheese

REHEATING INSTRUCTIONS

Let individual bags of taco meat thaw in the fridge for 24 hours, then reheat the meat in a saucepan, adding ¼ cup water if necessary for consistency.

—OR—

Lay a bag of frozen taco meat on a microwave-safe plate and defrost in the microwave according to your microwave's instructions. Transfer to a bowl (for the microwave) or a saucepan for reheating.

—OR—

Place a bag of frozen taco meat in a microwave-safe bowl and reheat according to your microwave's instructions.

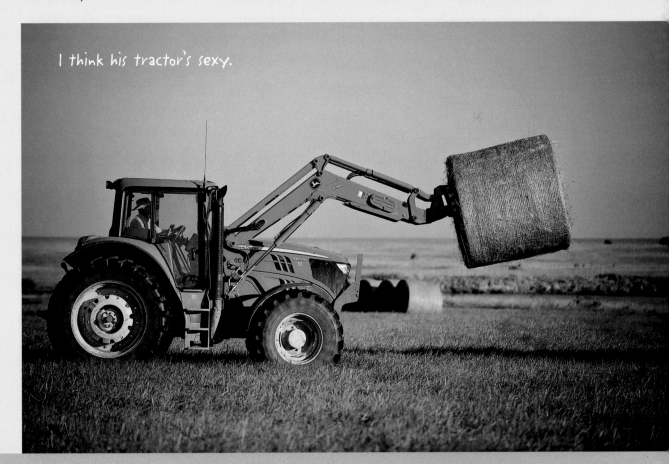

I think his tractor's sexy.

SALAD TACOS

MAKES 6 HARD SHELL TACOS, TO SERVE 2 OR 3

I call these "Salad Tacos" because lettuce features prominently and the tacos are topped with a simple salad dressing. Not much different than regular tacos, but they've got a little extra crunch and a super-fresh flavor that make my heart go pitter-pat.

¼ cup sour cream

¼ cup salsa

Several dashes of hot sauce (optional)

6 hard taco shells, crisped according to the package instructions

2 cups thinly sliced green-leaf lettuce

2 cups (1 packet) Ready-to-Go Beef Taco Filling (page 124), thawed and reheated

12 grape tomatoes, halved

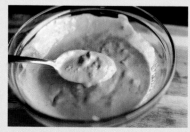

1. Mix together the sour cream, salsa, and hot sauce (if using) to make a dressing.

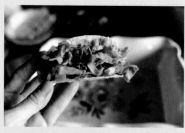

2. To assemble the tacos, fill the taco shells as full as you can with shredded lettuce . . .

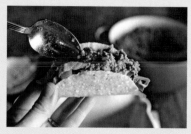

3. Then spoon on the warm taco meat . . .

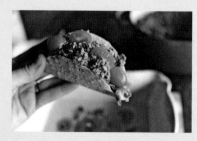

4. Add some tomato halves . . .

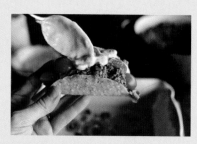

5. And spoon on plenty of dressing.

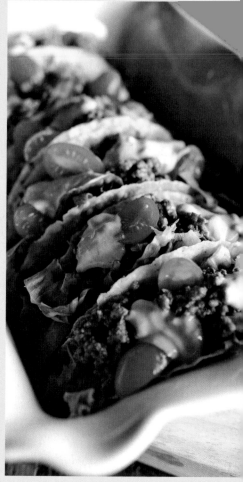

Crispy and crunchy as all get-out!

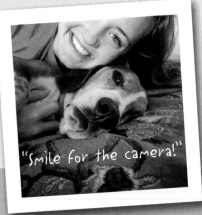

"Smile for the camera!"

BAKED ZITI

MAKES 12 SERVINGS

Before I begin with this recipe, I must make an important disclosure:

I did not use ziti to make this baked ziti. I used mostaccioli.

I'm truly sorry for this transgression. It's just that mostaccioli is all I had, and I did not want to call this dish "Baked Mostaccioli." Just doesn't have the same ring to it.

The next thing I need to say is this:

Oh my ever-loving goodness, is this good.

Baked ziti is a classic baked pasta dish. It's basically some kind of tomato or meat sauce baked in a dish with some kind of cheese and, of course, ziti noodles. Unless you're me, then you use mostaccioli noodles. Some people just use tomato/marinara sauce. That, of course, would never fly in this house. There must be meat. Meat there must be. As for the cheese, some people use only mozzarella, while others prefer to use a gooey cheese mixture stirred throughout.

I'm in the latter camp. I like baked ziti to be almost like lasagna that forgot to use lasagna noodles. Messy. Gooey. Decadent.

And it freezes really well!

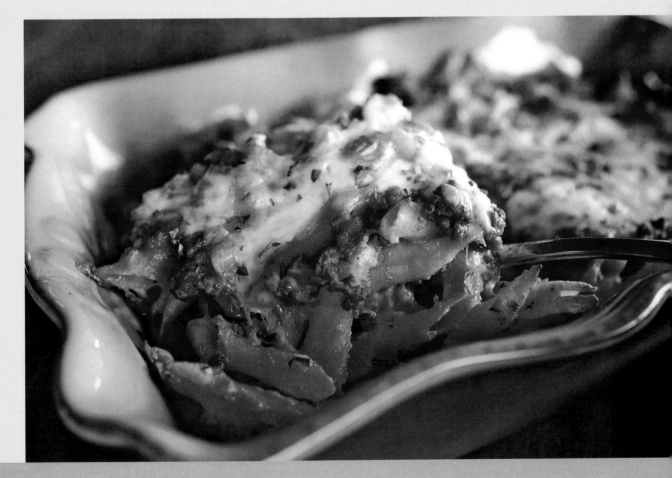

2 tablespoons olive oil

1 large onion, diced

3 garlic cloves, minced

1 pound Italian sausage

1 pound ground beef

One 28-ounce can whole tomatoes

One 24.5-ounce jar marinara sauce

2 teaspoons Italian seasoning

½ teaspoon red pepper flakes

1 teaspoon kosher salt

1 teaspoon black pepper

1 pound (16 ounces) ziti (or any short pasta!), cooked until not quite al dente

One 15-ounce container whole milk ricotta cheese

1½ pounds mozzarella cheese, grated

½ cup grated Parmesan cheese

1 large egg

2 tablespoons minced parsley, plus more for sprinkling

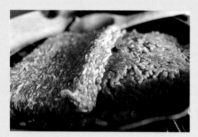

1. Heat the olive oil in a pot over medium heat. Add the onion, garlic, sausage, and ground beef . . .

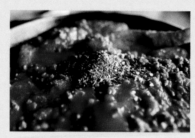

3. Add the tomatoes, marinara, Italian seasoning, red pepper flakes, ½ teaspoon of the salt, and ½ teaspoon of the black pepper.

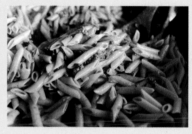

6. Then toss to coat the noodles. Set it aside to cool.

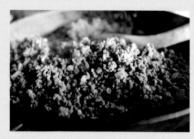

2. And cook until the meat is totally browned. Drain off and discard most of the fat from the pot, leaving a bit behind for flavor and moisture.

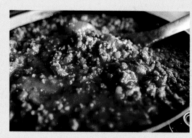

4. Stir to combine, then simmer the sauce for 25 to 30 minutes, stirring occasionally.

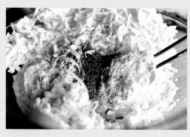

7. In a medium bowl, combine the ricotta, 2 cups of the grated mozzarella, the Parmesan, egg, parsley, and the remaining ½ teaspoon each salt and pepper.

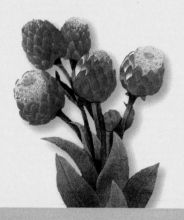

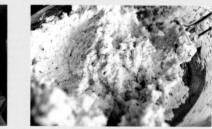

5. Place the pasta in a large bowl and ladle in 3 cups of the sauce mixture . . .

8. Stir the mixture together until combined.

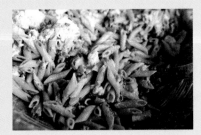

9. Toss the cheese mixture in with the sauce-and-pasta mixture. Do not overmix: You want to have some big chunks of the cheese mixture.

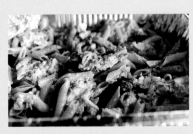

10. Add half the pasta mixture to a large casserole dish or disposable foil pan.

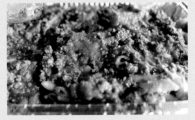

11. Spoon half the remaining sauce over the top . . .

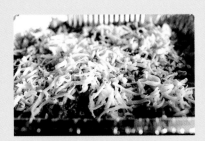

12. Then top with half the remaining mozzarella. Repeat with another round of pasta, sauce, and mozzarella.

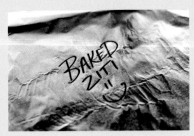

13. At this point, you can let the casserole cool, then cover and label it for the freezer! (See the freezer baking instructions below.)

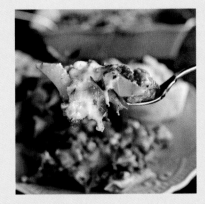

Or, if you're making it straight through, bake in a preheated 375°F oven for 25 to 30 minutes, or until bubbling and lightly browned. Remove from oven and let stand 5 minutes before serving. Sprinkle chopped parsley over the pasta before serving.

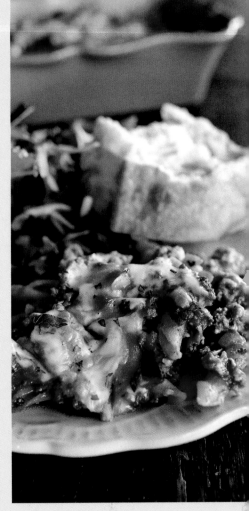

Serve up big platefuls while it's piping hot!

FREEZER INSTRUCTIONS

Cover the unbaked casserole tightly with heavy foil and freeze for up to 6 months.

To bake, place the frozen casserole straight into a 350°F oven, still covered, for 1 hour 45 minutes. Remove the foil and bake for anywhere from 10 to 30 minutes more, until hot and bubbly.

—OR—

Thaw the casserole in the refrigerator for 24 to 36 hours, until completely thawed. Bake according to the recipe instructions.

MEXICAN TORTILLA CASSEROLE

MAKES 12 TO 16 SERVINGS

This is based on a delicious, hearty casserole my friend Pastor Ryan shared with me several years ago. It's beyond satisfying and luscious, and it has served many a roomful of cowboys and teenagers in my house. Everyone loves it, and it's the perfect thing to have on standby in the freezer.

3 tablespoons olive oil

3 cups diced fresh tomatoes (from 5 to 7 whole, depending on size)

1 large onion, diced

3 garlic cloves, minced

4 teaspoons chili powder

2 teaspoons paprika

2 teaspoons ground cumin

½ teaspoon kosher salt, more to taste

2 boneless, skinless chicken breasts, cut into bite-size pieces

One 15-ounce can pinto beans, drained and rinsed

One 15-ounce can kidney beans, drained and rinsed

One 16-ounce jar salsa verde

12 large or 18 small flour or corn tortillas

3 cups cooked rice (from 1 cup uncooked)

One 11-ounce can corn, drained

1½ pounds grated Cheddar-Jack cheese

1 recipe Homemade Enchilada Sauce (page 8), or 2 cups red enchilada sauce

Sour cream, for serving

Cilantro, for serving

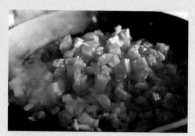

1. In a large skillet, heat 1 tablespoon of the oil over medium-high heat. Add the tomatoes, onion, and garlic, stir, and cook for a minute or two to soften the onion.

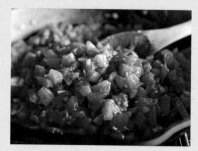

3. Stir and cook the mixture for another minute or two to release the flavors of the spices.

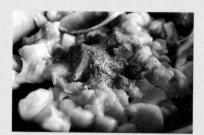

5. In the same skillet, heat the remaining 2 tablespoons oil. Add the chicken along with the remaining 2 teaspoons chili powder, 1 teaspoon paprika, 1 teaspoon cumin, and the salt . . .

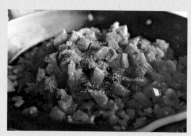

2. Add 2 teaspoons of the chili powder, 1 teaspoon of the paprika, and 1 teaspoon of the cumin.

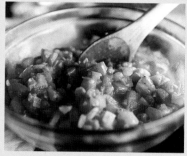

4. Remove the mixture to a bowl and set aside.

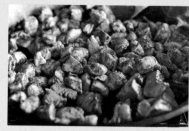

6. And sauté the chicken until it's deep golden brown and done in the middle, 4 to 5 minutes.

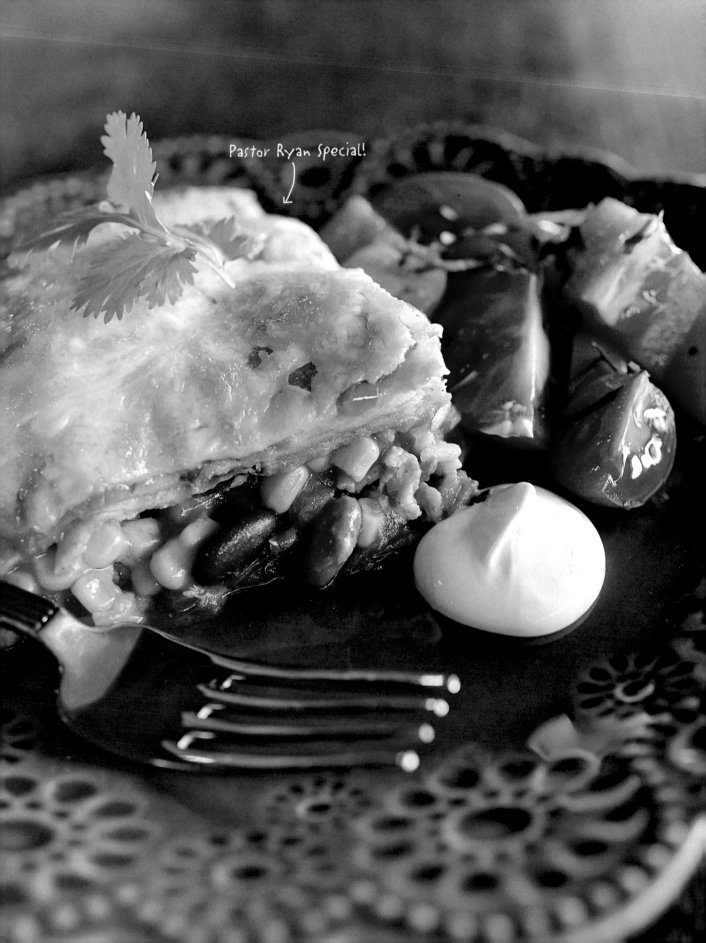

Pastor Ryan Special!

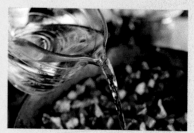

7. Add 1 cup water and stir to make a sauce. Bring the sauce to a boil and cook until it's reduced by half, 3 to 4 minutes.

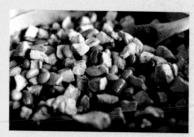

8. Stir in the beans and set aside.

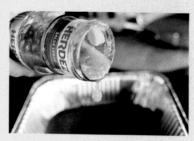

9. To assemble the casserole, pour half a jar (about 1 cup) of salsa verde in the bottom of a 9 x 13-inch casserole dish or disposable foil baking pan.

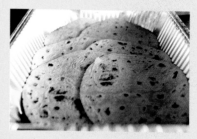

10. Add half the tortillas in a layer on top of the salsa verde, overlapping the edges.

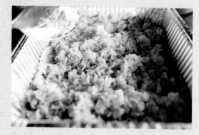

11. Spoon the rice over the tortillas . . .

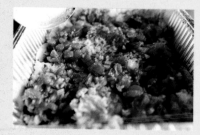

12. Spread the tomato mixture over the rice . . .

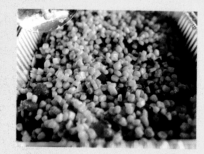

13. Then sprinkle the corn over the tomatoes.

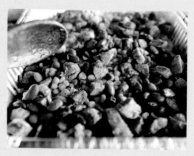

14. Next, add the chicken-and-bean mixture . . .

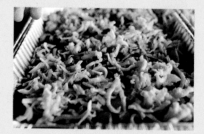

15. Then sprinkle on half the cheese . . .

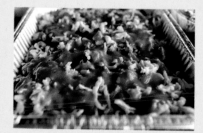

16. And pour over half the enchilada sauce.

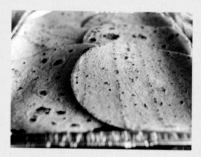

17. Next, add the rest of the tortillas . . .

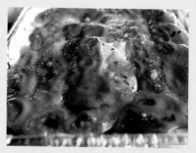

18. Then pour on the rest of the salsa verde and the rest of the enchilada sauce . . .

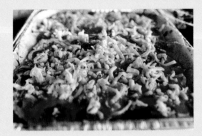

19. And sprinkle on the rest of the cheese. To freeze, see the instructions below.

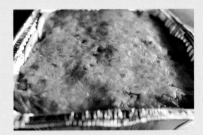

20. If you're baking the casserole right away, preheat the oven to 375°F and bake the casserole, covered in foil, for 20 minutes. Then remove the foil and continue baking for 15 to 20 minutes, or until hot and bubbly.

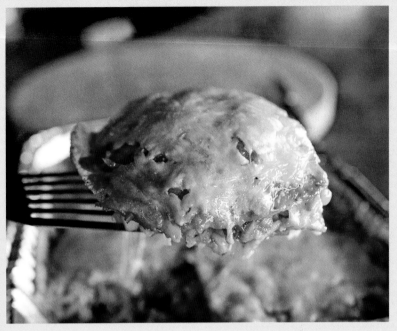

21. Serve up great big helpings!

FREEZER INSTRUCTIONS

Cover the unbaked casserole tightly in heavy foil and freeze for up to 6 months.

To bake the casserole, preheat the oven to 350°F. Bake the foil-covered pan for 2 hours. Remove the foil and bake for 10 to 30 minutes more, until hot and bubbly.

—OR—

Thaw the pan in the refrigerator for 24 to 36 hours, until completely thawed. Bake according to the recipe instructions.

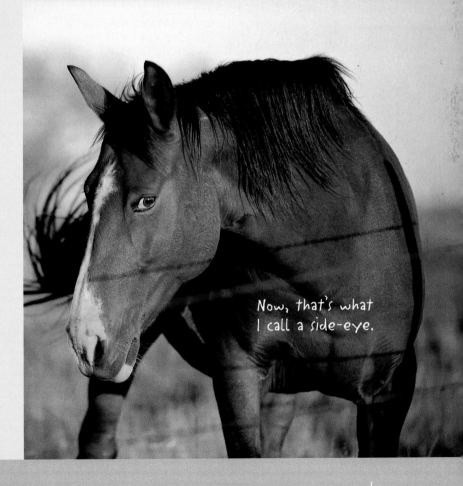

Now, that's what I call a side-eye.

RED, WHITE, AND GREEN STUFFED SHELLS

MAKES 12 SERVINGS

Stuffed shells are comfort food for me, and can be prepared in any number of ways. A creamy, herby white sauce topping the cheese-stuffed wonders is always delicious . . . but I also love the tang of a rich marinara. It's impossible decide which way is best.

The great thing about this version is that I don't have to choose!

I love it when a recipe enables my indecisiveness. (Or is it indecision? I can't decide.)

1 tablespoon olive oil

½ medium onion, diced

1 garlic clove, minced

10 ounces baby spinach

4 tablespoons (½ stick) butter

¼ cup all-purpose flour

2½ cups whole milk, more as needed

2 tablespoons chopped basil

2 tablespoons chopped parsley

Kosher salt and black pepper to taste

One 30-ounce container whole milk ricotta cheese

1 cup grated Parmesan cheese, plus more for sprinkling

1 large egg

12 ounces jumbo pasta shells (25 to 30 shells), cooked until slightly firmer than al dente

One 24-ounce jar marinara sauce

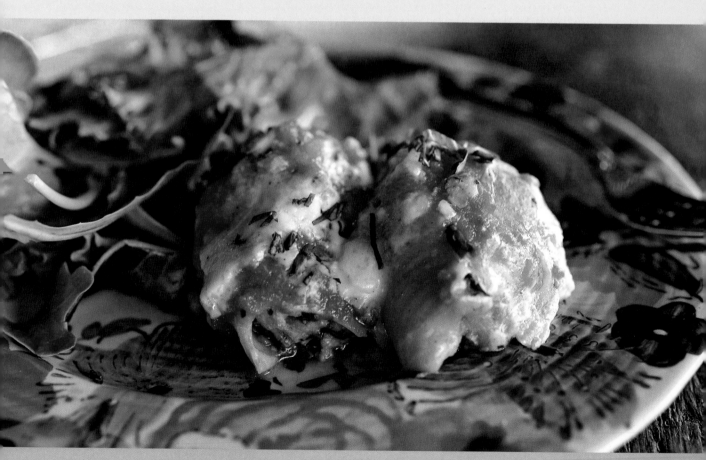

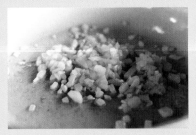

1. Heat the olive oil in large skillet over medium heat. Add the onion and garlic and sauté until the onion starts to soften, about 4 minutes.

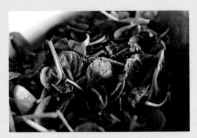

2. Add the spinach . . .

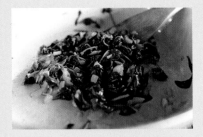

3. And cook, stirring continuously, until it's lightly wilted, about 2 minutes.

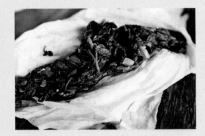

4. Remove the spinach from the pan and let it cool slightly, then place it inside a few paper towels and squeeze out as much liquid as you can.

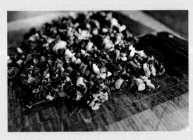

5. Give it a rough chop and set it aside.

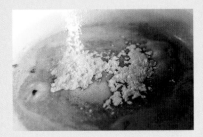

6. Turn the heat to medium-low, then, in the same skillet, melt the butter and sprinkle the flour over the top.

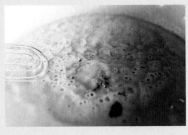

7. Whisk it together to make a roux, then cook it for a minute or two.

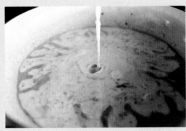

8. Slowly add the milk, whisking out lumps as you go . . .

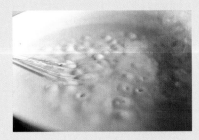

9. And cook it until the white sauce is thickened, 4 to 5 minutes.

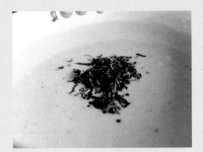

10. Turn off the heat and stir in half the basil, half the parsley, and salt and pepper to taste. (Add another ¼ cup milk if the white sauce is too thick.) Taste and adjust the seasonings.

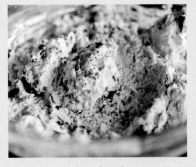

11. In a separate bowl, mix together the ricotta, Parmesan, egg, the rest of the basil, the rest of the parsley, and salt and pepper to taste until combined. Stir in the chopped spinach mixture.

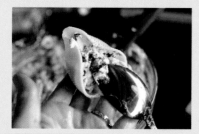

12. To assemble, use a spoon to fill the pasta shells with the cheese mixture. Stuff 'em generously!

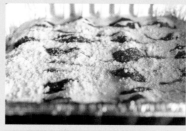

16. Finally, sprinkle on extra Parmesan! If you're making this for the freezer, see the freezer steps below.

FREEZER INSTRUCTIONS

Cover the pan of unbaked shells tightly with heavy foil and freeze for up to 6 months.

To bake the casserole, preheat the oven to 375°F. Bake the foil-covered pan for 1 hour 30 minutes. Remove the foil and bake for anywhere from 10 to 30 minutes more, until hot and bubbly.

—OR—

Thaw the pan in the refrigerator for 24 to 36 hours, until completely thawed. Bake according to the recipe instructions.

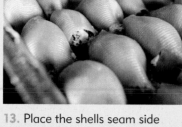

13. Place the shells seam side down in a 9 x 13-inch casserole dish or disposable foil baking pan.

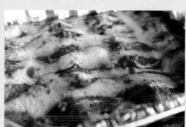

17. If you're baking it right away, preheat the oven to 375°F and bake the shells for 25 to 30 minutes, or until hot and bubbly.

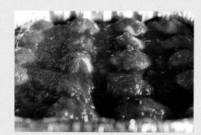

14. Pour the marinara evenly over the shells . . .

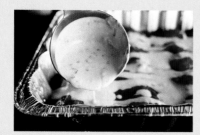

15. And then (this is my favorite part!), ladle the white sauce over the marinara in a zig-zag/line design.

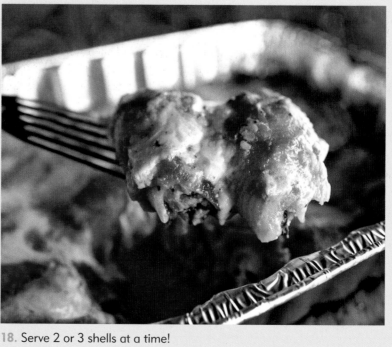

18. Serve 2 or 3 shells at a time!

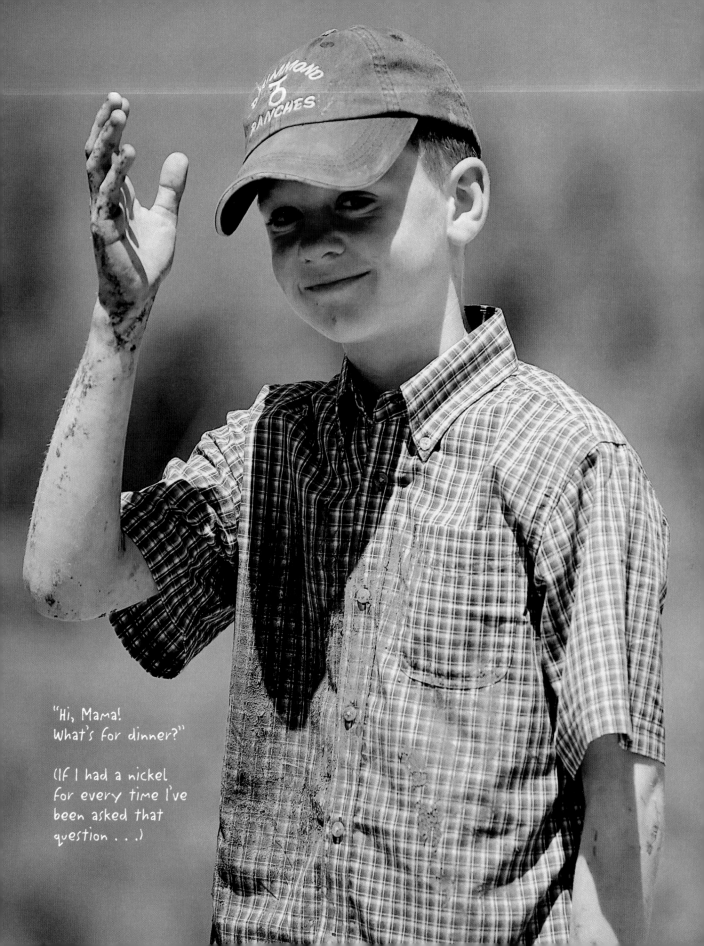

"Hi, Mama!
What's for dinner?"

(If I had a nickel
for every time I've
been asked that
question . . .)

INDIVIDUAL CHICKEN POT PIES

MAKES 4 LARGE INDIVIDUAL PIES

Chicken pot pies are the perfect freezer food, no matter what size they are. I've made plenty of full-size pies in disposable foil pie pans or casseroles, but I also love to whip up smaller versions using individual pie or tart pans.

Double, triple, quadruple this recipe to make as many as you'd like to have on hand!

4 tablespoons (½ stick) butter

1 medium onion, finely diced

2 medium carrots, finely diced

1 celery stalk, finely diced

¼ cup all-purpose flour

3 cups low-sodium chicken broth, more as needed

¼ cup dry white wine (or you may use chicken broth instead)

2 cups shredded or chopped cooked chicken breast

¼ teaspoon ground turmeric

Kosher salt and black pepper to taste

½ teaspoon dried thyme

¼ cup half-and-half

1 recipe All-Butter Pie Crust (recipe follows), or 2 store-bought crusts

1 large egg

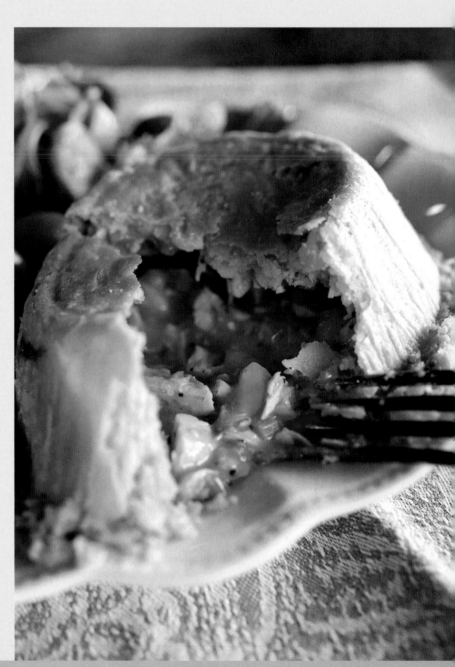

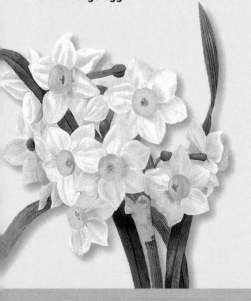

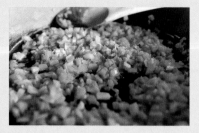

1. Melt the butter in a large skillet over medium-high heat, then add the onion, carrots, and celery. Cook, stirring the vegetables around, until they start to soften, about 3 minutes.

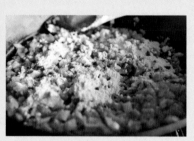

2. Sprinkle the flour over the veggies and stir to combine.

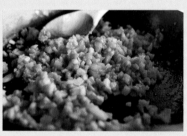

3. Cook the flour-coated veggies for 1 minute . . .

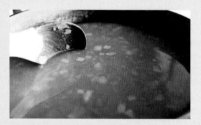

4. Then pour in the broth (and wine, if using!) and stir to combine. Let it heat up and start to bubble and thicken, about 3 minutes.

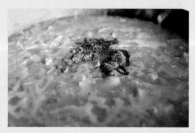

5. Stir in the chicken, then add the turmeric, salt and pepper to taste, and thyme.

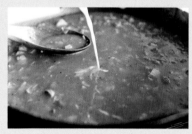

6. Add the half-and-half, then stir the mixture and let it bubble up and thicken, about 3 minutes. If it seems overly thick, splash in a little more broth.

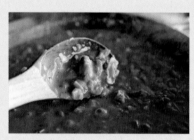

7. Turn off the heat and let the filling cool to room temperature.

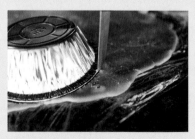

8. Meanwhile, roll out the pie crust(s) and cut out 8 dough circles just a bit larger than the pie pans.

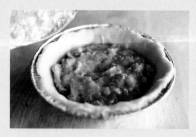

9. Press the dough into the pie pans, making sure the dough comes almost to the top of each pan. Fill the pies with the chicken mixture.

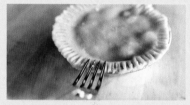

10. Lay a second round of dough over the top of each pie. Press the dough so that the edges meet, then use a fork to seal the edge.

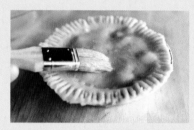

11. Mix the egg with 2 teaspoons water and brush it all over the surface of the crust. (Discard any extra egg wash.)

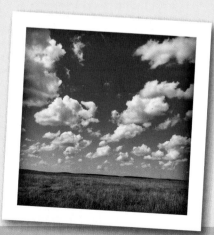

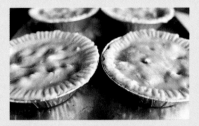

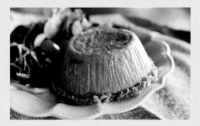

12. Cut small vents in the surface of the crusts, then place the pies on a baking sheet and flash freeze them for 45 minutes. After that, you can store them in large plastic freezer bags or wrap them tightly in foil. To bake them, see the freezer instructions below.

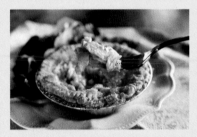

13. If you're baking the pies right away, preheat the oven to 350°F and bake them on a baking sheet for 25 to 30 minutes, until the crust is deep golden brown and the filling is bubbly. Serve them straight out of the pie pans . . .

Or turn them out of the pan and serve them upside down!

Ⓥ **VARIATIONS**

Use leftover Thanksgiving turkey instead of chicken.

Use rotisserie chicken for a nice shortcut!

Ⓢ **SERVE WITH**

Pretty green salad

Raw veggies with dip
(see pages 302–304)

Beautiful Roasted Vegetables
(page 290)

Kale Citrus Salad (page 40)

Store in plastic freezer bags or cover tightly with heavy foil and freeze for up to 6 months.

To bake, preheat the oven to 350°F, cover the pies with foil (if they aren't already covered), and bake them for 1 hour. Remove the foil and bake for 30 to 50 minutes more, until hot and bubbly.

—OR—

Thaw the pies in the refrigerator for 24 to 36 hours, until completely thawed. Bake according to the recipe instructions.

ALL-BUTTER PIE CRUST

1½ cups cold salted butter,
cut into pieces

3 cups all-purpose flour

1 large egg

5 tablespoons cold water

1 tablespoon white vinegar

1 teaspoon kosher salt

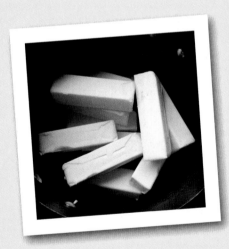

1. In a large bowl, gradually work the butter into the flour using a pastry cutter until the mixture resembles coarse crumbs.

2. In a small bowl, beat the egg with a fork and pour it into the flour mixture, stirring gently. Add the cold water, vinegar, and salt. Stir together gently until all of the ingredients are incorporated.

3. Divide the dough in half and place each portion in a plastic bag. Using a rolling pin, slightly flatten each ball of dough (about ½ inch thick) to make rolling easier later. Seal the bags and place them in the freezer until you need them. (If you will be using the dough immediately, it's still a good idea to put them in the freezer for 15 to 20 minutes to chill.)

LASAGNA ROLL-UPS

MAKES 20 ROLL-UPS, OR 5 LOAF PANS

Lasagna roll-ups are so perfectly convenient and handy, particularly for smaller households, because they can be easily assembled in small loaf pans and you can just grab the amount you need rather than bake off a huge pan at once. I can never have enough of these in the freezer!

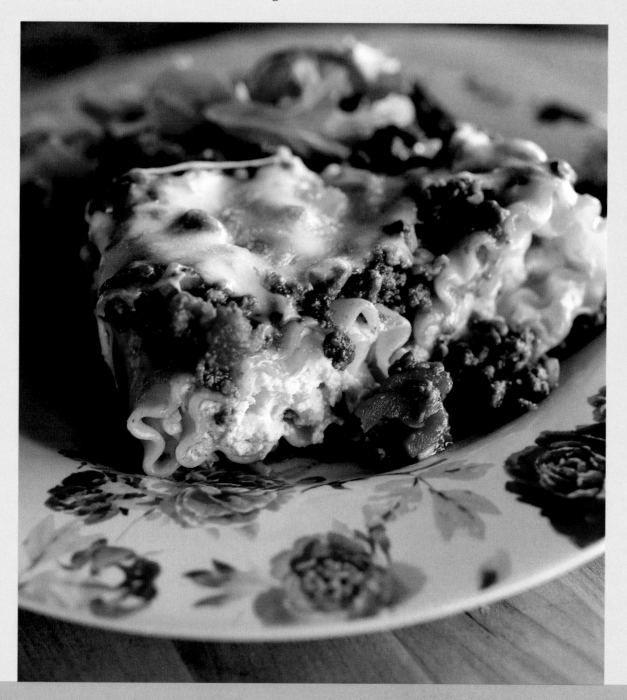

20 lasagna noodles

2 tablespoons olive oil

1 medium onion, diced

1 cup finely chopped mushrooms

1 green bell pepper, seeded and diced

3 garlic cloves, minced

2 pounds ground beef

One 28-ounce can diced tomatoes

One 6-ounce can tomato paste

1 teaspoon kosher salt

1 teaspoon black pepper

One 30-ounce container whole milk ricotta cheese

1 pound mozzarella, grated

1 cup grated Parmesan cheese

2 large eggs

¼ cup minced parsley

¼ cup minced basil

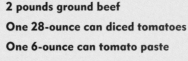

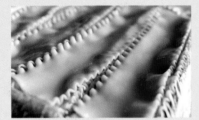

1. Boil the lasagna noodles in a large pot of salted water until al dente. Drain, rinse with cold water to cool, and lay flat on a sheet of foil. Set aside.

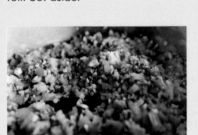

2. In a large pot, heat the olive oil over medium-high heat. Add the onion, mushrooms, bell pepper, and garlic and sauté for 4 to 5 minutes, until the vegetables are starting to soften.

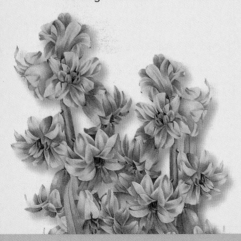

3. Remove the veggie mixture from the pan . . .

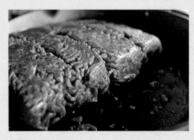

4. Then add the ground beef to the pan and cook, stirring occasionally, until it's totally browned. Drain the excess fat . . .

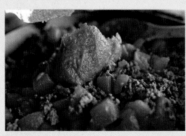

5. Then add the diced tomatoes, tomato paste, ½ teaspoon of the salt, and ½ teaspoon of the pepper . . .

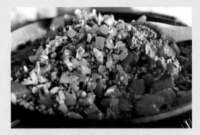

6. And the veggie mixture . . .

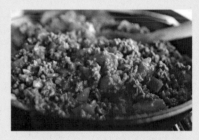

7. And stir to combine. Let the mixture simmer on low heat for 30 minutes.

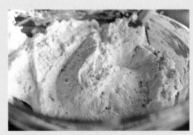

8. To make the filling, combine the ricotta, ½ cup of the mozzarella, ¾ cup of the Parmesan, the eggs, the remaining ½ teaspoon salt and ½ teaspoon pepper, the parsley, and the basil. Stir to combine.

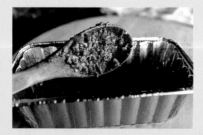

9. To assemble, spoon a thin layer of sauce into the bottom of a 9 x 13-inch baking pan OR five 6-inch disposable foil loaf pans.

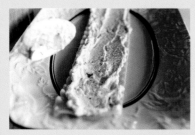

10. Spread 2 to 3 tablespoons of the ricotta filling on each noodle . . .

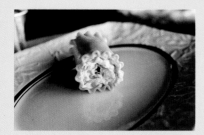

11. Then roll them up so that the cheese is on the inside of the roll.

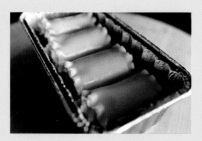

12. Lay them sideways in the pans (four will fit in each loaf pan, or you can fill a 9 x 13-inch pan with the roll-ups).

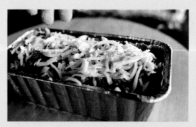

13. Top evenly with the remaining sauce, mozzarella, and Parmesan.

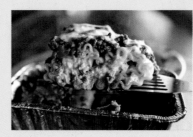

14. Follow the instructions to freeze at right. If you're making the roll-ups right away, preheat the oven to 375°F, place the pan(s) on a baking sheet, and bake for 20 minutes, until hot and bubbly.

FREEZER INSTRUCTIONS

Cover the unbaked pans tightly with heavy foil and freeze for up to 4 months.

To bake the roll-ups, preheat the oven to 350°F. Place the pans on a baking sheet and bake the foil-covered pans for 1 hour 30 minutes. Remove the foil and bake for anywhere from 30 to 45 minutes more, until hot and bubbly.

—OR—

Thaw the pans in the refrigerator for 24 to 36 hours, until completely thawed. Bake according to the recipe instructions.

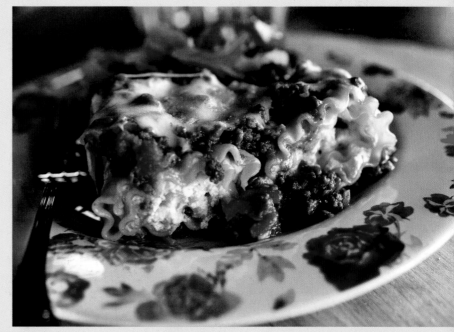

15. Serve with salad and a hunk of bread. Convenient and wonderfully good!

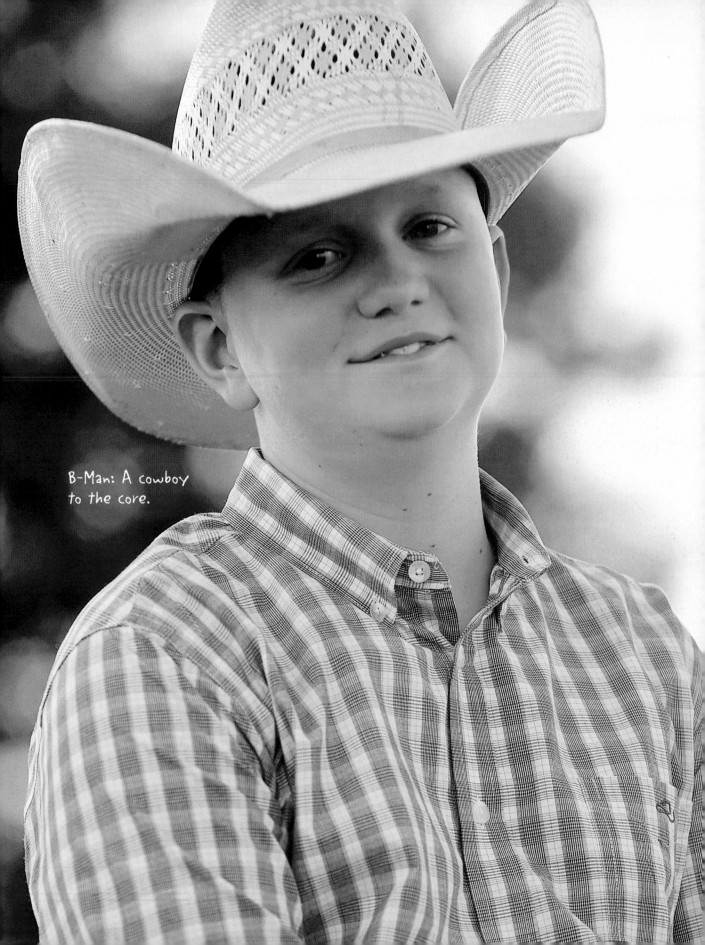

B-Man: A cowboy to the core.

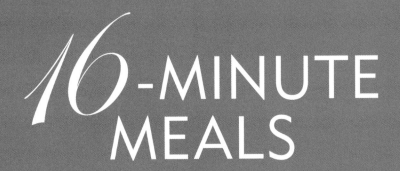

16-MINUTE MEALS

Loosely translated, "16-Minute" is the same thing as "Darn-Tootin' Fast," in which case I wonder why I don't just call this section "Darn-Tootin' Fast Meals"? I guess I'll have to think about that for the next cookbook, but for now I'll just leave it at 16-Minute Meals and encourage you to make every single one of them as soon as humanly possible. They are some of the quickest, easiest, and most well-received dinners in my toolbox, and they'll become lifesavers for you. (And a couple of them might even take you 15.92284 minutes instead! A bonus!)

CHICKEN WITH MUSTARD CREAM SAUCE

MAKES 8 SERVINGS

This chicken, with its delectable, tangy, creamy pan sauce, is one of my favorite quick dinners ever, and I'm getting ready to tell you why. Are you ready? Here goes:

It's delectable, tangy, and creamy! That's why.

But really, guys. So good. Instantly transforms plain ol' chicken breasts.

Make it for someone you love sometime soon.

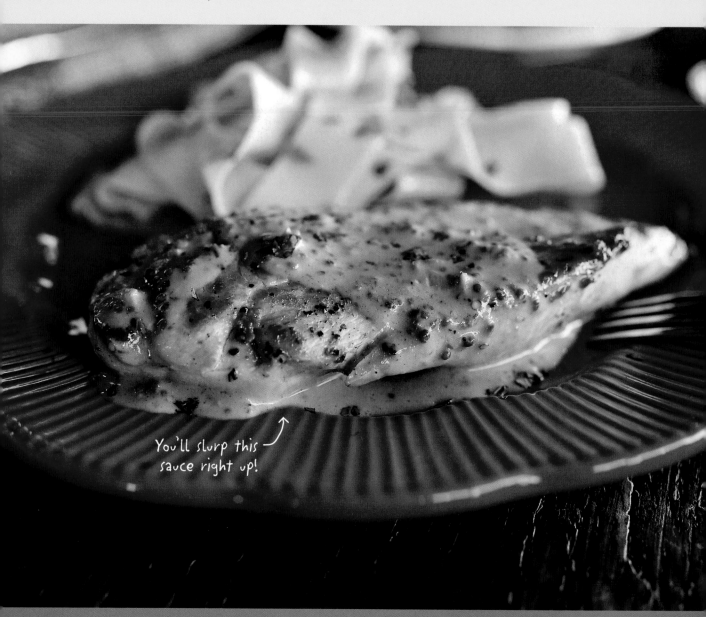

You'll slurp this sauce right up!

4 boneless, skinless chicken breasts

Kosher salt and black pepper to taste

2 tablespoons olive oil

2 tablespoons butter

3 garlic cloves, minced

1 cup brandy, white wine, or low-sodium chicken broth

1 heaping tablespoon Dijon mustard

1 heaping tablespoon grainy brown mustard

½ cup chicken broth, more as needed

⅓ cup heavy cream

Chopped parsley, for garnish

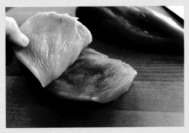

1. Use a sharp knife to slice the chicken breasts in half horizontally, giving you 8 thinner chicken breast pieces. Salt and pepper the chicken on both sides.

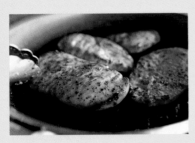

2. Heat the olive oil and butter in a large skillet over medium-high heat. Working in batches, add the chicken and cook until it is golden brown and done in the middle, about 2 to 3 minutes per side. Remove the chicken to a plate.

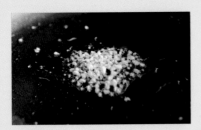

3. Add the garlic to the pan and stir it around for a minute so it won't burn.

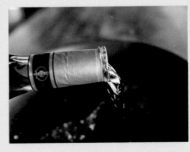

4. Turn off the heat for a moment and pour in the brandy.

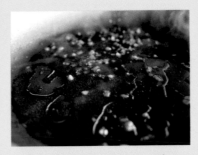

5. Turn the heat back to medium-high. Stir the mixture and let the liquid bubble up to deglaze the pan. Cook until the liquid has reduced by half, about 3 minutes.

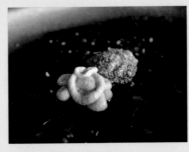

6. Add the mustards . . .

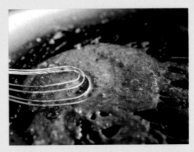

7. Then whisk them around and let them bubble up a bit.

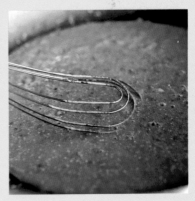

8. Pour in the broth . . .

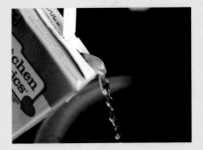

9. And whisk as the sauce heats up . . .

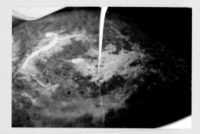

10. Then pour in the delicious cream!

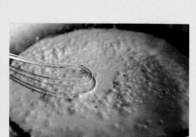

11. Whisk the sauce around, add salt and pepper to taste, and let it come to a gentle simmer. Turn off the heat. (If the sauce seems too thick, splash in a little extra chicken broth as needed.)

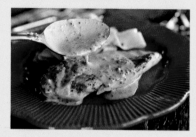

12. Place one or two chicken pieces on a plate, then spoon on a generous amount of sauce.

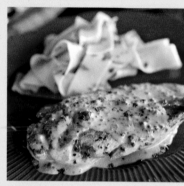

13. Top it with a sprinkling of parsley.

Ⓥ VARIATIONS

Use thin pork chops or thin steaks instead of chicken.

Omit the cream for a deeper mustard flavor.

Add 2 tablespoons chopped herbs (parsley, thyme, oregano, or whatever you like) to the sauce for delicious flavor.

Ⓢ SERVE WITH

Buttered Parsley Noodles (page 324)

Polenta (page 322)

Kale Citrus Salad (page 40)

Lemony Green Beans (page 292)

Roasted Carrots with Vinaigrette (page 300)

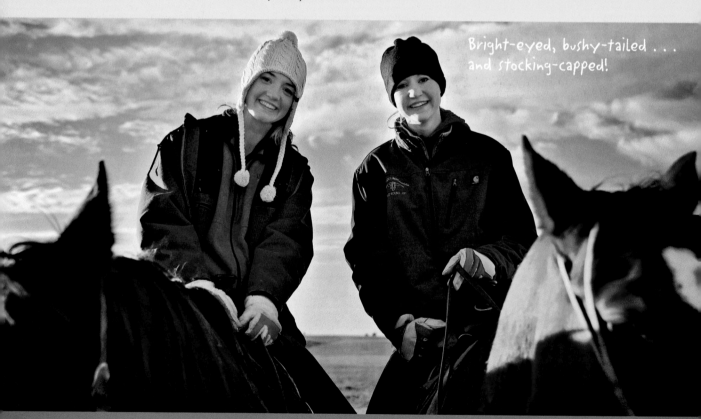

Bright-eyed, bushy-tailed . . . and stocking-capped!

BLACK BEAN BURGERS

MAKES 4 BURGERS

My husband and I have been married for many years, and I'd say as marriages go, ours is pretty darn good. We have four kids, work pretty hard, and spend a lot of time together, which is just fine with us since we really like each other and all that.

   Now, I will confess that there has been one steady source of marital conflict through the years, and that is the fact that I gosh darn *love* a good meatless burger. I can't really explain it. It must be a throwback to my vegetarian days. I don't know . . . I just love them. I'll never, ever forget the time, very early in our marriage, that Ladd and I went out to eat and I ordered—gasp—a *veggie burger* from the menu. The look on his face—it is etched in my memory. From where he stood, he didn't even know burgers without meat existed. In his experience, a burger *was* meat, much like rain was water. It sent shockwaves through his being, and rattled the very foundation of our marriage.

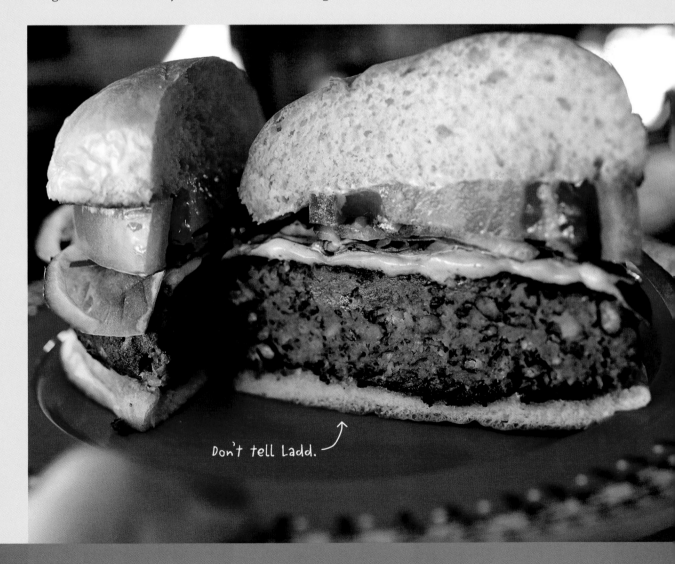

Don't tell Ladd.

Over the years, I've tried to help my beloved cattle rancher husband understand my position: that my love of meatless burgers has no hidden meaning. It doesn't mean I don't also love big, beefy burgers. It doesn't mean I'm going to start making the family drink shots of wheatgrass juice every morning. I just like the taste of weird, mushy concoctions meant to resemble hamburger patties. Call me wacky!

I love you, Ladd.

But I also love meatless burgers.

And I know in my heart that those two things can coexist.

Two 14.5-ounce cans seasoned black beans, drained (or use 3 cups Black Bean Soup, page 77, drained)

1 cup seasoned breadcrumbs

¼ cup grated white onion

1 large egg

½ teaspoon chili powder, more to taste

Kosher salt and black pepper to taste

Several dashes of hot sauce, such as Cholula, plus more for serving

2 tablespoons olive oil, for frying

2 tablespoons butter, for frying, plus more for grilling the buns

8 slices Swiss cheese (or any cheese you'd like)

4 kaiser rolls or good hamburger buns

Mayonnaise, for serving

Lettuce or other greens, for serving

Thinly sliced red onion, for serving

Sliced tomato, for serving

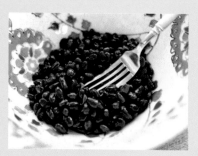

1. Place the beans in a medium bowl and mash them with a fork . . .

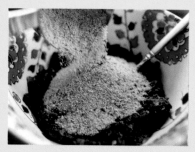

3. Pour in the breadcrumbs . . .

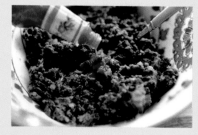

5. Stir the mixture around until everything is combined, then add the hot sauce and stir it in. Let the mixture sit for 5 minutes.

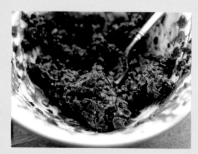

2. Until they're mostly broken up, but with a few large pieces still visible.

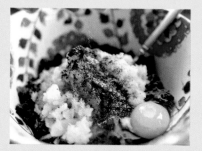

4. Then add the grated onion, egg, chili powder, and salt and pepper to taste.

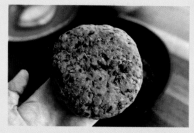

6. Heat the olive oil and butter in a skillet over medium-low heat. Form the bean mixture into 4 equal-size patties that are a little larger in circumference than the burger buns (the patties won't shrink when cooking).

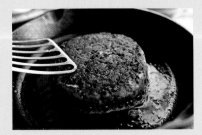

7. Cook the patties for 5 minutes on the first side, or until nicely browned, then flip them to the other side.

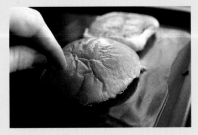

9. Meanwhile, heat a separate skillet or griddle over medium heat and butter the surface. Split the buns and grill them until golden brown on the surface.

M MAKE AHEAD

Make the bean mixture up to 24 hours ahead of time and store in the fridge.

V VARIATIONS

Use a mix of beans to change things up a bit.

Add ½ cup grated sharp Cheddar cheese to the bean mixture.

Add ¼ cup chopped cilantro to the bean mixture.

Add ¼ cup jarred salsa to the bean mixture.

S SERVE WITH

Thin Fries (page 318)

Sweet Potato Fries (page 308)

Beautiful Roasted Vegetables (page 290)

Colorful Coleslaw (page 294)

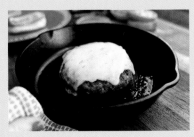

8. Place 2 slices of cheese on each patty and cook for 5 minutes more, or until the burgers are thoroughly heated through. (Place a lid on the skillet if the cheese needs help melting.)

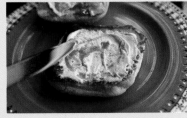

10. To serve, spread a mixture of mayonnaise and hot sauce on both sides of the buns.

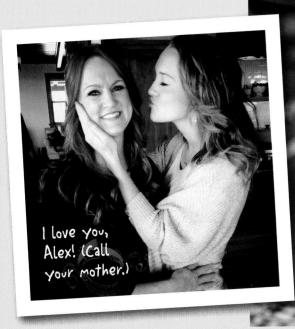

I love you, Alex! (Call your mother.)

11. Then lay on the lettuce, onion, and tomato and serve them up!

HAWAIIAN BURGERS

MAKES 4 BURGERS

This is a loose interpretation of what an official Hawaiian burger would look like if there was such a thing as an official Hawaiian burger, and I don't know if there is or not, because how in the world would I ever find something like that out? I suppose I could Google "Official Hawaiian Burger" and spend the rest of the day researching it and determining the authentic elements of what one would involve. . . .

(But I think I'd rather just eat this one instead.)

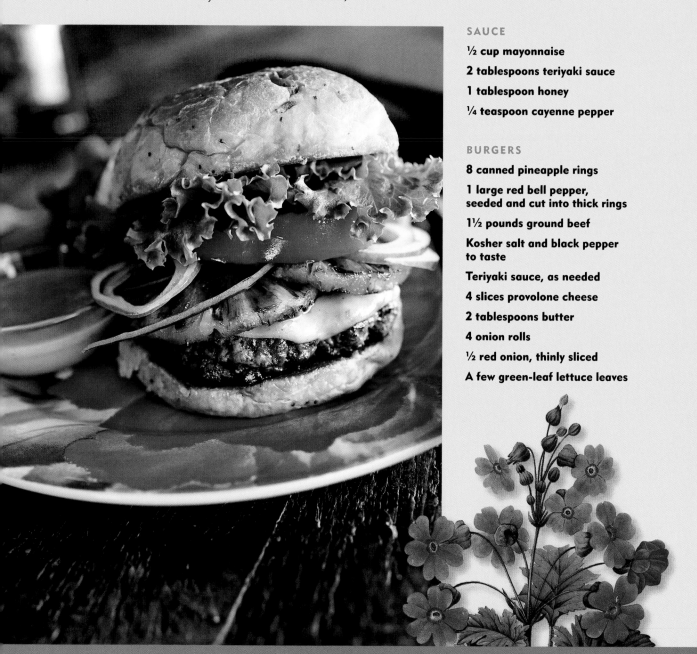

SAUCE

½ cup mayonnaise

2 tablespoons teriyaki sauce

1 tablespoon honey

¼ teaspoon cayenne pepper

BURGERS

8 canned pineapple rings

1 large red bell pepper, seeded and cut into thick rings

1½ pounds ground beef

Kosher salt and black pepper to taste

Teriyaki sauce, as needed

4 slices provolone cheese

2 tablespoons butter

4 onion rolls

½ red onion, thinly sliced

A few green-leaf lettuce leaves

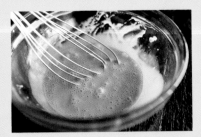

1. To whip up the mysterious delicious sauce, in a bowl, whisk together the mayonnaise, teriyaki sauce, honey, and cayenne until smooth. Set aside.

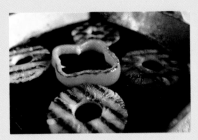

2. To make the burgers, on a grill pan (or an outdoor grill), quickly grill the pineapple and bell pepper rings until they have great marks on both sides. Remove and set aside.

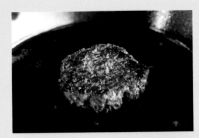

3. Season the ground beef with salt and pepper and form it into 4 equal-size patties. Cook them on the grill pan (or grill) or in a skillet over medium heat for 4 to 5 minutes on the first side, then flip them over . . .

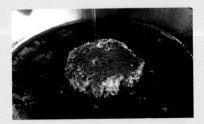

4. And add a splash of teriyaki sauce on top of each one.

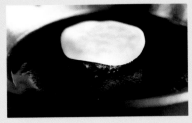

5. Place a slice of provolone on each patty and let it melt while the burger cooks through, 4 minutes or so more, until no longer pink in the middle.

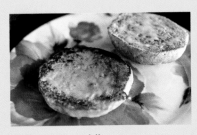

6. Butter a griddle or separate skillet and grill the buns over medium heat until golden brown. Spoon a little bit of the sauce on the cut side of the buns and allow it to slightly soak into the bread.

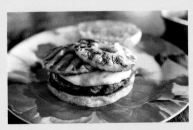

7. Place the patties on the bottom buns and top each one with two pineapple slices . . .

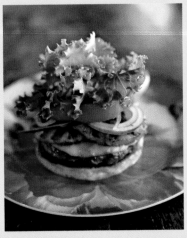

8. Along with red onion slices, a grilled bell pepper slice, and lettuce.

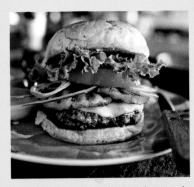

9. Then smash it all together and serve with dishes of extra sauce for dipping. (The dipping sauce absolutely makes this burger!)

V VARIATIONS

Add some jalapeño slices to the burger for a little spice.

Add a thin slice of ham or Canadian bacon to the burger. Weird but delicious!

S SERVE WITH

Thin Fries (page 318)
Sweet Potato Fries (page 308)
Colorful Coleslaw (page 294)

SUPREME PIZZA BURGERS

MAKES 4 BURGERS (OR 8 SERVINGS IF YOU SPLIT THEM! THEY'RE HUGE.)

Anything that can go on a slice of pizza can go on a pizza burger! I love this lusciously loaded version.

1½ pounds ground beef

½ pound Italian sausage

½ teaspoon Italian seasoning

12 slices mozzarella or provolone cheese

Pepperoni slices (about 24)

½ red onion, very thinly sliced

1 green bell pepper, seeded and sliced into thick rings

⅓ cup sliced pitted black olives

½ cup jarred marinara sauce, plus more as needed

4 white mushrooms, thinly sliced

4 kaiser rolls or good hamburger buns

Butter, for toasting

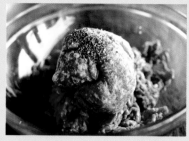

1. Combine the ground beef, sausage, and Italian seasoning in a large bowl . . .

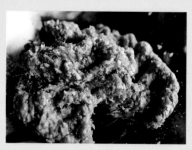

2. And mix thoroughly until it's all combined. Form the mixture into 4 equal-size patties.

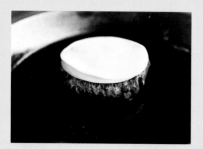

3. In a large skillet, cook the burgers over medium heat for 4 to 5 minutes on the first side, then flip them, reduce the heat to low, and lay 2 slices of the cheese on each one.

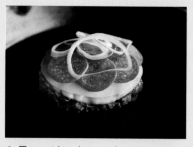

4. Top with a layer of pepperoni slices, along with some red onion slices.

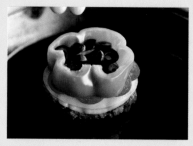

5. Next, place a bell pepper ring on top and sprinkle in a few olive slices.

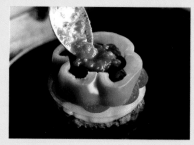

6. Spoon in a little marinara sauce . . .

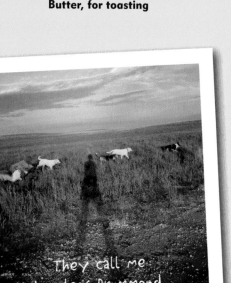

They call me Longlegs Drummond.

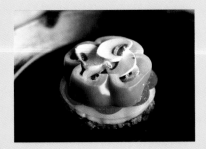

7. Fill the rest of the bell pepper with sliced mushrooms . . .

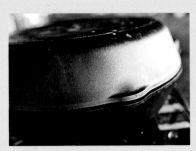

8. And lay a third slice of cheese on top.

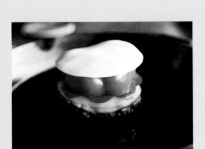

9. Place a lid (or a second inverted skillet as shown) on top of the skillet and cook the burger for 3 to 4 minutes more, to let the cheese really melt.

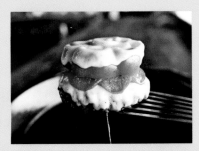

10. I'd say that's really melted!

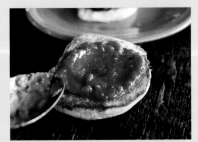

11. Meanwhile, toast the buns with a little butter on a separate skillet or griddle until golden brown. Spread both sides with a little marinara . . .

Ⓥ VARIATIONS

Add/substitute any pizza topping—Canadian bacon, pineapple—whatever floats your boat!

Use any kind of cheese you'd like!

Ⓢ SERVE WITH

Thin Fries (page 318)

Sweet Potato Fries (page 308)

Colorful Coleslaw (page 294)

Beer. Ha.

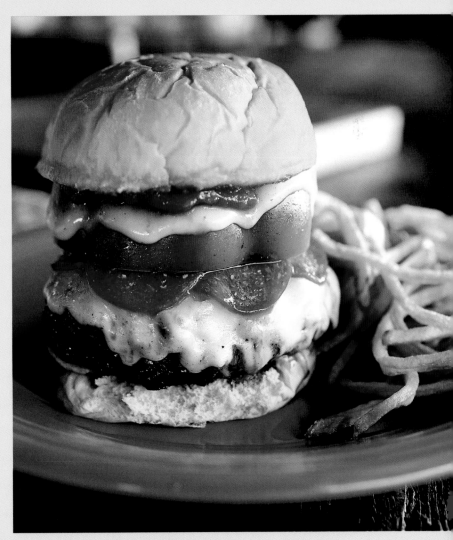

12. Then bring all the craziness together!

PAN-FRIED PORK CHOPS

MAKES 6 SERVINGS

These pork chops are *not* rocket science! They're the simplest, most delightful little numbers—easy to prepare, flavorful, and unapologetically man-pleasing. In fact, I wrote a poem about them. Here it is! (Thank you, Helen Reddy, for the inspiration.)

I am woman.
Hear me roar.
But my husband's taste buds
I can't ignore.
And if I make the pork chops,
he will smile.

Man, can I write a bad poem.
I really should be fired.

2 cups all-purpose flour

**2 teaspoons kosher salt,
more as needed**

**1 teaspoon black pepper,
more as needed**

1 teaspoon seasoned salt

1 teaspoon garlic powder

**12 thin bone-in pork chops
(also called breakfast chops)**

1 cup vegetable oil

4 tablespoons (½ stick) butter

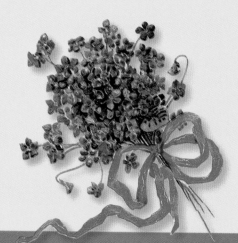

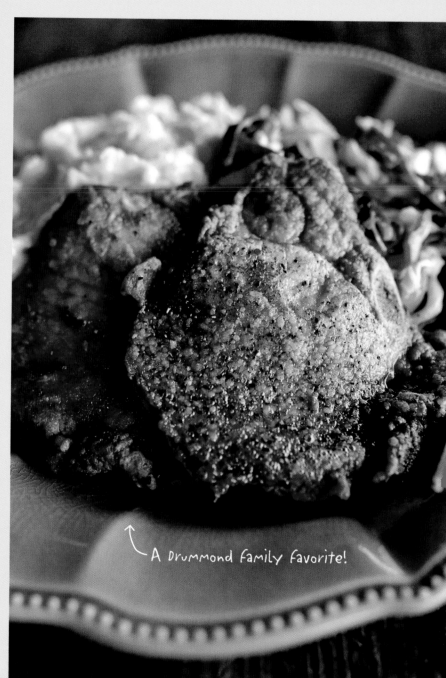

A Drummond family favorite!

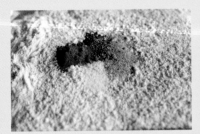

1. Combine the flour, kosher salt, pepper, seasoned salt, and garlic powder in a shallow pan . . .

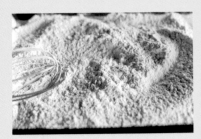

2. And whisk it together.

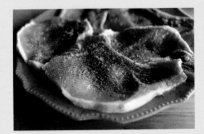

3. Sprinkle both sides of the chops with kosher salt and pepper . . .

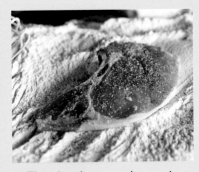

4. Then lay them one by one in the flour mixture . . .

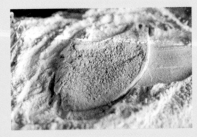

5. Turning them over to dredge them.

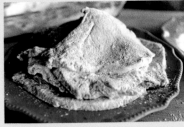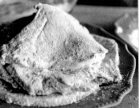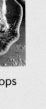

6. Keep going until all the chops are coated in flour.

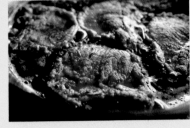

7. Heat the oil and butter in a large skillet over medium heat, then fry the chops in batches until they're golden on both sides and cooked through, about 2 minutes per side.

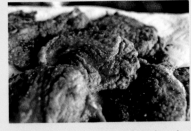

8. Remove them to a plate lined with a paper towel to remove the excess grease . . .

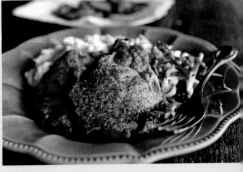

9. And serve them to your hungry crew.

Ⓥ VARIATIONS

Use any thickness of chops you'd like; just adjust the cooking time accordingly so they are fully cooked through.

To make a heavier breading, dredge the chops in the flour, then in a mixture of 3 eggs beaten with 2 tablespoons milk, then back in the flour.

Make gravy with the pan drippings: Stir 2 to 3 tablespoons all-purpose flour into the grease, let it brown slightly, then stir in 2 to 3 cups whole milk and whisk until thickened. Season with salt and pepper and serve over the chops.

Ⓢ SERVE WITH

Stovetop Mashed Potatoes (page 310)

"Slice-Baked" Potatoes (page 314)

Colorful Coleslaw (page 294)

Lemony Green Beans (page 292)

Roasted Carrots with Vinaigrette (page 300)

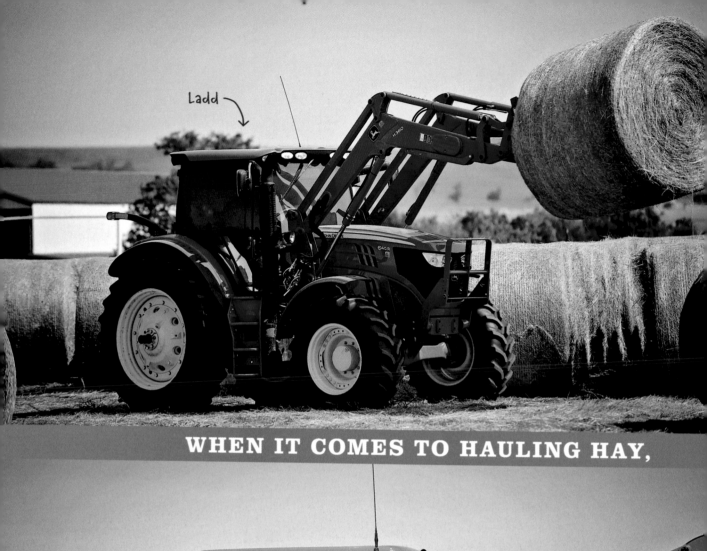

Ladd

WHEN IT COMES TO HAULING HAY,

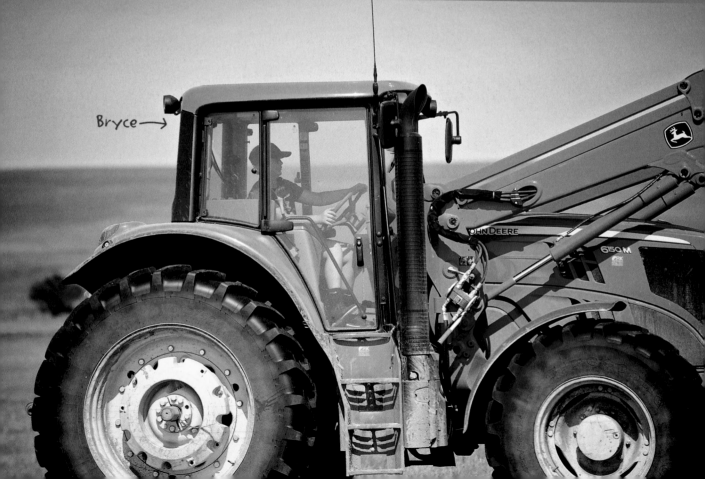

Bryce

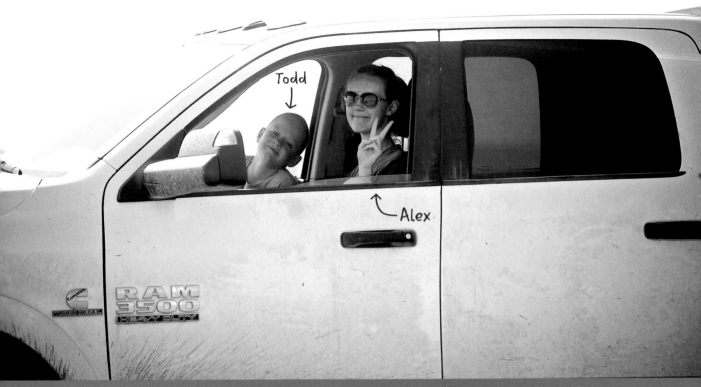

IT'S DEFINITELY ALL HANDS ON DECK!

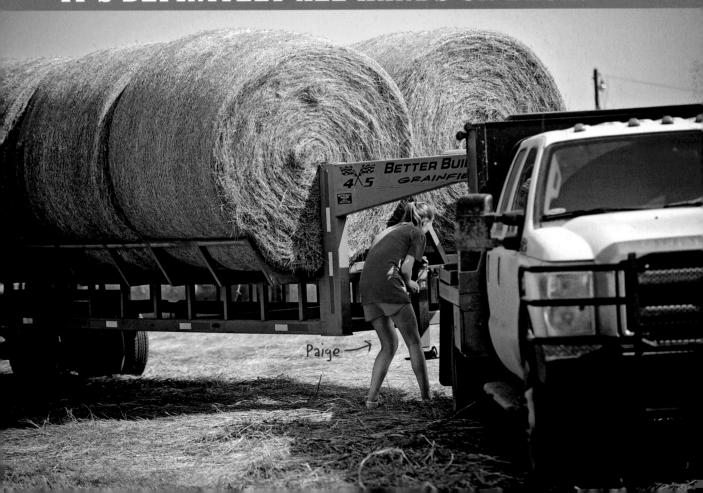

ORANGE CHICKEN

MAKES 4 SERVINGS

One of the motivating factors to get me to drive nearly ninety minutes every Friday morning to take my kids to our homeschooling co-op in the city is the promise that I'll get to have Chinese takeout for lunch that day. I'm such a selfless mom in that way!

I love it all: Beijing Beef, Kung Pao Chicken, Crab Rangoon . . . the works. Orange Chicken is always Paige's choice, and this make-at-home version is a treat!

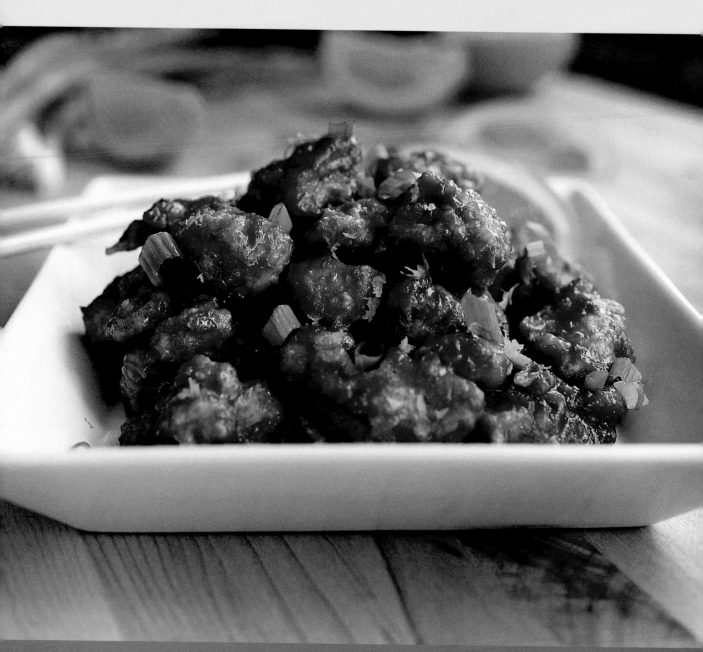

Vegetable or peanut oil, for frying

4 egg whites

3 tablespoons cornstarch

4 boneless, skinless chicken thighs, cut into bite-size pieces

½ cup orange juice

1 tablespoon soy sauce

1 tablespoon packed brown sugar or honey

1 tablespoon rice vinegar or white vinegar

¼ teaspoon sesame oil

Dash of kosher salt

Pinch of red pepper flakes, more to taste

1 garlic clove

One 2-inch piece fresh ginger, peeled

Zest of 1 orange

2 green onions, sliced

1. Heat about 2 inches of oil in a heavy-bottomed pot over medium-high heat until a deep-fry thermometer registers 350°F.

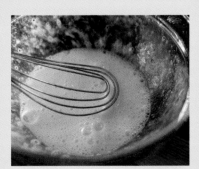

2. In a bowl, whisk together the egg whites and 2 tablespoons of the cornstarch until they're completely combined and slightly frothy.

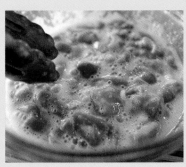

3. Add the chicken pieces to the mixture and let them sit for about 5 minutes.

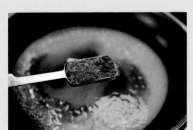

4. Meanwhile, in a skillet (nonstick is best if you have one), combine the orange juice, soy sauce, brown sugar, vinegar . . .

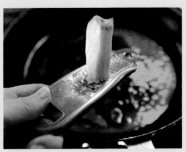

5. Sesame oil, salt, and red pepper flakes . . .

6. Then grate in the garlic and ginger.

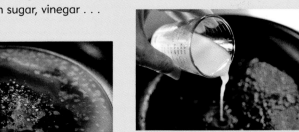

7. Finally, add the orange zest, reserving a little extra for the end!

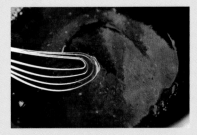

8. Bring the mixture to a gentle boil over medium-high heat, then whisk together the remaining 1 tablespoon cornstarch and ¼ cup water to make a slurry and pour it in.

9. Cook the sauce for 1 minute, or until it's very thick. Turn off the heat and set it aside. (Add a little more water if it gets too thick!)

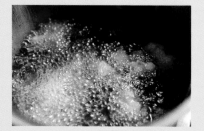

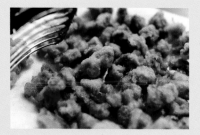

10. In batches, drop a few of the chicken pieces into the hot oil. (Use tongs to drop them one by one—you don't want them sticking together.) Cook the pieces for 2 to 2½ minutes, or until light golden brown and cooked through, moving them around a bit as they cook.

13. Make sure the oil is back to the right temperature, then return the chicken in batches to cook a second time, 1 minute per batch. This will just help solidify and crisp up the coating a bit.

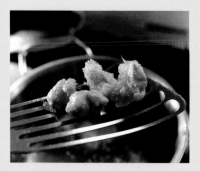

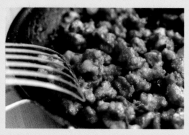

11. Use a slotted spatula to remove them from the oil . . .

14. Remove them and let them drain on a fresh paper towel.

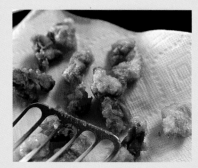

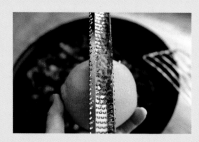

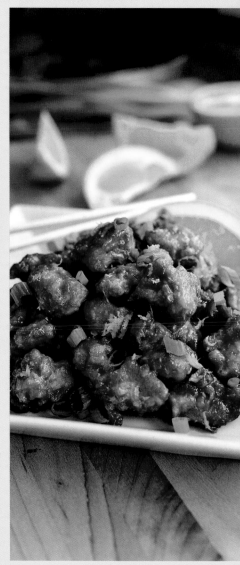

12. And drain them on a paper towel. Repeat with the rest of the chicken pieces.

15. Immediately throw the chicken into the skillet and toss it in the sauce . . .

17. Serve it with a sprinkling of green onion (and heck . . . a little extra zest never hurt anyone!).

Ⓥ VARIATIONS

Use a mix of orange and lemon juice/zest.

Double the sauce for a saucier dish.

Ⓢ SERVE WITH

Pineapple Fried Rice (page 261)

Chow Mein (page 174)

Cooked long-grain or jasmine rice

16. Then grate in the rest of the zest.

BEEF WITH SNOW PEAS

MAKES 6 SERVINGS

It came to me in a vision a few years ago. I saw it written on a bright white wall. "Ree," the wall read, "you must make beef with snow peas tonight. It is your destiny."

I have long since stopped trying to ignore visions of words written on bright white walls. Every time I follow what the words on the wall tell me to do, things have always worked out okay in my life!

You do the same, right? *(Right?)*

(Oh, never mind.)

½ cup low-sodium soy sauce, plus more for serving

3 tablespoons sherry

2 tablespoons packed brown sugar

2 tablespoons cornstarch

1 tablespoon minced fresh ginger

1½ pounds flank steak, trimmed of fat and sliced very thin against the grain

3 tablespoons peanut oil

8 ounces snow peas, ends trimmed

2 cups cooked white or jasmine rice

Red pepper flakes, for sprinkling

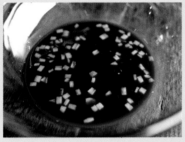

1. In a bowl, mix together the soy sauce, sherry, brown sugar, cornstarch, and ginger to make a marinade.

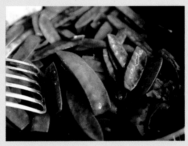

3. Heat the oil in a heavy skillet or wok over high heat. Add the snow peas and stir them around for 1 minute.

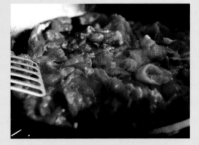

5. Let the pan get very hot again. Add half the meat to the pan and spread it out, but do not stir or disturb it for at least 1 minute.

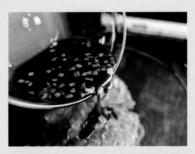

2. Place the sliced meat in a bowl and pour half the marinade on top. Toss with your hands and set aside.

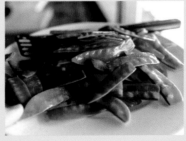

4. Remove to a plate and set aside.

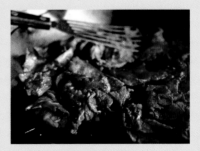

6. Turn meat to the other side and cook for 30 seconds more . . .

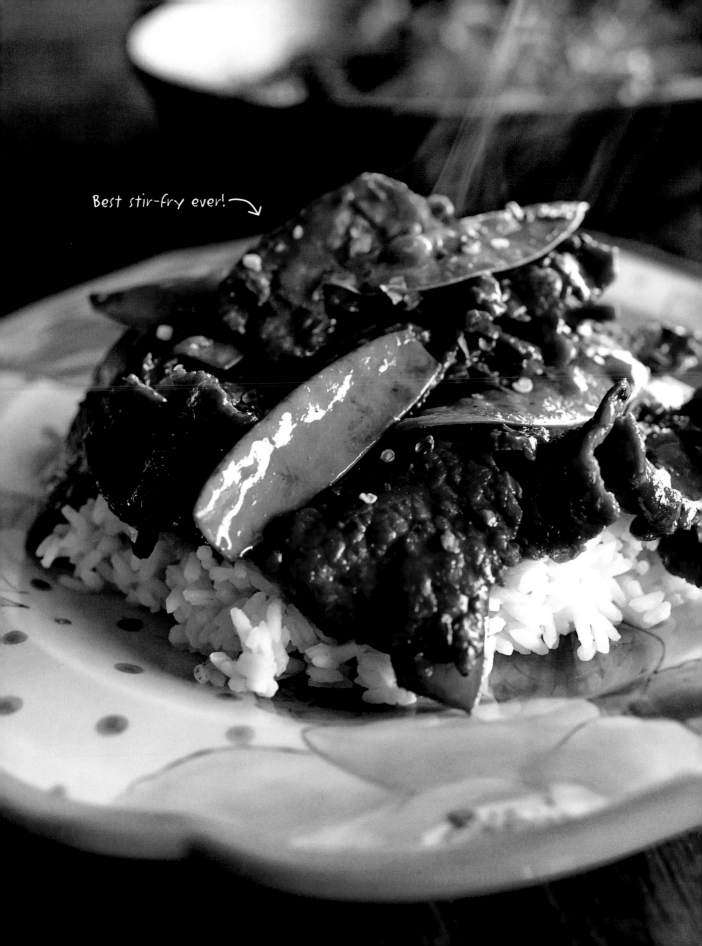

Best stir-fry ever!

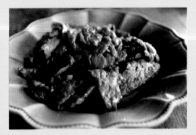

7. And remove it to a clean plate. Repeat with other half of the meat.

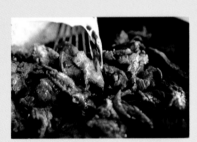

8. Return all the meat to the pan and pour in the rest of the marinade.

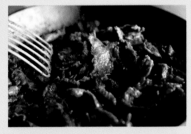

9. Stir it around, then pour in ½ cup hot water . . .

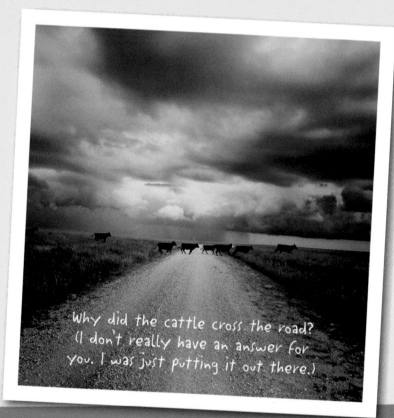

10. And let the sauce thicken for 30 to 45 seconds.

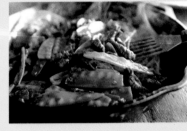

11. Turn off the heat and stir in the snow peas . . .

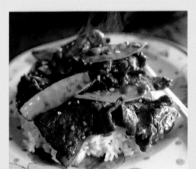

12. Then serve the mixture over rice, with red pepper flakes sprinkled over the top as desired.

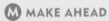

M MAKE AHEAD

Slice the meat and mix the marinade up to 8 hours before cooking the dish. Store in separate containers in the fridge until dinnertime.

V VARIATIONS

Double the amount of sauce if you'd like the dish to have a saucier consistency.

Add 1 chopped red or green bell pepper to the pan with the snow peas.

Substitute 3 cups broccoli florets for the snow peas.

Add 1 can baby corn, drained and cut into large pieces, to the finished dish.

S SERVE WITH

Chow Mein (page 174)

Pineapple Fried Rice (page 261)

Why did the cattle cross the road? (I don't really have an answer for you. I was just putting it out there.)

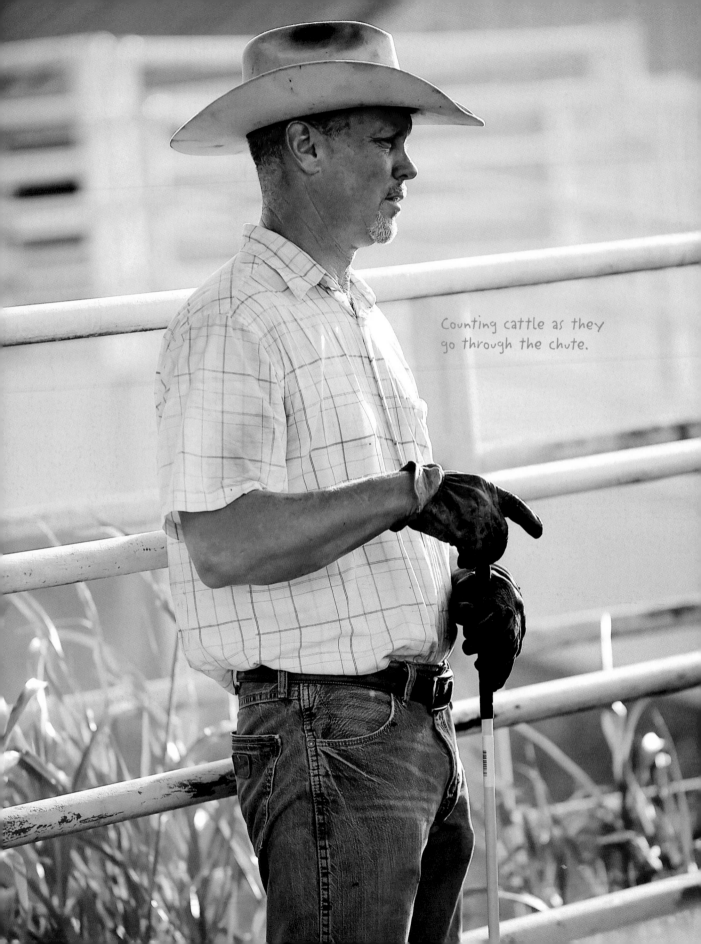

Counting cattle as they
go through the chute.

CASHEW CHICKEN

MAKES 8 SERVINGS

Aw, this recipe reminds me of China Garden, the old restaurant in my hometown of Bartlesville, Oklahoma, where my friends and I used to go out for dinner, back when my jean size was six and my curfew was exactly ten. Isn't it funny the things we remember? I remember that I would drive my friends and myself to China Garden in my mom's Jeep Wagoneer, I remember the way the restaurant's tables were arranged, I remember that I used to spray my bangs with Stiff Stuff before we all went out for dinner, and I remember that a big platter of Cashew Chicken was the only thing we ever ordered.

This is why I can't seem to remember where I put my sunglasses today. I'm too mired in the memories of yesterday.

½ cup low-sodium soy sauce

1 tablespoon rice vinegar

1 tablespoon packed brown sugar

2 tablespoons oyster sauce

½ teaspoon sesame oil

3 tablespoons vegetable oil

6 boneless, skinless chicken thighs, cut into small cubes

Kosher salt to taste

1 tablespoon chopped garlic

1 tablespoon chopped fresh ginger

1 green bell pepper, diced

¼ cup sherry or low-sodium chicken broth

2 tablespoons cornstarch

⅓ cup drained canned water chestnuts, coarsely chopped

1 cup unsalted cashews (be sure to use unsalted, or the dish will be overly salty)

2 green onions, thinly sliced

Cooked rice or noodles, for serving (if desired)

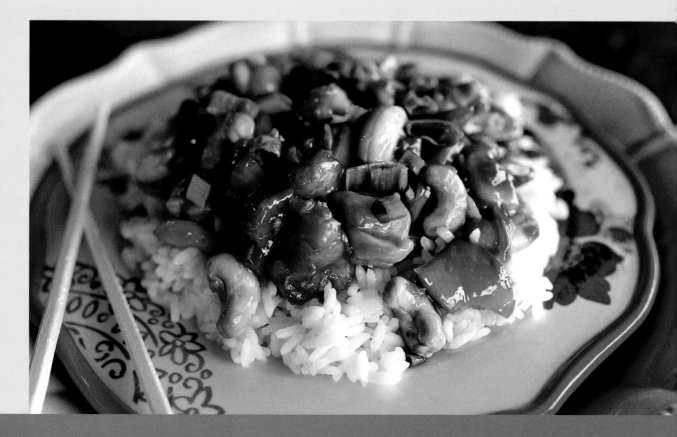

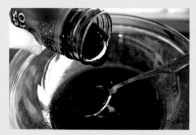

1. In a bowl, mix together the soy sauce, vinegar, brown sugar, oyster sauce, and sesame oil. Set aside.

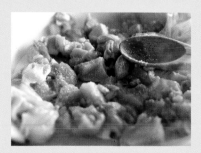

2. Heat the vegetable oil in a large skillet over high heat and add the chicken in a single layer. Sprinkle with a small amount of salt, then leave it alone for at least a couple of minutes to give the chicken a chance to brown.

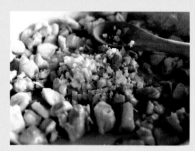

3. When the chicken has turned golden, stir it around so that it can brown on all sides. Throw in the garlic and ginger and stir to combine . . .

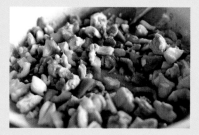

4. Then stir in the bell pepper and let it cook for 2 to 3 minutes.

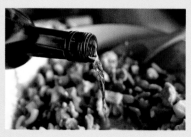

5. While the pan is still hot, pour in the sherry . . .

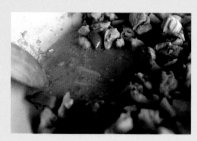

6. And stir it around, scraping the bottom of the pan to loosen all the flavorful bits.

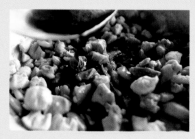

7. Turn the heat to medium-low and pour in the sauce mixture . . .

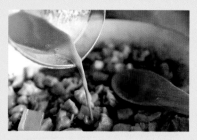

8. Then mix the cornstarch with ¼ cup water to make a slurry and pour it in.

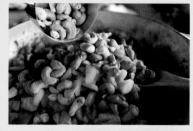

9. Stir the sauce for 1 to 2 minutes to thicken, then add the water chestnuts and cashews . . .

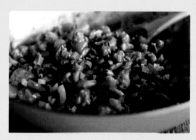

10. And stir to coat everything with the sauce, adding a splash of water if the sauce is too thick.

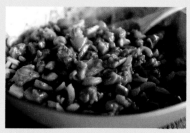

11. Finally, sprinkle on the green onions. Done!

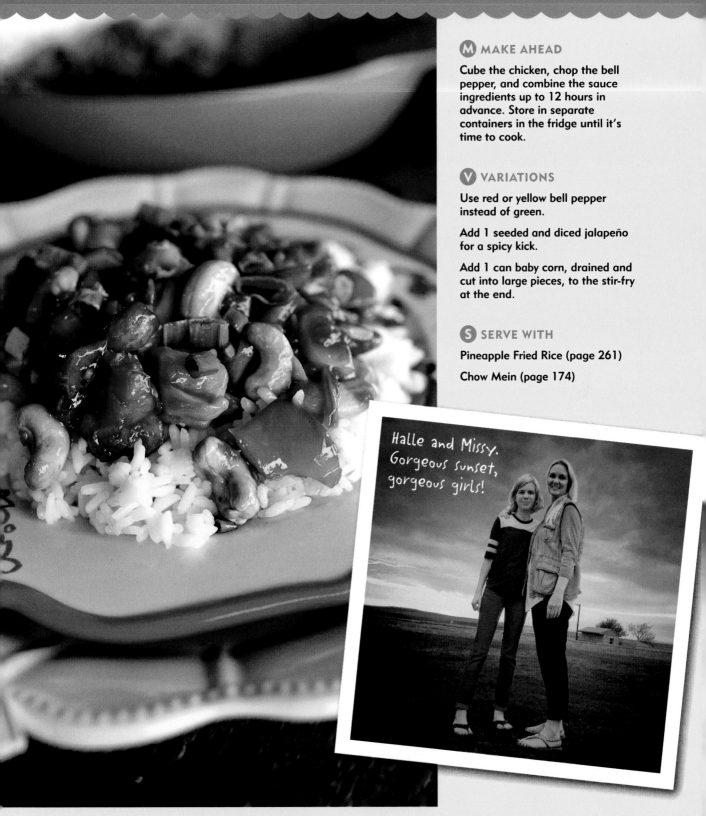

M MAKE AHEAD

Cube the chicken, chop the bell pepper, and combine the sauce ingredients up to 12 hours in advance. Store in separate containers in the fridge until it's time to cook.

V VARIATIONS

Use red or yellow bell pepper instead of green.

Add 1 seeded and diced jalapeño for a spicy kick.

Add 1 can baby corn, drained and cut into large pieces, to the stir-fry at the end.

S SERVE WITH

Pineapple Fried Rice (page 261)

Chow Mein (page 174)

Halle and Missy.
Gorgeous sunset,
gorgeous girls!

12. Serve it over rice, noodles . . . or just by itself.

SPICY CAULIFLOWER STIR-FRY

MAKES 2 TO 4 SERVINGS

Ohhhhhhhhhh, is this good. So simple, so delightful, so delicious. I first made it one dark and stormy night a while back when I was in the mood to eat something light and veggie-licious, but I was a day away from going on a big grocery shopping trip and my food supply was low. So here were my choices:

* 4 somewhat wrinkly grape tomatoes
* Half of a very sad-looking zucchini wrapped in plastic
* A carrot that had lost its will to live
* A respectable head of cauliflower

I opted for the cauliflower, and I just let my soul take me where it wanted to go.

It was so good, it's taken me back to the same place several times since!

Come along with me on my cauliflower journey, my friends. I promise you won't be sorry.

2 teaspoons vegetable oil

1 cauliflower head, broken into very small florets

2 garlic cloves, minced

2 tablespoons soy sauce

1 lime, plus lime wedges for serving

2 green onions, thinly sliced

1 tablespoon sriracha or other hot sauce, or to taste

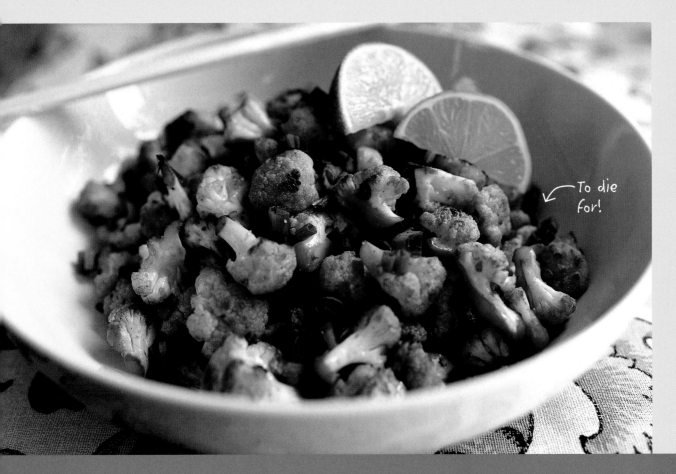

To die for!

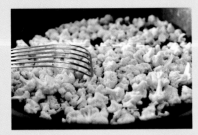

1. Heat the oil in a large skillet over medium-high heat. Add the cauliflower and garlic . . .

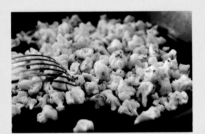

2. And stir them around. Cook for 2½ to 3 minutes, until there are some very dark brown areas on the cauliflower, then turn the heat to low.

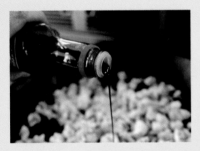

3. Add the soy sauce . . .

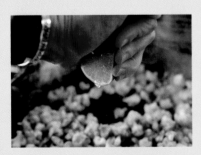

4. Squeeze in the juice of the whole lime . . .

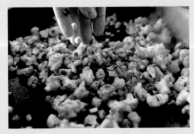

5. And add most of the green onions, reserving a sprinkle for serving.

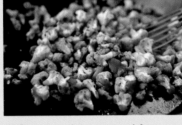

6. Stir everything around for another minute.

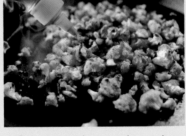

7. Squeeze in the sriracha and stir the cauliflower until it's all combined.

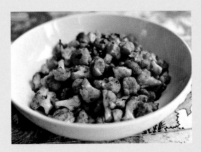

8. Then serve it up . . .

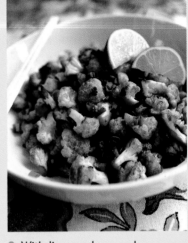

9. With lime wedges and a sprinkling of green onions.

You won't believe how deliciously addictive this is!

Ⓥ VARIATIONS

Use butter instead of vegetable oil for deeper flavor and color.

Add a sprinkling of chili powder or red pepper flakes for a little kick.

Use rice vinegar instead of lime juice for a slightly different bite.

Ⓢ SERVE WITH

Chow Mein (page 174)

Pineapple Fried Rice (page 261)

Any beef, chicken, pork, or seafood main dish

VEGGIE STIR-FRY

MAKES 8 SERVINGS

This gorgeous, luscious stir-fry will knock your socks off! I could eat it every day for the rest of my life.

½ cup low-sodium soy sauce

3 tablespoons sherry or low-sodium vegetable broth

2 tablespoons packed brown sugar

2 tablespoons cornstarch

2 tablespoons sriracha

1 tablespoon minced fresh ginger

3 tablespoons peanut oil

1 yellow onion, cut into large chunks

1 red bell pepper, seeded and cut into large chunks

1 yellow bell pepper, seeded and cut into large chunks

2 garlic cloves, minced

2 medium zucchini, cut into large wedges

One 15-ounce can baby corn, drained and halved crosswise

1 broccoli head, cut into florets

Cooked noodles or rice, for serving

Sesame seeds, for serving

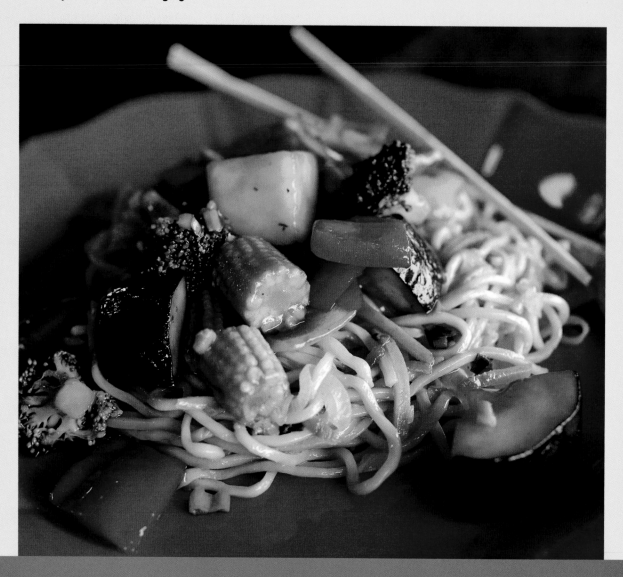

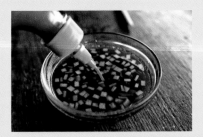

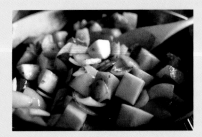

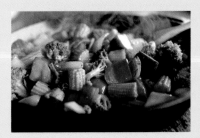

1. In a bowl, mix together the soy sauce, sherry, brown sugar, cornstarch, sriracha, and ginger. Set aside.

5. Add the zucchini and stir it around. Cook for 2 minutes more.

9. And stir. Cook for 1 to 2 minutes more, or until the sauce is very thick. If it needs a little more sauce, stir in ½ cup hot water.

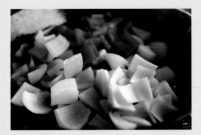

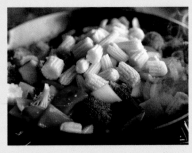

2. Heat the oil in a large skillet over medium-high heat. Add the onion and peppers . . .

6. Add the baby corn . . .

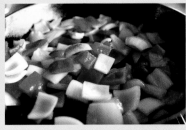

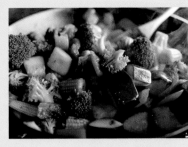

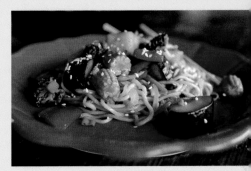

3. And stir, then cook for 2 to 3 minutes.

7. Then toss in the broccoli and let it cook for a couple of minutes.

10. Serve over noodles or rice, with a sprinkling of sesame seeds.

Ⓜ MAKE AHEAD

Prep all the veggies and make the sauce up to 24 hours ahead of time. Keep in separate containers in the fridge.

Ⓥ VARIATIONS

Add 8 ounces quartered cremini mushrooms to the skillet with the onions and peppers.

Substitute any other veggies you'd like; just add them to the skillet according to how tender they are (tender veggies get added later in the cooking process).

Ⓢ SERVE WITH

Chow Mein (page 174)

Pineapple Fried Rice (page 261)

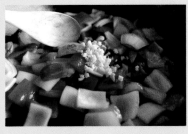

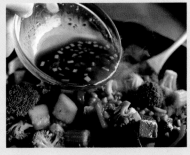

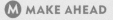

4. Add the garlic and cook for 30 seconds to 1 minute more, stirring continuously.

8. Then, while the veggies are still firm, pour in the sauce . . .

CHOW MEIN

MAKES 6 SERVINGS

You'll love this quick, easy noodle dish, which can be a main course or side dish (or midnight snack . . . whatever you've got going on in your life!).

1 tablespoon peanut oil

1 large onion, halved and thinly sliced

1 cup julienned carrots

4 green onions, sliced

½ head napa cabbage, thinly sliced

8 ounces thin Chinese noodles, cooked according to the package directions

¼ cup low-sodium soy sauce

1 teaspoon sesame oil

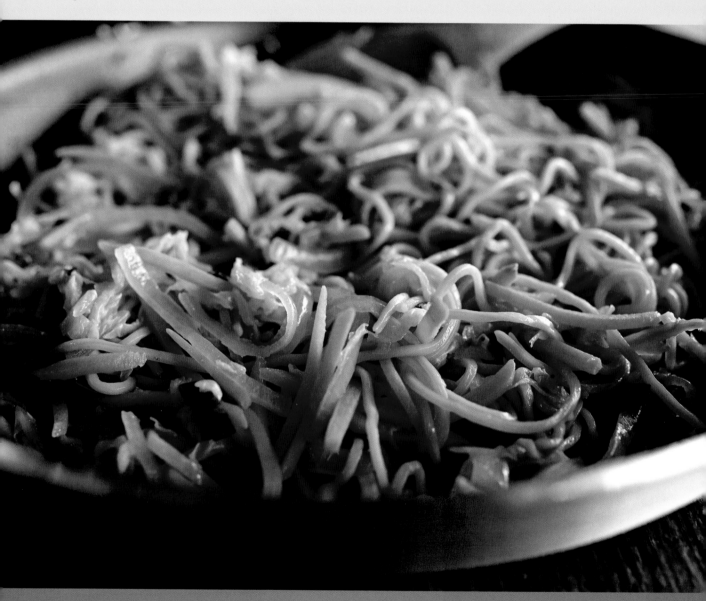

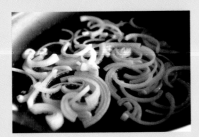

1. Heat the peanut oil in a large skillet or wok over medium-high heat. Add the onion and cook for a couple of minutes, until it starts to soften.

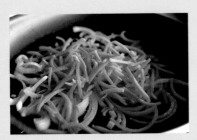

2. Add the carrots . . .

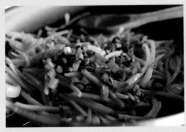

3. And half the green onions, then stir and let the veggies cook for 2 minutes.

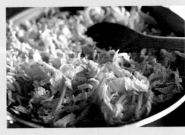

4. Stir in the cabbage and cook for 2 minutes more . . .

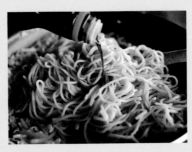

5. Then add the noodles, soy sauce, and sesame oil.

V VARIATIONS

Add mushrooms, zucchini, broccoli, baby corn, or any other veggie you'd like.

Use cooked thin spaghetti instead of Chinese noodles.

Stir in cooked chicken, beef, or shrimp for a protein-packed Chow Mein.

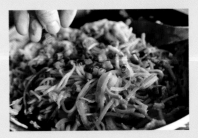

6. Toss it together, then add the rest of the green onions . . .

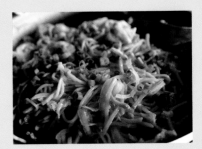

7. And toss them in. Serve hot.

S SERVE WITH

Beef with Snow Peas (page 163)

Orange Chicken (page 160)

Cashew Chicken (page 167)

Veggie Stir-Fry (page 172)

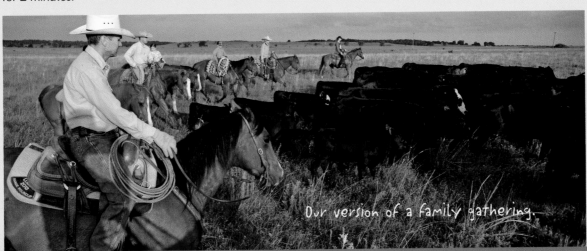

Our version of a family gathering.

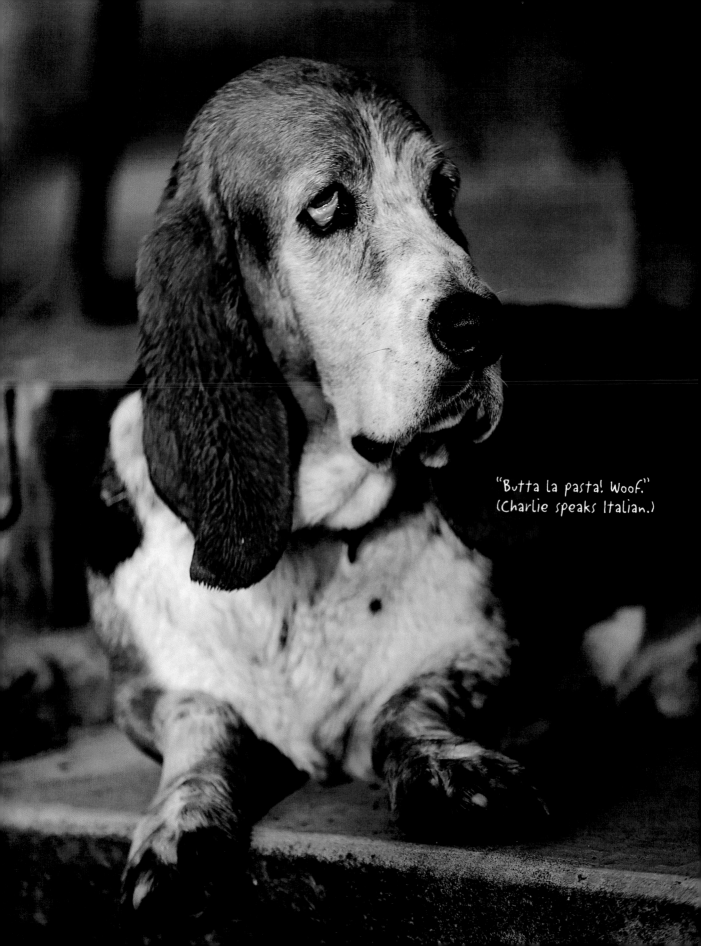
"Butta la pasta! Woof."
(Charlie speaks Italian.)

PASTA PRONTO

I've never not loved pasta. I've not ever not loved pasta. I've never loved not loving pasta. You get the idea. Just gimme a noodle, and I'm a noodle in your hands. Want to win friends and influence people? Serve one of these simple-and-scrumptious pasta dishes! In my world, pasta cures just about anything that ails ya . . . even ails ya don't even have. And if that didn't make any sense, it's only because I haven't had my pasta yet today.

PASTA PUTTANESCA

MAKES 6 TO 8 SERVINGS

I'm not going to go into the history of Puttanesca or where it comes from or what the name translates to, because this is a family-friendly cookbook and *Puttanesca* sounds a lot nicer than its English translation. Unless, of course, your native language is Italian. And if that's the case, I'm in big trouble at any rate.

What's in a name, anyway? This simple, throw-together pasta is so delicious, it makes it impossible to care.

2 garlic cloves

4 anchovy fillets

1 cup assorted pitted olives (different colors are great!)

2 tablespoons olive oil

½ red onion, thinly sliced

1½ cups grape tomatoes, halved

½ cup low-sodium chicken broth

½ cup white wine

Kosher salt and black pepper to taste

8 ounces (½ pound) bucatini or spaghetti, cooked to al dente

½ cup freshly grated Parmesan cheese

6 to 8 basil leaves

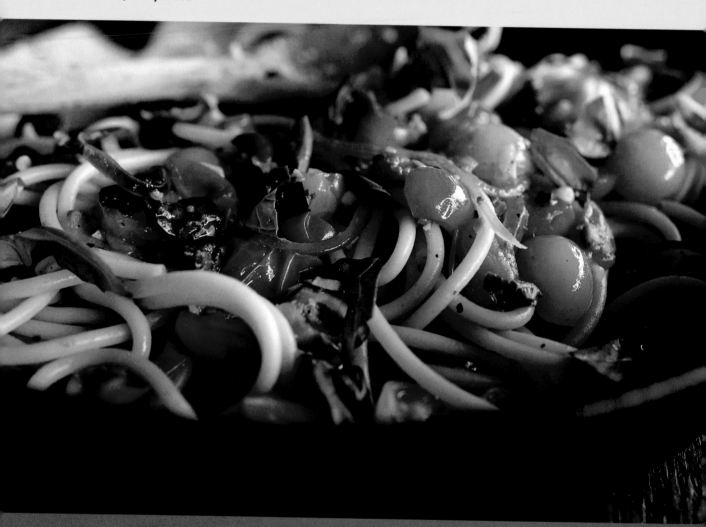

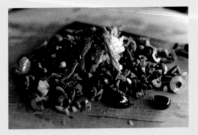

1. Begin by making a pile of the garlic, anchovies, and olives on a cutting board.

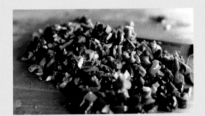

2. Chop until you have a mixture of finely chopped pieces and larger chunks. Set aside.

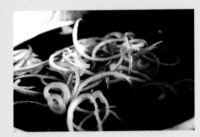

3. Heat the olive oil in a large skillet over medium-high heat. Add the onion and cook, stirring occasionally, until it starts to turn golden brown, about 5 minutes.

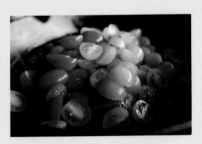

4. Throw in the tomatoes and cook them for a couple of minutes, stirring occasionally.

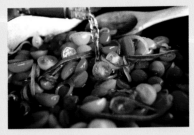

5. Then pour in the broth and wine . . .

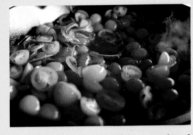

6. And cook for another couple of minutes, until the liquid starts to reduce.

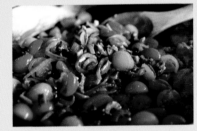

7. Add the delicious garlic-anchovy-olive mixture. Stir and cook for several minutes, until the sauce is nice and reduced and wonderful. Add salt and pepper to taste.

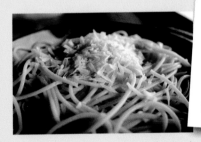

8. Add the pasta to the skillet and sprinkle the Parmesan on top.

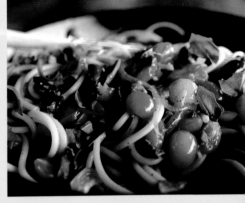

9. Toss everything together to coat the pasta, then tear the basil into pieces and toss it in.

V VARIATIONS

Add thinly sliced mushrooms to the skillet with the red onion.

Add cooked chicken or shrimp if desired.

Stir in crumbled feta cheese. Yum!

Use all broth in place of wine.

S SERVE WITH

The Bread (page 336)

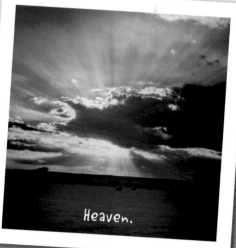

Heaven.

BOW-TIE CHICKEN ALFREDO

MAKES 6 TO 8 SERVINGS

As far as my four children are concerned, dinner doesn't get any better than this.

It's creamy!

It's cheesy!

It . . . it . . . it has chicken in it!

And that's all there is to say about that.

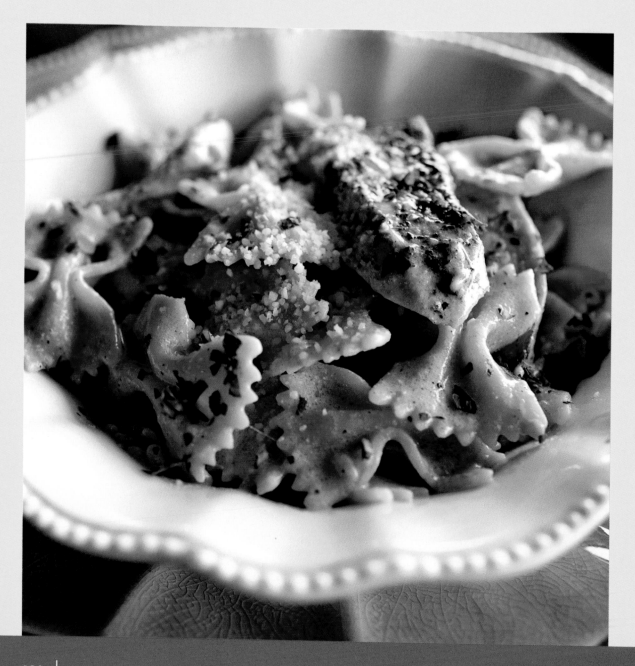

2 boneless, skinless chicken breasts

1 tablespoon Italian seasoning

Kosher salt and black pepper to taste

1 tablespoon butter

1 tablespoon olive oil

2 garlic cloves, minced

½ cup dry white wine

½ cup low-sodium chicken broth, more as needed

½ cup half-and-half

¼ cup heavy cream

1 cup freshly grated Parmesan cheese, plus more for serving

12 ounces bow-tie pasta (farfalle), cooked to al dente

2 tablespoons minced parsley

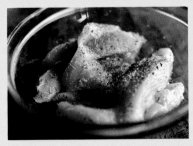

1. Slice the chicken into strips and season with Italian seasoning and salt and pepper to taste.

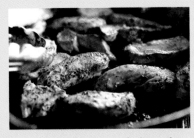

2. Heat the butter and olive oil in a large skillet over medium heat. Add the chicken and cook until it is deep golden brown on both sides and done in the middle, 6 to 7 minutes.

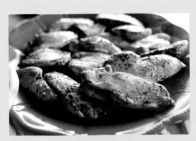

3. Remove the chicken to a plate and set it aside.

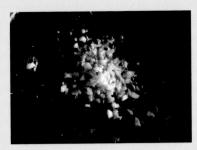

4. Add the garlic to the pan and quickly stir it around, letting it cook and release its flavors for 30 seconds . . .

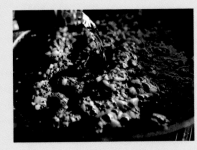

5. Then pour in the wine . . .

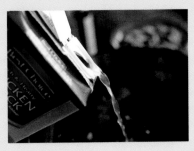

6. And the broth.

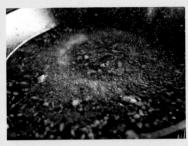

7. Scrape the bottom of the pan, then let the liquid bubble up and reduce by half, 2 to 3 minutes.

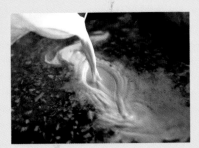

8. And now for the fun part! Add the half-and-half . . .

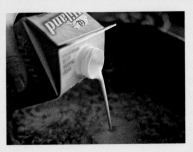

9. And cream.

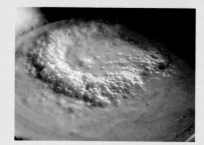

10. Let the sauce heat up and thicken for a few minutes.

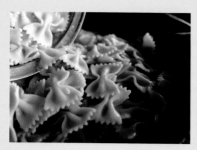

11. When the sauce has thickened, remove it from the heat. Add the Parmesan to the pan . . .

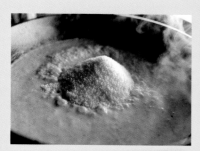

12. Then the pasta . . .

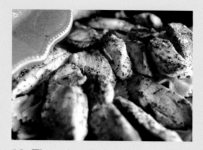

13. Then the chicken!

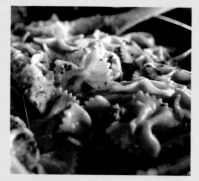

14. Toss it around, then taste it and add more salt and pepper as needed. Top with the parsley and extra Parmesan. Serve immediately!

V VARIATIONS

Omit the chicken for a meat-free pasta dish.

Add 1 heaping tablespoon prepared pesto to the sauce before adding the pasta, chicken, and Parmesan.

Add 8 ounces sautéed mushrooms to the dish.

Use all broth in place of wine.

S SERVE WITH

The Bread (page 336)

Roasted Grape Tomatoes (page 281)

Lemony Green Beans (page 292)

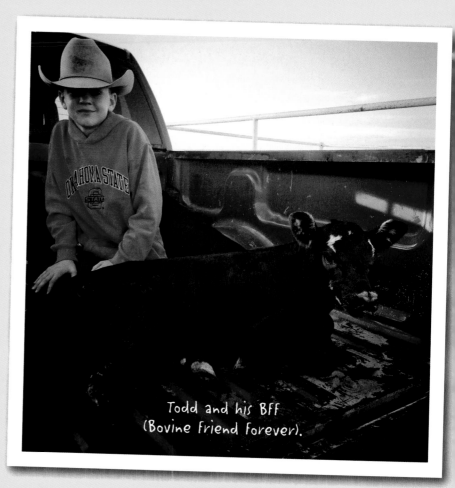

Todd and his BFF (Bovine Friend Forever).

PUMPKIN WONTON RAVIOLI

MAKES 6 SERVINGS

I love making ravioli with ready-to-go wonton wrappers. It's so much easier than making homemade pasta dough from scratch, and once you master the basic steps, you'll be making "homemade" ravioli all the time!

I'll devour pretty much any and every ravioli filling there is—meat, cheese, seafood, veggies—but this pumpkin filling is out of this world. Serve 'em as an appetizer or main course. Just serve 'em . . . as soon as humanly possible!

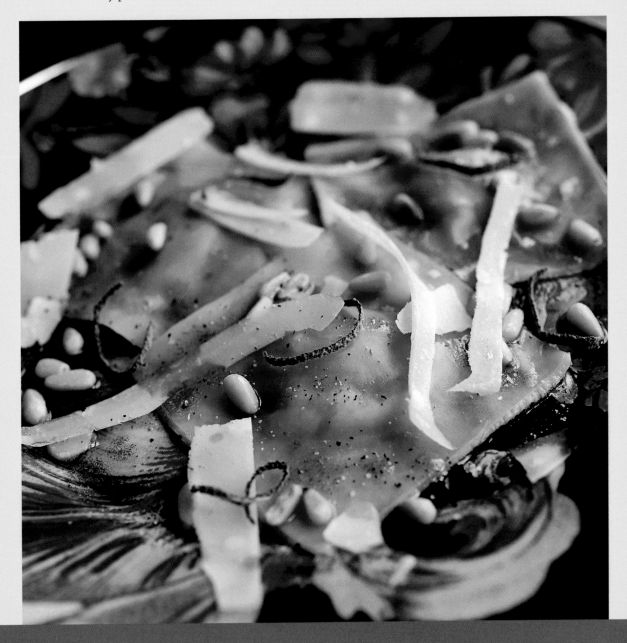

6 tablespoons (¾ stick) butter

2 garlic cloves, minced

One 15-ounce can pumpkin puree

¼ teaspoon kosher salt

¼ teaspoon chili powder

¼ cup pine nuts

1 egg

36 wonton wrappers

1½ cups Parmesan shavings

6 sage leaves, rolled and very thinly sliced

Black pepper to taste

1. Bring a pot of water to a boil.

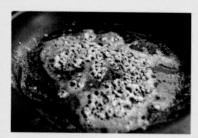

2. Melt 2 tablespoons of the butter in a large skillet over medium heat. Add the garlic and heat it for a couple of minutes (don't brown it).

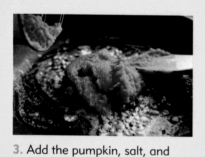

3. Add the pumpkin, salt, and chili powder.

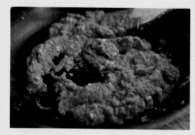

4. Cook this filling for a few minutes, stirring occasionally, to warm it and cook off some of the excess liquid. Remove from the heat and let it cool slightly while you get the other components ready!

5. Toast the pine nuts in a small skillet over medium-low heat, tossing and stirring occasionally, until golden. Remove them to a plate and set aside.

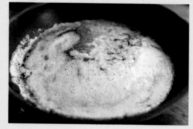

6. Next you'll make browned butter. In the same small skillet, melt the remaining 4 tablespoons butter over medium-high heat . . .

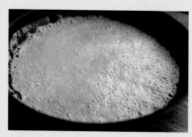

7. And let it cook and bubble up for an additional minute or so, until the foam is golden brown. Watch it carefully and take the pan off the heat as soon as it's ready!

8. Finally, beat the egg with 1 tablespoon cold water. Now you're ready for Operation Ravioli!

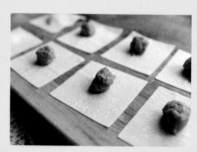

9. Lay out a few wonton wrappers at a time and place a teaspoon-size scoop of the pumpkin mixture in the middle of each one.

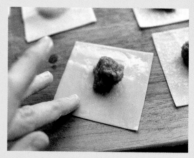

10. Then, one at a time, dab your finger into the egg wash mixture and "paint" around the pumpkin on the wrapper.

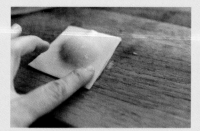

11. Lay a second wonton wrapper on top of each one, match up the edges, and press the two wrappers together.

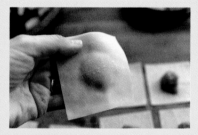

12. Gently press out any air bubbles as you go.

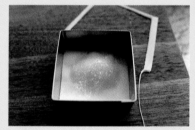

13. To seal the ravioli, use a knife or square cutter to neatly trim the edges.

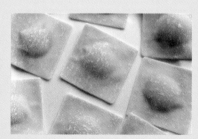

14. Set them aside while you work on the rest!

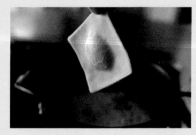

15. Drop a few ravioli at a time into the boiling water. Boil them for 1½ to 2 minutes . . .

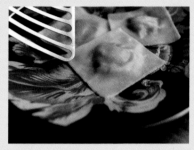

16. Then place them on serving plates.

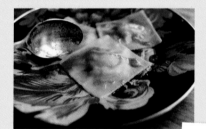

17. Spoon a little bit of the browned butter over the ravioli . . .

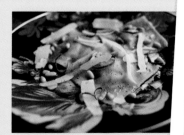

18. Then sprinkle on the Parmesan shavings, sage, toasted pine nuts, and a little pepper.

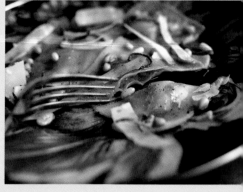

19. You'll absolutely adore every bite!

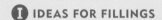

I IDEAS FOR FILLINGS

**Ricotta cheese mixture
(as on page 128)**

Chopped sautéed mushrooms

Spinach-ricotta mixture

Crabmeat-ricotta mixture

**Cooked Italian sausage–ricotta
mixture**

I IDEAS FOR SAUCES

Marinara

Alfredo (see page 181)

Puttanesca (see page 179)

Meat sauce

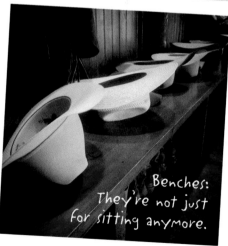

Benches:
They're not just
for sitting anymore.

PASTA WITH VODKA SAUCE

MAKES 8 SERVINGS

Pasta alla vodka. How can I adequately describe to you my love for this tomato-and-cream-based dish of delight? I'm a raging tomato-cream-sauce fiend anyway, but this one . . . Lord, have mercy. Normally, I'd use white wine in a pasta sauce rather than vodka, and that's also scrumptious. It's difficult for me to describe the difference between the flavor of this dish when you use vodka versus wine, but I'll try:

When you cook this sauce with wine, it leaves that delicious "winey" aftertaste—that satisfying "mmmm . . . wine" flavor that's unmistakable and wonderful. But when you use vodka, there's a cleanness to it—a slight sharpness. Not a bitterness at all; in fact, I'm always surprised at how mild the final sauce really is, considering it has a cup of the sharp stuff in it. But it is! It's mild. And each bite has a really clean finish, a perfect ending.

Here! Let me prove it to you!

Note: For those avoiding alcohol (or for kids), you may substitute 1 cup low-sodium vegetable or chicken broth for the vodka. You'll be left with a beautiful pasta with tomato-cream sauce, and you'll love it!

2 tablespoons olive oil

2 tablespoons butter

2 garlic cloves, minced

1 medium onion, finely diced

1 cup vodka or low-sodium chicken broth

One 14-ounce can tomato puree or tomato sauce

Pinch of red pepper flakes

½ teaspoon kosher salt, more to taste

Black pepper to taste

1 cup heavy cream

1 pound fusilli or any pasta of your choice, cooked to al dente

Freshly grated Parmesan cheese, for serving

Basil leaves, torn, for serving

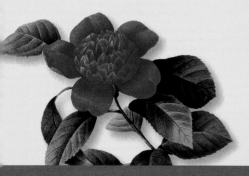

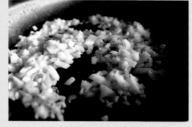

1. In a large skillet, combine the olive oil, butter, and garlic and cook over medium heat for a minute or two to soften the garlic. Add the onion and stir it around to soften, about 3 minutes.

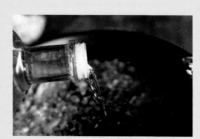

2. Turn off the burner and pour in the vodka . . .

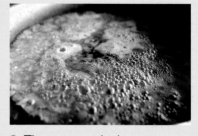

3. Then turn on the heat to medium-high and let the liquid bubble up and cook for 1 to 2 minutes.

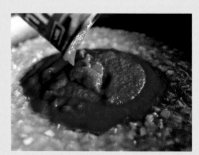

4. Turn the heat to medium-low and add the tomato puree.

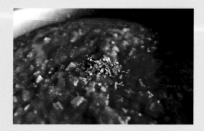

5. Stir it around, add the red pepper flakes, salt, and pepper, and let it simmer for a couple of minutes.

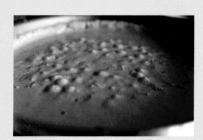

6. Slowly add the cream, stirring continuously until it's combined.

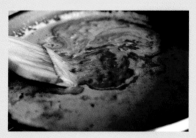

7. Reduce the heat to low and let the sauce simmer for another minute or two, until it is heated through. Taste and add more salt if needed. (This sauce often requires a little extra salt.)

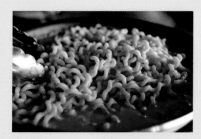

8. Pour in the pasta . . .

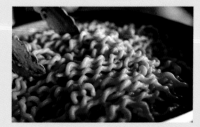

9. And gently toss it until every single noodle is coated!

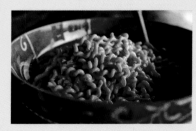

10. There are few things in life that get me more excited than this.

V VARIATIONS

Make the same sauce using dry white wine instead of vodka. Of course, you won't be able to call it vodka sauce . . .

Stir in cubed cooked chicken or cooked shrimp for a decadent dish.

Add 8 ounces sliced white mushrooms to the skillet with the onions and garlic.

S SERVE WITH

Sliced Ready-to-Go Grilled Chicken (page 110)

Salisbury Steak (page 216)

Lemony Green Beans (page 292)

Beautiful Roasted Vegetables (page 290)

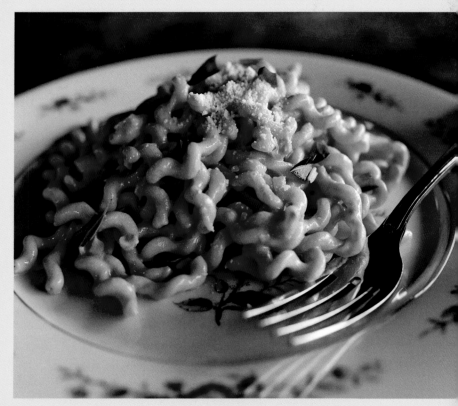

11. A little sprinkle of Parmesan and a few pieces of torn basil?

Stick a fork in me. I'm done.

CAJUN CHICKEN PASTA

MAKES 8 SERVINGS

This one of the most popular recipes on my cooking website, and there's a reason for that: It's an exceedingly yummy, decadent pasta with chicken, vegetables, and lots and lots of scrumptious carbs. It's a cinch to throw together, and you can add Cajun extras to this dish—things like Andouille sausage, crawfish, or shrimp.

Just remember: Part of the deliciousness of this pasta dish is the spicy kick. So don't wimp out on me, baby.

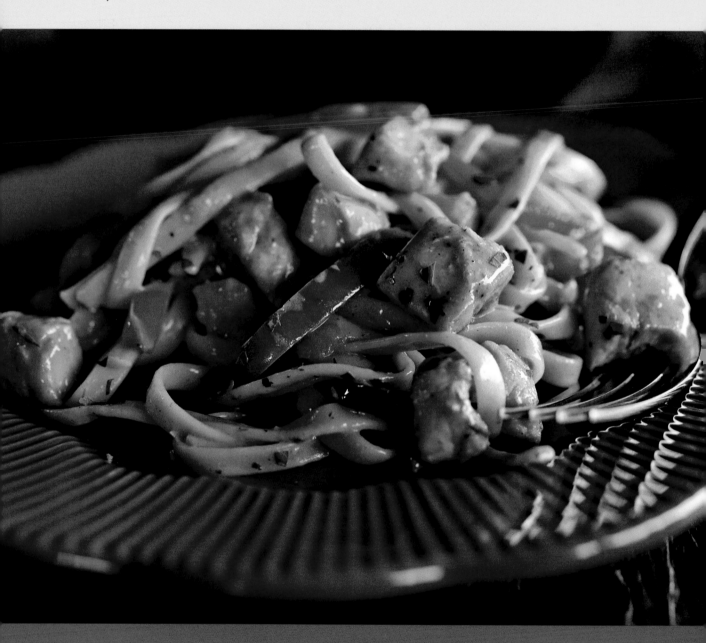

2 tablespoons olive oil

2 tablespoons butter

3 boneless, skinless chicken breasts, cut into cubes

4 teaspoons Cajun spice mix, more to taste

1 green bell pepper, seeded and sliced into strips

1 red bell pepper, seeded and sliced into strips

½ large red onion, halved and thinly sliced

3 garlic cloves, minced

2¼ cups low-sodium chicken broth

½ cup white wine

1 tablespoon cornstarch

½ cup heavy cream

Kosher salt and black pepper to taste

1 pound fettuccine, cooked to al dente

6 Roma tomatoes, diced

Chopped parsley, to taste

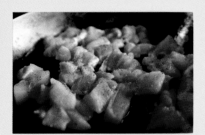

1. Heat 1 tablespoon of the olive oil and 1 tablespoon of the butter in a large skillet over high heat. Add the chicken in a single layer and sprinkle on 2 teaspoons of the Cajun spice mix. Do not stir the chicken at first; allow it to brown on the first side for a minute or two.

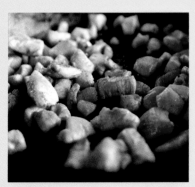

2. Flip to the other side and cook for about 1 minute, then stir the chicken around and continue to cook it until it's totally done, about 2 minutes more. Remove the chicken to a plate and set aside.

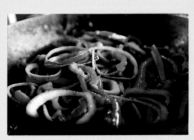

3. To the same skillet, add the peppers, onion, and garlic. Sprinkle on the remaining 2 teaspoons Cajun spice mix and cook the vegetables over very high heat for 1 minute, stirring gently and trying to get as much color on the veggies as possible.

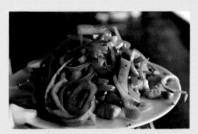

4. Remove the vegetables to the plate with the chicken.

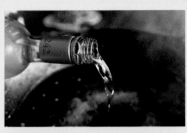

5. Reduce the heat to medium-high and pour in 2 cups of the chicken broth and the wine.

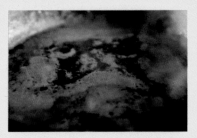

6. Cook and let the liquid bubble up and cook for 3 to 4 minutes, until reduced by half, scraping the bottom of the pan to deglaze. Turn the heat to medium-low.

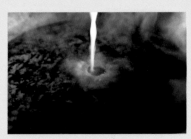

7. Make a slurry by whisking the cornstarch with the remaining ¼ cup chicken broth. Pour it into the skillet and stir to combine.

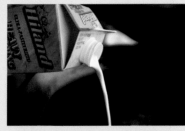

8. Pour in the cream, stirring or whisking continuously.

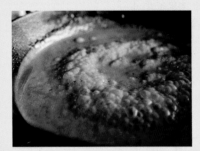

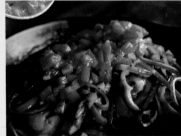

9. Cook the sauce over medium-low heat for a few minutes, stirring occasionally, until the mixture thickens.

11. Add the pasta, chicken, and veggies to the skillet, along with all the juices from the plate. Add the tomatoes on top . . .

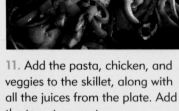

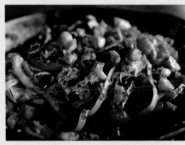

10. Taste and add salt, black pepper, or more Cajun spice mix . . . whatever you think it needs!

12. And toss it all together to heat through, adding the parsley at the end.

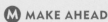 MAKE AHEAD

Cut up the chicken, slice the onion and pepper, and mince the garlic up to 24 hours in advance. Store in separate containers in the fridge.

Ⓥ VARIATIONS

Use more broth in place of the wine.

Add Andouille sausage, crawfish, and/or peeled, deveined shrimp to give it an authentic Cajun flavor.

Add 8 ounces sliced mushrooms with the onions and peppers.

Stir in 1 cup grated Parmesan cheese at the end.

Serve the chicken/veggies mixture over Polenta (page 322) or Stovetop Mashed Potatoes (page 310) instead of pasta.

Ⓢ SERVE WITH

The Bread (page 336)

Refrigerator Rolls (page 334)

Cheese Biscuits (page 332)

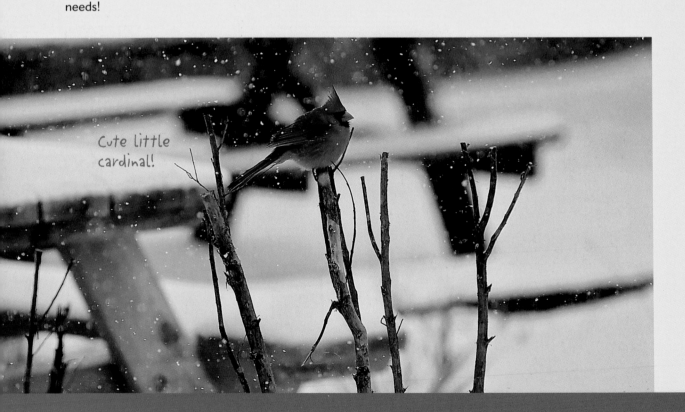

Cute little cardinal!

SEAFOOD PASTA IN A FOIL PACKAGE

MAKES 6 TO 8 SERVINGS

Now, *this* is a fun meal to cook. Yummy, delicious, scrumptious . . . and fun, fun, fun for company. Basically, you sauté seafood, make a simple sauce, throw it into a foil package with pasta, and bake it. It turns into a big, beautiful packet of yum. The seafood cooks in the foil, which means all the juices and aroma stay in there . . . and when you open it up, the heavens open up, too.

1 pound scallops, rinsed

3 tablespoons butter

3 tablespoons olive oil

1 pound jumbo or large shrimp, peeled, deveined, and rinsed

4 garlic cloves, minced

½ cup dry white wine

Three 14.5-ounce cans diced tomatoes

Kosher salt and black pepper to taste

¼ teaspoon red pepper flakes, more to taste

1 pound linguine, fettuccini, fusilli, or riccia pasta, cooked just short of al dente

½ cup heavy cream, warmed

Basil leaves, torn

Parsley leaves, torn

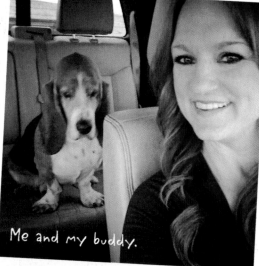

Me and my buddy.

1. Preheat the oven to 350°F.

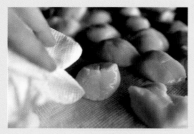

2. Place the scallops on a couple of paper towels and pat them dry with another paper towel. (This will help them sear better.)

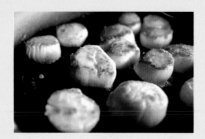

3. In a large skillet (I used non-stick), heat 1 tablespoon of the butter and 1 tablespoon of the olive oil over medium-high heat. Sear the scallops on both sides until they have nice color on the surface, 1 to 1½ minutes per side.

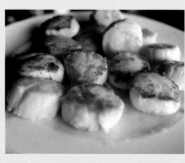

4. Remove them to a plate (and try not to sneak one of them! They're irresistible). . . .

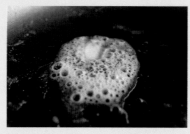

5. In the same skillet, keeping the heat at medium high, heat 1 tablespoon of the butter and 1 tablespoon of the olive oil . . .

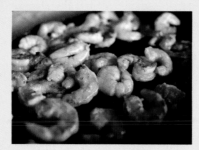

6. And throw in the shrimp, cooking them quickly until they're nicely opaque and browned, 1½ to 2 minutes. Remove them to a plate and set aside.

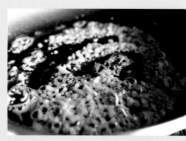

7. Reduce the heat to medium. Add the remaining 1 tablespoon butter and 1 tablespoon olive oil to the skillet and throw in the garlic. Stir it quickly to prevent it from burning . . .

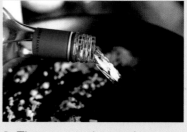

8. Then pour in the wine!

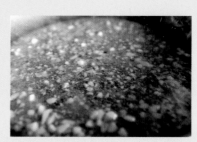

9. Stir the liquid and let it reduce for a couple of minutes . . .

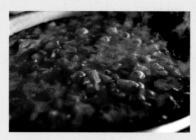

10. Then add the tomatoes with their juices, salt, black pepper, and red pepper flakes. Stir the sauce and let it simmer for 10 minutes.

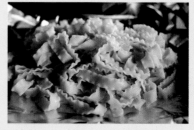

11. Grab two large sheets of heavy aluminum foil and overlap them by about 8 inches on a rimmed baking sheet. Pour the drained pasta onto the foil.

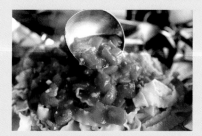

12. Spoon the sauce over the pasta . . .

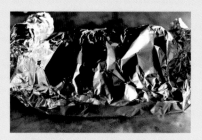

13. Then slide the sautéed seafood on top, making sure you include all the juices from the plate.

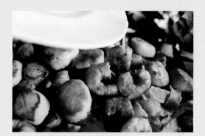

14. Tightly wrap the foil into a package, rolling up the sides so it won't leak. Bake for 15 minutes.

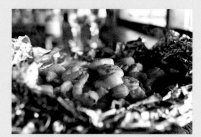

15. To serve, carefully transfer the foil package onto a platter. Open it right before serving . . .

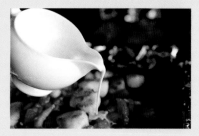

16. Drizzle warm cream over the top . . .

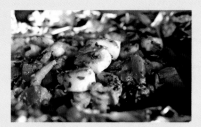

17. And sprinkle with torn basil and parsley.

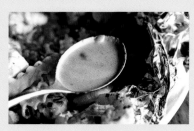

18. As you serve it up, be sure to give everyone a spoonful of the sauce! It's heavenly.

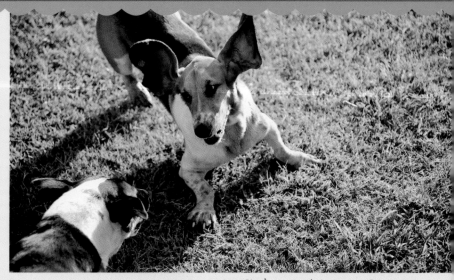

The Flying Nun! I mean Basset.

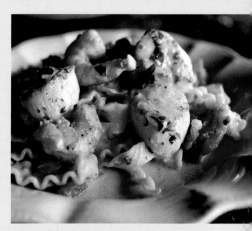

This. This is what they serve in Paradise.

Ⓥ VARIATIONS

Use mussels, lobster, or any other seafood you like!

Add Parmesan shavings to the finished pasta.

Substitute seafood or vegetable broth for the wine.

Ⓢ SERVE WITH

The Bread (page 336)

Cheese Biscuits (page 332)

Refrigerator Rolls (page 334)

SKILLET LASAGNA

MAKES 6 SERVINGS

A million versions of skillet lasagna exist, but I love this simple-but-scrumptious one based on a recipe from Rozanie, a member of my recipe site, Tasty Kitchen. Rather than ricotta, it uses sour cream, and the result is a lovely, mild, family-friendly skilletful of yum.

(Thank you, Rozanie!)

2 tablespoons olive oil

1½ pounds ground beef

2 garlic cloves, minced

One 24-ounce jar marinara sauce

1 tablespoon Italian seasoning

Kosher salt and black pepper to taste

½ cup sour cream, at room temperature

½ cup grated fresh mozzarella (Hint: it helps if the mozzarella is very cold before grating)

12 ounces cooked bow-tie pasta (farfalle), cooked to al dente

8 basil leaves, chopped

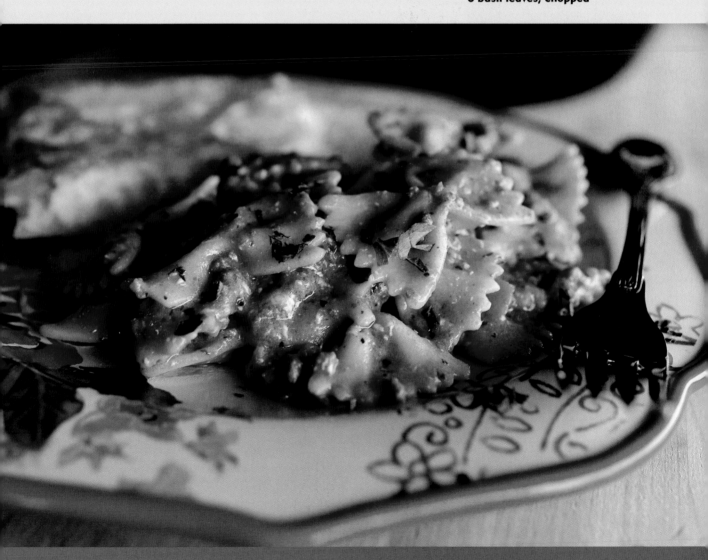

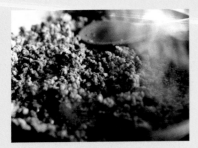

1. Heat the olive oil in a large skillet over medium-high heat. Cook the beef with the garlic until it's completely browned, then drain off the excess fat.

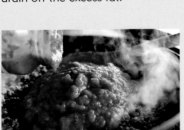

2. Pour in the marinara sauce . . .

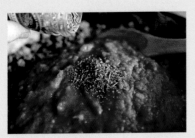

3. Then add the Italian seasoning and salt and pepper to taste.

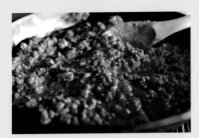

4. Stir, reduce the heat to low, and simmer for 15 minutes.

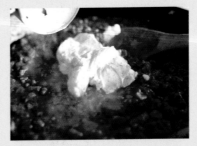

5. Add the sour cream . . .

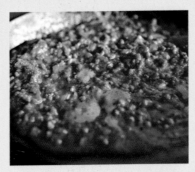

6. And stir until it's all combined.

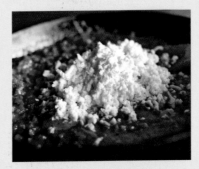

7. Throw in the mozzarella . . .

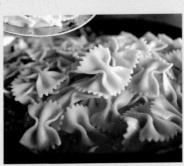

8. And the cooked pasta . . .

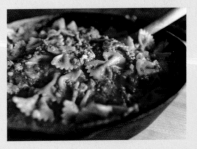

9. And stir it all around to combine.

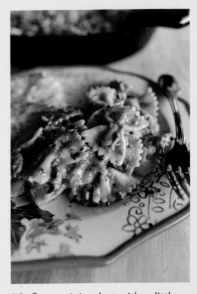

10. Serve piping hot with a little chopped basil on top!

Ⓥ VARIATIONS

Use ground turkey or Italian sausage in place of the beef.

Add 8 ounces chopped mushrooms to the meat mixture.

Add chopped onion and bell pepper to the meat mixture.

Ⓢ SERVE WITH

The Bread (page 336)

Roasted Grape Tomatoes (page 281)

Lemony Green Beans (page 292)

CHICKEN KALE PASTA

MAKES 8 SERVINGS

If the world of pasta were a beauty pageant, this looker of a dish would be in the list of contenders for Most Gorgeous.

(Is "Most Gorgeous" a category in beauty pageants? Can someone get back to me on this?)

Anyway, you will love, adore, and stare at this dish. Not only is it beautiful and healthy, it's really fun to look at, too.

2 tablespoons butter

2 tablespoons olive oil

3 boneless, skinless chicken breasts, cut into bite-size pieces

Kosher salt and black pepper to taste

4 garlic cloves, minced

¾ cup dry white wine

¾ cup low-sodium chicken broth, more as needed

1 bunch kale, stalks removed, leaves torn into small pieces

2 cups grape tomatoes, halved lengthwise

1 pound penne, cooked to al dente and kept hot

1 cup Parmesan cheese shavings

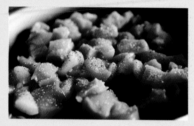

1. Heat the butter and olive oil in a large skillet over high heat. Add the chicken pieces in a single layer and sprinkle with salt and pepper. Don't stir for a minute or two in order to let the chicken brown a bit.

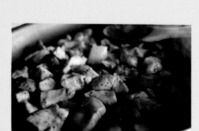

2. Turn the chicken and brown it on the other side. After 30 seconds, stir it around and cook it until it's done, a couple of minutes more . . .

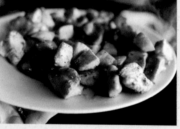

3. Then remove the chicken to a plate and set it aside.

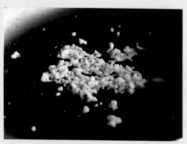

4. Reduce the heat to medium. Add the garlic and quickly stir it to avoid burning.

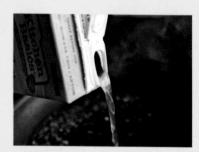

5. After about 30 seconds, pour in the wine . . .

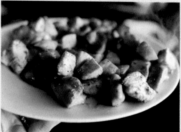

6. And broth.

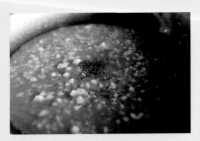

7. Stir the liquid, scraping to deglaze the pan. Let it bubble up, then continue cooking until the liquid has reduced by at least half, about 4 to 5 minutes.

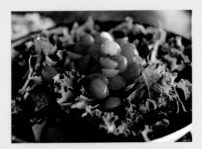

8. Turn off the heat, then add the kale, tomatoes . . .

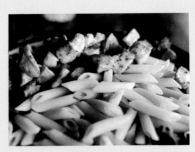

9. Pasta, and chicken . . .

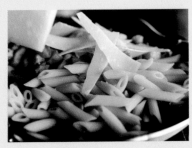

10. And finally, the Parmesan shavings. Sprinkle in more salt and pepper to taste.

M MAKE AHEAD

Cut up the chicken, stem and tear the kale, mince the garlic, and halve the tomatoes up to 24 hours ahead of time. Store them in separate containers in the fridge.

V VARIATIONS

Use all broth if you prefer to omit the wine.

Use baby spinach instead of kale.

Stir in 1 cup crumbled feta cheese instead of Parmesan shavings.

Use peeled, deveined shrimp instead of chicken.

S SERVE WITH

The Bread (page 336)

Refrigerator Rolls (page 334)

Cheese Biscuits (page 332)

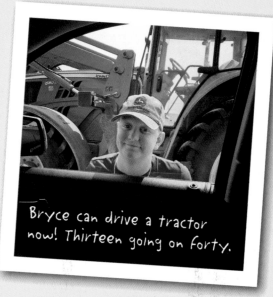

Bryce can drive a tractor now! Thirteen going on forty.

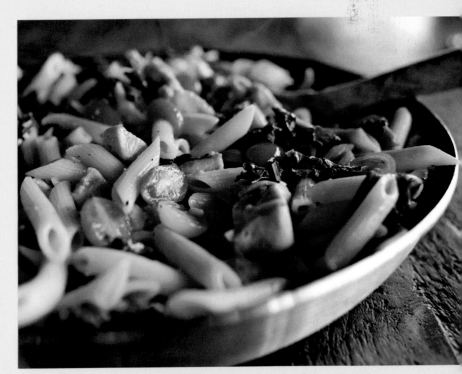

11. Toss it to combine; the kale will start to wilt and soften as it mixes with the other ingredients. Serve it right out of the skillet to hungry folks! Such a gorgeous and satisfying dish.

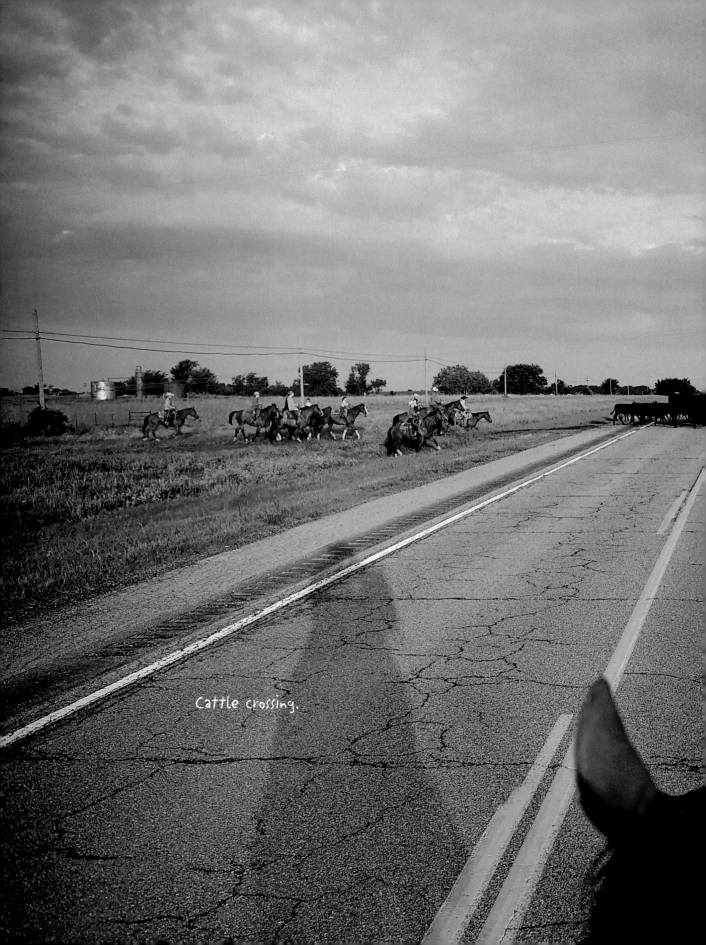

Cattle crossing.

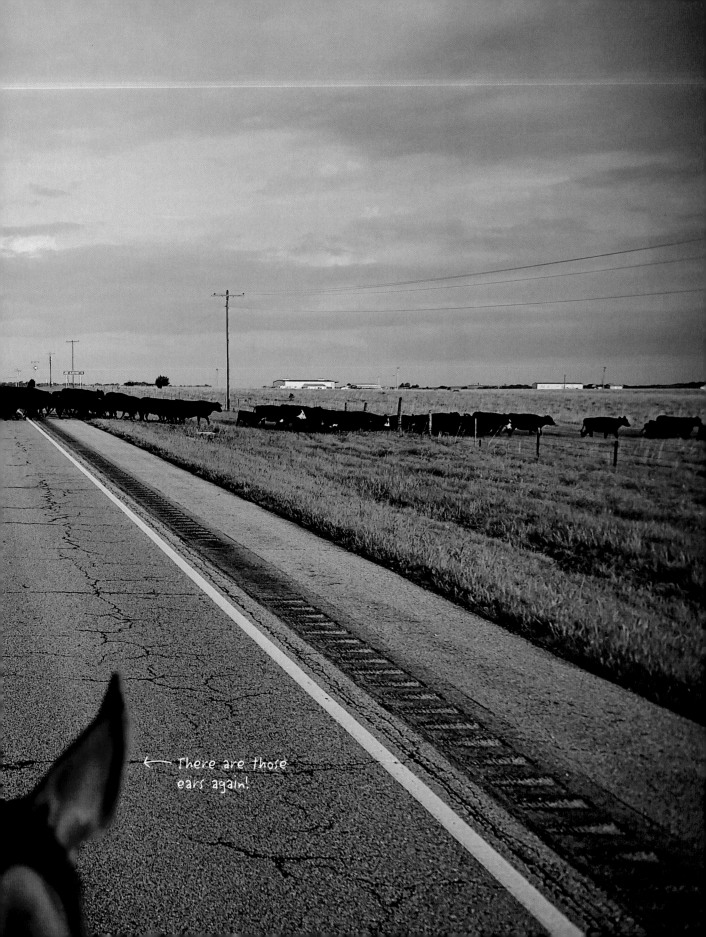

← There are those
ears again!

CHICKEN MOZZARELLA PASTA

MAKES 6 TO 8 SERVINGS

This pasta really is the total package: hearty, easy, full of cheese, and bursting with carbs! All the qualities I look for in a friend.

That made no sense. Sorry.

Anyway, you'll absolutely love this pasta, as you get a bunch of deliciousness without a whole lot of effort. It's the perfect weeknight meal and also makes a great presentation if you're having company over. (Does anyone have company over anymore? Do people still call guests "company"? Or is that just another old term I've hung on to through the years, along with "television set" and "fella"?)

**2 tablespoons olive oil,
more for drizzling**

**2 boneless, skinless chicken
breasts, cut into small pieces**

**Kosher salt and black pepper
to taste**

1 large onion, finely diced

2 garlic cloves, minced

**One 25-ounce jar good-quality
marinara sauce**

½ teaspoon red pepper flakes

2 tablespoons minced parsley

**1 pound penne, cooked to
al dente and kept hot**

**¼ cup Parmesan shavings,
plus more for serving**

**8 ounces (½ pound) fresh
mozzarella, cubed**

**12 basil leaves, cut into
chiffonade**

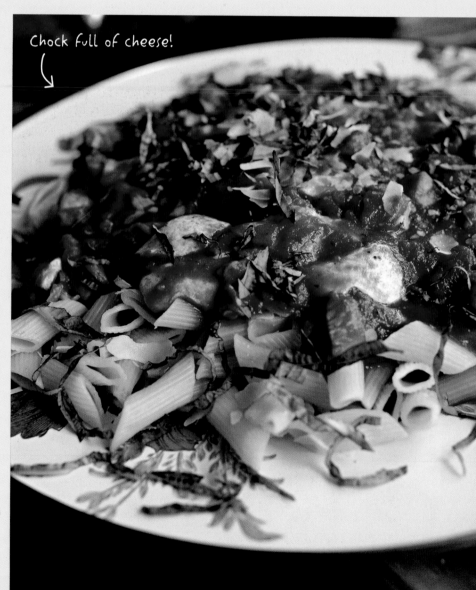

Chock full of cheese!

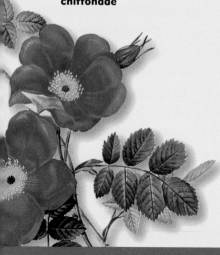

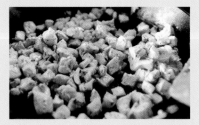

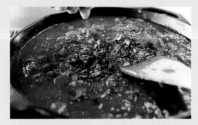

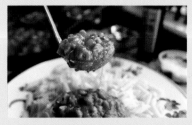

1. Heat the olive oil in a large skillet over medium-high heat. Add the chicken, season it with salt and pepper, and cook for 2 minutes on the first side, until golden brown, then flip and cook for 2 minutes more, until totally done. Remove the chicken to a plate.

5. Stir the sauce, then add the parsley and stir it through. Let the sauce simmer for 7 to 8 minutes more, stirring occasionally.

9. Before the cheese fully melts, ladle the sauce onto the pasta. It'll keep softening and melting as you go and will pretty much look like a miracle.

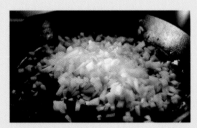

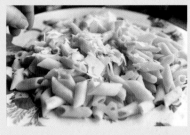

2. Add the onion and garlic to the pan.

6. Place the pasta on a large platter, drizzle on a little olive oil, and sprinkle on some Parmesan shavings.

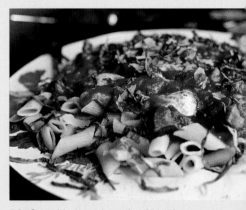

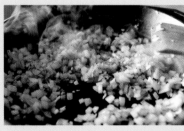

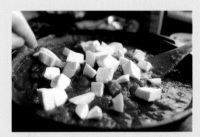

3. Cook, stirring, for 3 to 4 minutes, or until the onions are golden brown.

7. And now, for the moment we've all been waiting for: Throw the mozzarella into the piping-hot sauce . . .

10. Sprinkle on a bunch of basil at the end, then dig in! It's a cheesy wonderland in there.

Ⓥ VARIATIONS

Use any kind of pasta you'd like: spaghetti, penne, fettuccine, and so on.

Pour ½ cup heavy cream into the sauce after you add the parsley for a richer dish.

Brown 1 pound ground beef instead of the chicken for a beefy version.

Omit the chicken and double the amount of mozzarella for a meat-free dish.

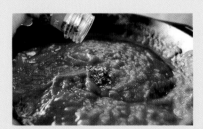

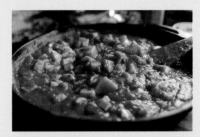

4. Reduce the heat to low and add the marinara sauce, red pepper flakes, and ½ cup water.

8. And stir it through, allowing the cheese to begin to soften and melt.

Ⓢ SERVE WITH

The Bread (page 336)

Cheese Biscuits (page 332)

Refrigerator Rolls (page 334)

SHRIMP SCAMPI

MAKES 6 SERVINGS

(I apologize in advance for the following rant.)

Shrimp scampi reminds me of khaki shorts. And little silver hair clips threaded with thin satin ribbon, finished with a neat little bow at the end. I had red, pink, purple, and white. What colors did you have?

Shrimp scampi also reminds me of Foreigner. Seriously, try this exercise with me: *Listen to "Waiting for a Girl Like You." Ingest it. Feel it. Remember slow dancing with Matthew at the youth group dance. You're wearing a Gunne Sax dress and he loves Julie and not you. This dance is a sympathy dance. Matthew likes you as a friend, nothing more. Your red bangs are frizzy. Julie is tan.*

Anyway (*shaking it off*) the whole thing just reminds me of shrimp scampi, the classic late seventies/early eighties throw-together meal of shrimp, butter, garlic, and lemon. I add wine (of course) and a dash or two of hot sauce in an effort to be weird, but it's hard to do too much to improve on the original.

Oh, and about shrimp scampi: I think I ate it with Matthew once. Probably at Julie's house.

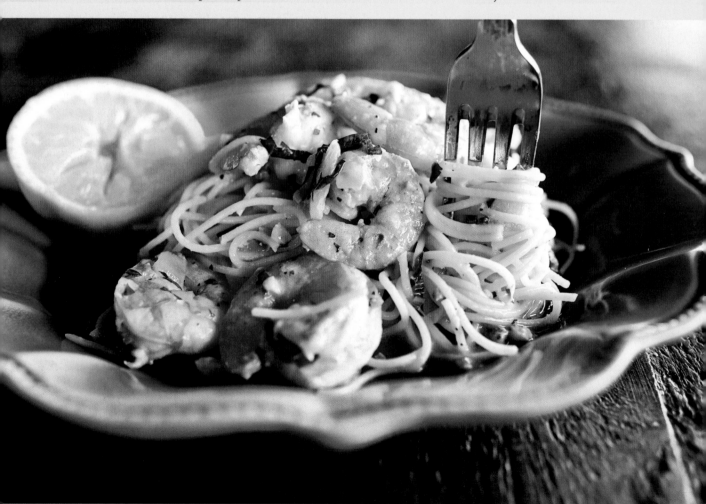

2 tablespoons olive oil

4 tablespoons (½ stick) butter

½ medium onion, finely diced

4 garlic cloves, minced or pressed

1 pound large shrimp, peeled and deveined

Kosher salt and black pepper to taste

½ cup white wine

Juice of 2 lemons, plus extra lemon wedges for serving

4 dashes hot sauce

8 ounces angel hair pasta

½ cup grated Parmesan cheese

Chopped basil to taste

Chopped parsley to taste

1. Boil a big pot of water for the pasta so it will be ready.

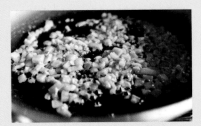

2. Heat the olive oil and 2 table-spoons of the butter in large skillet over medium heat. Add the onion and garlic and cook for 2 to 3 minutes, or until the onion is translucent.

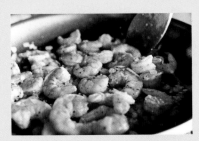

3. Add the shrimp, sprinkle them with salt and pepper, and sauté them for a couple of minutes. When they're done they'll be pink and opaque throughout. They'll go fast!

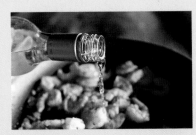

4. Add the wine . . .

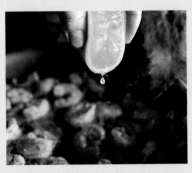

5. Lemon juice . . .

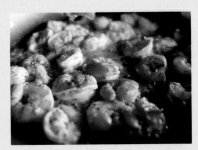

6. And hot sauce. Stir and reduce the heat to a low simmer. Throw the pasta in the boiling water and cook until al dente (this will take a very short time).

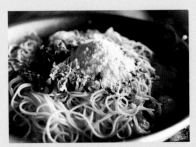

7. Turn the heat off under the skillet and add the remaining 2 tablespoons butter, the pasta, Parmesan, and basil and parsley to taste.

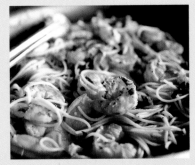

8. Toss it all around until it's a skillet of absolute bliss.

Enjoy every bite!

V VARIATIONS

Use all broth if you prefer to omit the wine.

Use small scallops instead of (or in addition to!) the shrimp.

Add a splash of cream when you add the pasta, cheese, and herbs for a little decadence.

S SERVE WITH

The Bread (page 336)

Refrigerator Rolls (page 334)

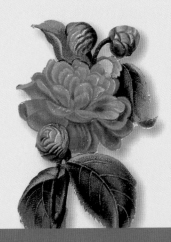

TORTELLINI PRIMAVERA

MAKES 6 TO 8 SERVINGS

This is a cheesy, delicious play on the classic pasta primavera recipe my mom always used to make.
   And actually, I think she still makes it. I'll have to ask her.
   Mom? Do you still make the same pasta primavera you always used to make?
   (I won't make you wait for her to respond. I'll let you know what I find out.)

2 tablespoons butter

1 onion, finely diced

3 garlic cloves, minced

3 medium carrots, diced

1 cup small cauliflower florets

¼ cup white wine

¼ cup low-sodium chicken broth

⅓ cup heavy cream

½ cup freshly grated Parmesan cheese, plus more for serving

1 cup frozen peas

¾ cup small-diced cooked ham

12 basil leaves, chopped, plus more for serving

Kosher salt and black pepper to taste

1 pound cheese or spinach tortellini, cooked according to the package instructions

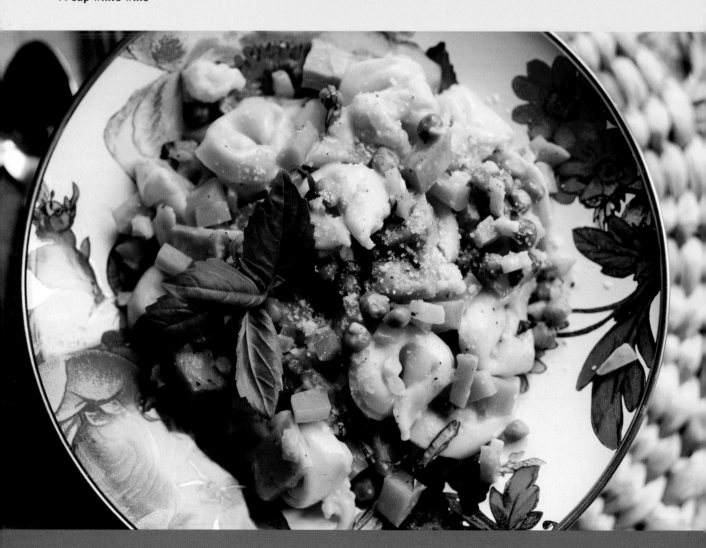

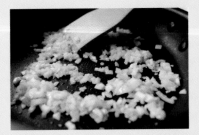

1. Melt the butter in a large skillet over medium-high heat. Add the onion and garlic and sauté for 1 minute.

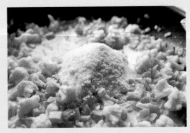

5. Turn the heat to low and add the cream and Parmesan. Stir the sauce and let it bubble up and thicken for 2 to 3 minutes more.

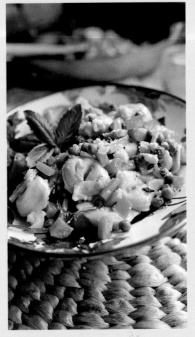

9. And serve it up with extra Parmesan and basil.

Deliciously delightful! (And delightfully delicious.)

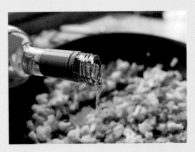

2. Add the carrots and cauliflower and stir, then cook for another minute.

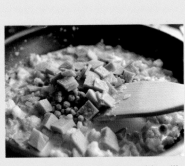

6. Pour in the frozen peas (they'll start to thaw immediately!) and the ham.

Ⓜ MAKE AHEAD

Prep all the vegetables and dice the ham up to 48 hours ahead of time and store in the fridge.

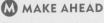

3. Splash in the wine and broth . . .

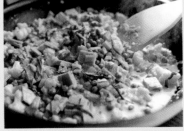
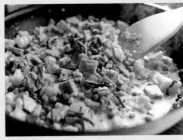

7. Stir it all around, then add the basil and salt and pepper to taste.

Ⓥ VARIATIONS

Add cooked shrimp instead of the ham.

Use any variety of vegetables: asparagus pieces, diced zucchini, diced yellow squash, diced red bell pepper, whatever you like!

Try a different pasta: angel hair, penne, linguine . . .

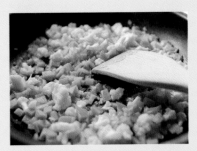

4. Then cook for 2 to 3 minutes, until the liquid has reduced a bit.

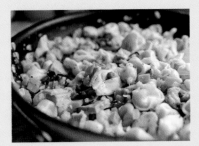
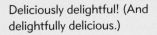

8. Finally, toss in the tortellini . . .

Ⓢ SERVE WITH

The Bread (page 336)

Cheese Biscuits (page 332)

Refrigerator Rolls (page 334)

ROASTED RED PEPPER PASTA

MAKES 8 SERVINGS

This exceedingly excellent pasta dish is a throwback to my vegetarian days in Los Angeles, and I still love it every bit as much today as I did then. Okay, so a few things about me have changed slightly. I was neither a wife nor a mother then. I am now. I wore small jeans then. I don't now. I wore neon scrunchies in my hair then. I don't now.

And based on that last one alone, I totally win!

4 tablespoons (½ stick) butter

1 medium onion, diced

3 garlic cloves, minced

One 15.5-ounce jar roasted red peppers, drained and coarsely chopped

1 cup low-sodium vegetable or chicken broth

½ teaspoon kosher salt, more to taste

½ teaspoon black pepper

½ cup heavy cream

3 tablespoons minced parsley, plus more for serving

12 ounces rigatoni or other short pasta, cooked to al dente

½ cup Parmesan shavings, plus more for serving

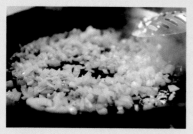

1. Heat the butter in a large skillet over medium-high heat. Add the onion and garlic and sauté for 2 to 3 minutes, until slightly softened.

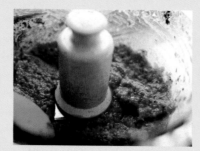

3. Transfer the mixture to a food processor or blender . . .

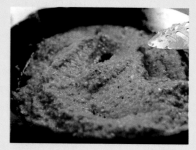

5. Return the puree to the same skillet over medium heat.

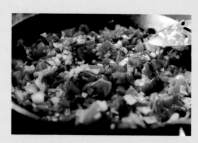

2. Add the peppers and sauté for 2 to 3 minutes, until the peppers are nice and piping hot. Remove the pan from the heat to cool slightly.

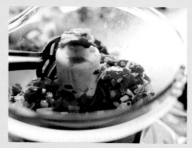

4. And process until it's totally pureed.

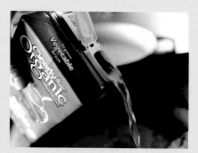

6. Pour in the broth . . .

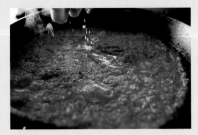

7. Then add the salt and black pepper and stir until heated.

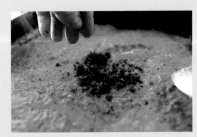

9. Add the parsley, then taste and add more salt as needed.

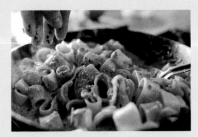

11. Stir it around to coat the pasta, adding more salt and pepper if needed.

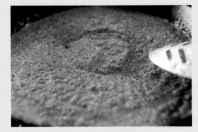

8. Stir in the cream. It'll be a gorgeous light orange color at this point.

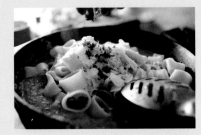

10. Pile in the pasta, Parmesan shavings, and a little more parsley if you'd like!

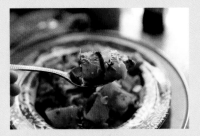

12. Then serve it up and dig right in!

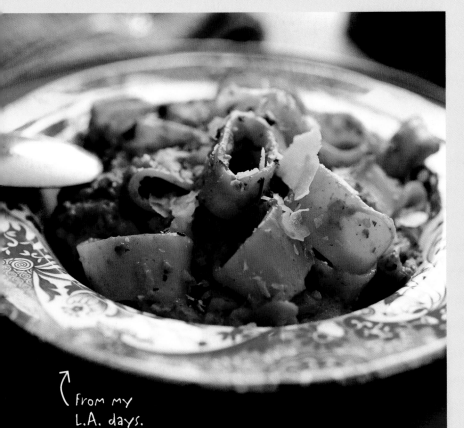

from my L.A. days.

Ⓜ MAKE AHEAD

The sauce can be made up until the addition of the cream and kept in the fridge for up to 48 hours. To serve, reheat the sauce in a skillet, add the cream, and proceed with the recipe.

Ⓥ VARIATIONS

Add sliced Ready-to-Go Grilled Chicken (page 110).

Add cooked spicy sausage.

Add sautéed mushrooms.

Add sautéed shrimp.

Forgo the pasta and spoon the roasted red pepper sauce over grilled chicken! Yum.

ZUCCHINI NOODLES

MAKES 2 SERVINGS

Zucchini . . . *noodles*? What is the world coming to? But wait! Before you run off: These are delicious! A light alternative to pasta, and while I added a light tomato-garlic sauce to mine, you can pretty much use any sauce you'd normally put on pasta. So delightful, and so fun to make!

2 medium zucchini

1 tablespoon butter

1 tablespoon olive oil

2 garlic cloves, minced

Kosher salt and black pepper to taste

2 or 3 Roma tomatoes, diced

2 to 3 tablespoons shredded Parmesan cheese

2 or 3 basil leaves, cut into chiffonade

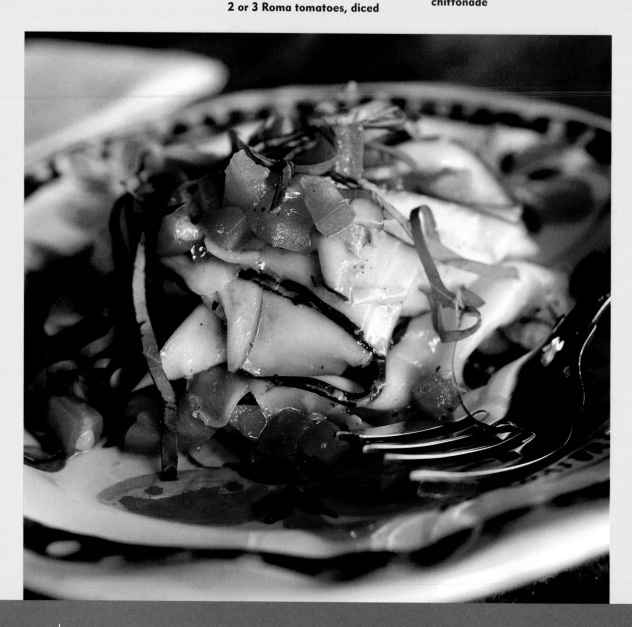

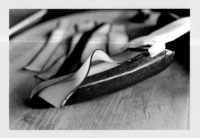

1. Using a vegetable peeler, cut the zucchini into long, thin ribbons . . .

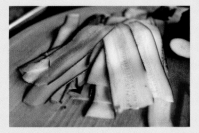

2. Until you have a big pile.

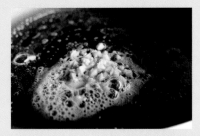

3. Heat the butter and olive oil in a large skillet (I used nonstick) over medium heat. When the butter has melted, add the garlic and cook it for 1 minute, stirring.

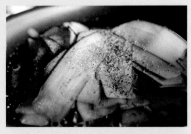

4. Drop the zucchini ribbons into the skillet separately so that they don't stick together, sprinkle on salt and pepper to taste . . .

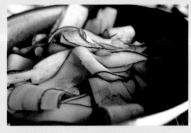

5. And gently toss them around to lightly cook them for about 1 minute.

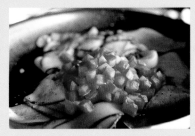

6. Add the tomatoes . . .

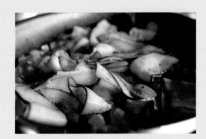

7. And toss them gently . . .

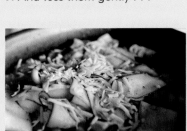

8. Then add the Parmesan and toss it in! Both the tomatoes and Parmesan will warm up almost instantly.

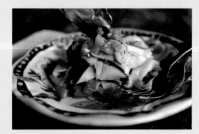

9. Serve the zucchini noodles in a pretty pile, with some of the tomatoes on top . . .

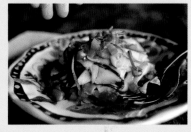

10. And a sprinkle of basil.

V VARIATIONS

Stir in crumbled feta cheese instead of (or in addition to) the Parmesan.

Saute ½ cup diced onion in the skillet for 4 to 5 minutes before adding the zucchini.

S SERVE WITH

Ready-to-Go Grilled Chicken (page 110)

Italian Meatloaf (page 212)

Oven-Barbecued Chicken (page 234)

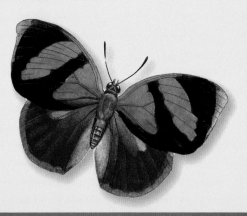

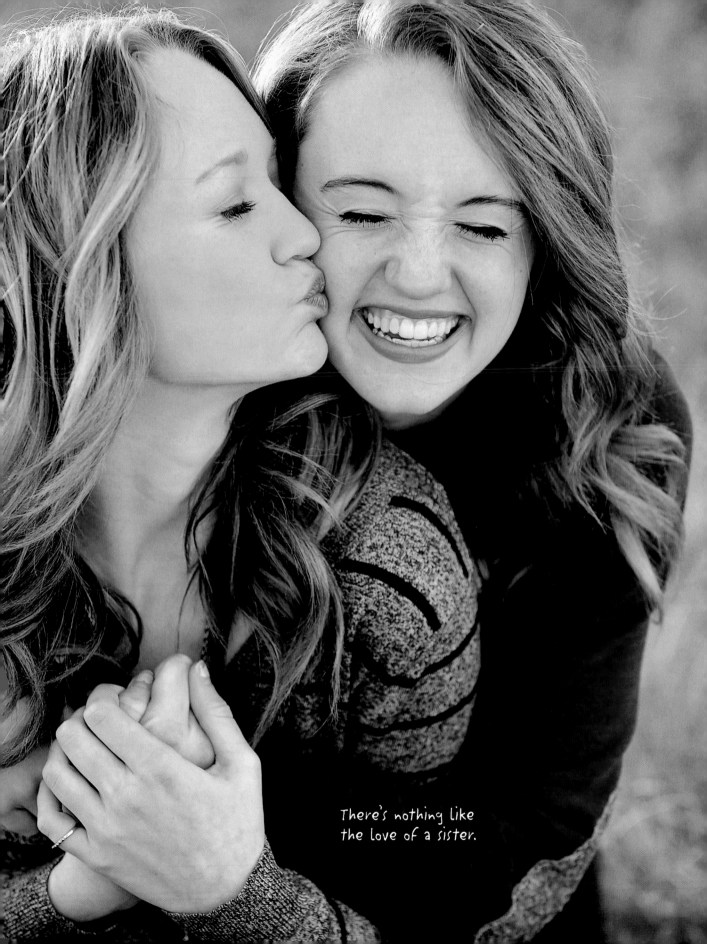

There's nothing like
the love of a sister.

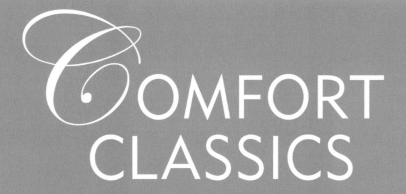COMFORT CLASSICS

Comfort food is called comfort food because eating it makes you feel safe, warm, loved, nourished . . . and twelve. Whether it's Salisbury steak from the seventies or beef Stroganoff from, well, the seventies, these classic comfort dishes will remind you of your school cafeteria, your grandma's house, and your childhood home all at once. (Note: You do not have to have grown up in the seventies to make these recipes. Sorry to bring my own decadist bias into this.)

ITALIAN MEATLOAF

MAKES 8 TO 12 SERVINGS

I can't draw to save my life. I can't paint a pretty picture. I can't write a sonnet, sing an aria, or sculpt. But I can make meatloaf. And this Italian version will make you feel like you can do all of the above.

6 slices crusty Italian bread

1 cup milk

2 pounds ground beef

1 cup freshly grated Parmesan cheese

4 large eggs

⅓ cup minced parsley

1 tablespoon Italian seasoning

1 teaspoon kosher salt

½ teaspoon black pepper

Two 14.5-ounce cans diced tomatoes, drained

¼ cup packed brown sugar

1 teaspoon dry mustard

Pinch of cayenne pepper

A few dashes of Worcestershire sauce

12 to 16 thin slices pancetta (about 4 ounces)

1. Preheat the oven to 350°F.

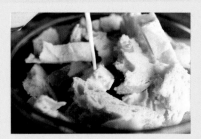

2. Tear the bread into chunks and place it in a bowl. Pour the milk over the bread, toss it around, and let it soak in for several minutes.

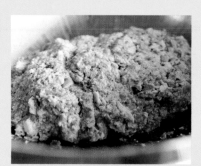

4. And smush and knead it around with your hands until everything is completely mixed.

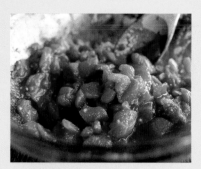

6. And stir it together.

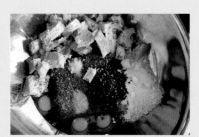

3. Place the ground beef, milk-soaked bread, Parmesan, eggs, parsley, Italian seasoning, salt, and black pepper in a large bowl . . .

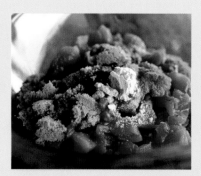

5. Meanwhile, in a separate bowl, combine the tomatoes, brown sugar, mustard, cayenne, and Worcestershire . . .

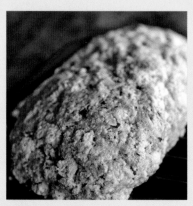

7. Place the meat mixture on a drip pan (a pan with a slotted tray on top) and form it into a big honkin' loaf shape.

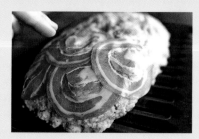

8. Arrange the pancetta slices in an overlapping pattern all over the surface . . .

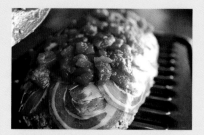

9. Then spoon the tomato mixture all over the top. (Leave any excess juices in the bowl.)

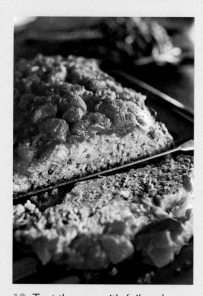

10. Tent the pan with foil and bake the meatloaf for 50 minutes. Remove the foil and continue baking for 20 to 30 minutes more, or until done in the middle. (Be careful not to let the pancetta burn.) Cut it into thick slices . . .

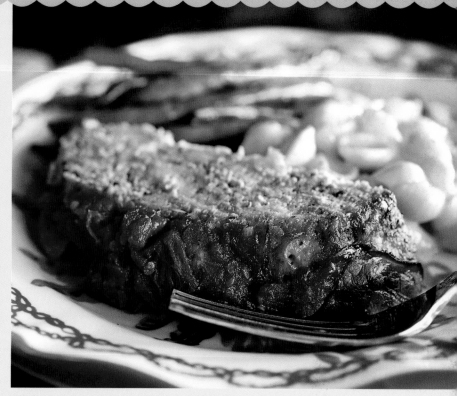

11. And serve it with your favorite sides.

This takes meatloaf to a whole new level!

N NOTE

It's best to form a loaf that isn't too thick; this way the meatloaf has a better chance of cooking more thoroughly. Long and somewhat flat is my preferred meatloaf shape!

V VARIATIONS

Use a combination of ground beef and ground turkey.

Use a combination of ground beef and Italian sausage.

Add 12 to 15 roasted garlic cloves (see page 247) to the meat mixture. Mmmm . . . the flavor!

Add a mixture of chopped fresh herbs (oregano, basil, parsley . . .) instead of Italian seasoning.

Add 1 cup grated Asiago cheese instead of Parmesan for a sharper flavor.

S SERVE WITH

Lemony Green Beans (page 292)
Quick Shells and Cheese (page 214)
Stovetop Mashed Potatoes (page 310)
Buttered Parsley Noodles (page 324)
Peas and Carrots (page 293)
Beautiful Roasted Vegetables (page 290)

QUICK SHELLS AND CHEESE

MAKES 6 TO 8 SERVINGS

Everyone needs a little dose of shells and cheese every now and again. Whether it's served alongside meatloaf or just in a bowl by itself, you'll go back to this beauty again and again.

And again. And again. And again!

2 cups whole milk

1 tablespoon butter

2 cups grated sharp Cheddar cheese

8 ounces processed cheese (Velveeta!), cut into cubes

1 teaspoon black pepper

½ teaspoon kosher salt

¼ teaspoon seasoned salt

1 pound small pasta shells, cooked to al dente

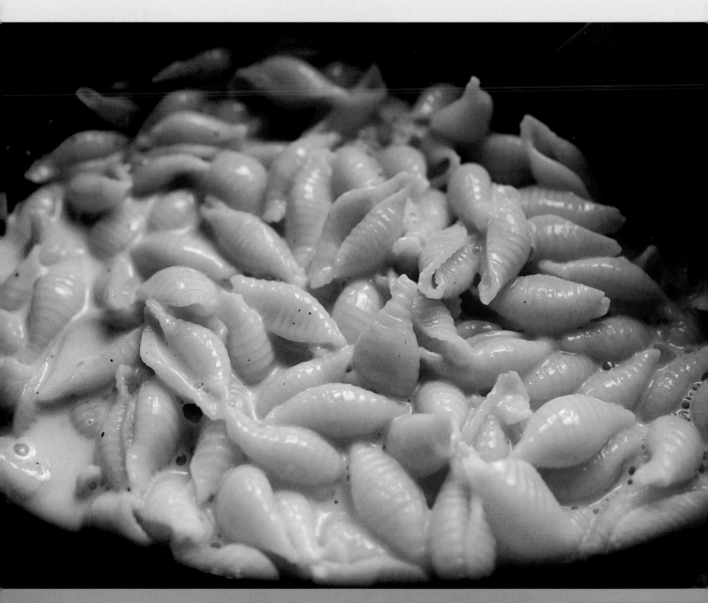

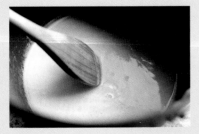

1. Heat the milk and butter in a medium pot over medium heat, until hot.

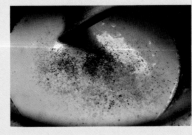

3. When the cheeses start to melt, stir in the pepper, kosher salt, and seasoned salt.

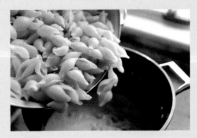

5. Finally, pour in the cooked shells . . .

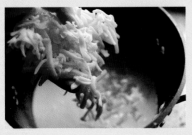

2. Then add the cheeses and stir them around a bit.

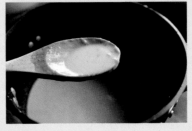

4. Keep stirring until it's nice and smooth!

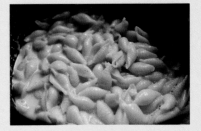

6. And stir until it's all combined. Come to Mama!

V VARIATIONS

Use pepper Jack, grated Fontina, grated Parmesan, and/or goat cheese for a different cheese flavor.

Stir in caramelized onions.

Stir in frozen peas. They'll thaw instantly!

S SERVE WITH

Italian Meatloaf (page 212)

Salisbury Steak (page 216)

Classic Pulled Pork (page 228)

Oven Barbecued Chicken (page 234)

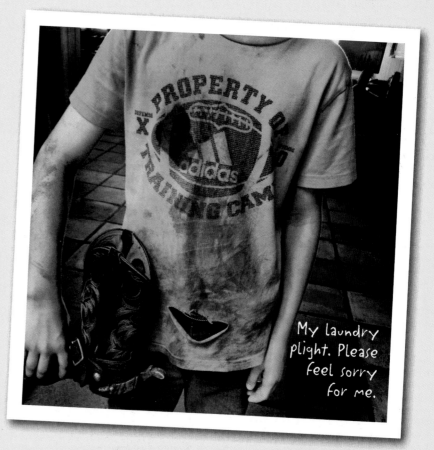

My laundry plight. Please feel sorry for me.

SALISBURY STEAK

MAKES 6 SERVINGS

Salisbury steak is a 1970s school cafeteria fave, which automatically secures it a permanent spot on any list of classic comfort foods.

STEAKS

1½ pounds lean ground beef

½ cup seasoned breadcrumbs

2 tablespoons heavy cream

2 teaspoons dry mustard

1 beef bouillon cube, crumbled

4 dashes of Worcestershire sauce

1 tablespoon ketchup

½ teaspoon kosher salt

½ teaspoon black pepper

1 tablespoon olive oil

1 tablespoon butter

GRAVY

½ onion, halved and thinly sliced

2¼ cups beef broth

4 dashes of Worcestershire sauce

1 tablespoon ketchup

1 teaspoon Kitchen Bouquet browning sauce (optional)

2 tablespoons cornstarch

Kosher salt and black pepper to taste

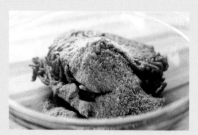

1. To make the steaks, combine the beef, breadcrumbs, cream, mustard, bouillon, Worcestershire, ketchup, salt, and pepper in a bowl.

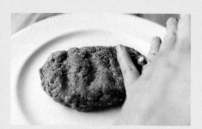

2. Knead the mixture until it's evenly combined, then form it into 6 oblong patties. Use your little finger to press indentations all down the patties. (This is just for fun, to give them a "steak" appearance!)

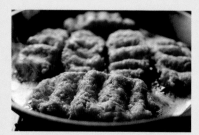

3. Heat a large skillet over medium-high heat and add the olive oil and butter. Fry the patties on both sides . . .

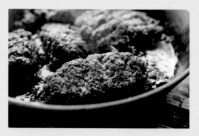

4. Until nicely crusty outside and no longer pink in the middle, 3 to 4 minutes per side. Remove the patties to a plate.

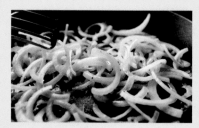

5. To make the gravy, add the onion to the pan.

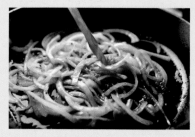

6. Sauté the onion for several minutes, until golden, then add 2 cups of the beef broth, the Worcestershire, ketchup, and Kitchen Bouquet (if using).

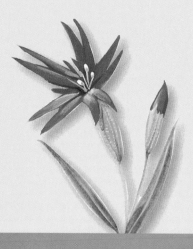

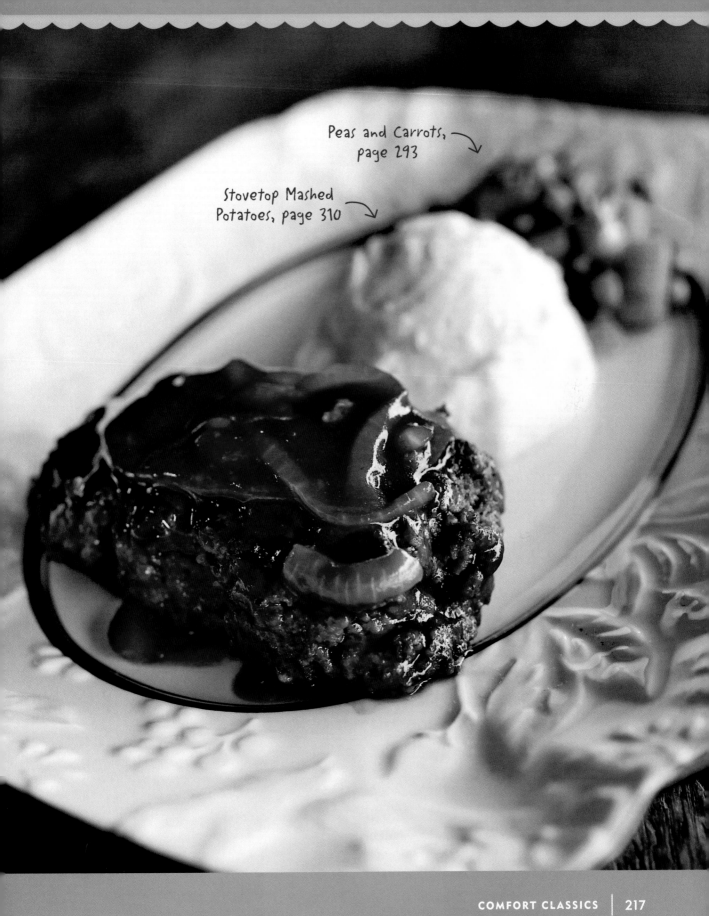

Peas and Carrots,
page 293

Stovetop Mashed
Potatoes, page 310

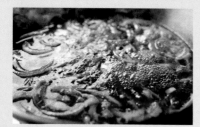

7. Stir and cook for 2 to 3 minutes to reduce the liquid slightly.

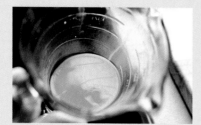

8. Make a slurry by mixing together the cornstarch and remaining ¼ cup broth.

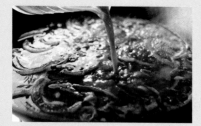

9. Pour the slurry into the gravy, then stir and let it bubble up and thicken for 3 to 4 minutes. Taste and adjust the seasonings, adding salt and pepper if the flavors need more pop.

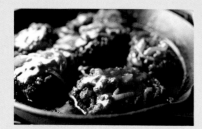

10. Nestle the steaks into the skillet and spoon the gravy over the top. Let it simmer for a couple more minutes.

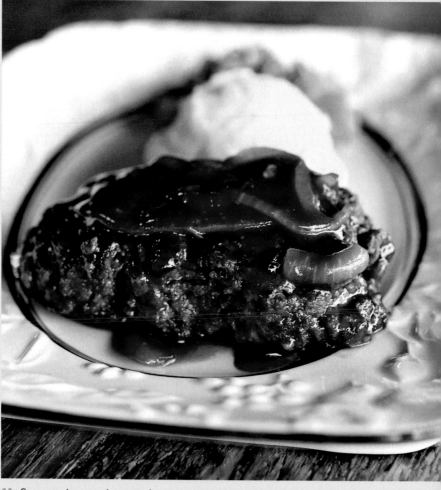

11. Serve to hungry humans!

Ⓜ MAKE AHEAD

Make the meat mixture and slice the onions up to 24 hours in advance.

Ⓥ VARIATIONS

Use ground turkey and chicken broth instead of beef and beef broth if you prefer.

Substitute ½ cup dry sherry for ½ cup of the broth in the gravy. Yum!

Add 6 ounces sliced white mushrooms to the skillet with the onions.

Ⓢ SERVE WITH

Stovetop Mashed Potatoes (page 310)

Peas and Carrots (page 293)

Quick Shells and Cheese (page 214)

Broccoli with Cheese Sauce (page 286)

Broccoli Cauliflower Casserole (page 152)

Roasted Carrots with Vinaigrette (page 300)

Lemony Green Beans (page 292)

CHICKEN CACCIATORE

MAKES 6 TO 8 SERVINGS

I am a lover of braised meats, whether it's pot roast or short ribs or beef brisket . . . or this beautiful stewed chicken dish. Just give me some meat, a pot with a lid, and some combination of liquid ingredients, and I'll be eating out of your hand . . . as long as your hand is holding braised meat.

That might have been the weirdest introductory sentence of any recipe I've ever written.

Chicken cacciatore generally involves browning chicken pieces in a pot over high heat, then sautéing a mix of vegetables—onions, peppers, mushrooms, tomatoes—in the same pot. Spices are added, followed by a little wine and broth, and the chicken and veggies are allowed to cook together in the oven long enough for magic to happen . . .

And magic does happen.

I use chicken thighs for this recipe because I happen to love chicken thighs. But you can use a cut-up whole chicken or a mix of your favorite pieces. Just be sure to leave the skin on or you'll regret it the rest of your life.

Not that I'm dramatic or anything.

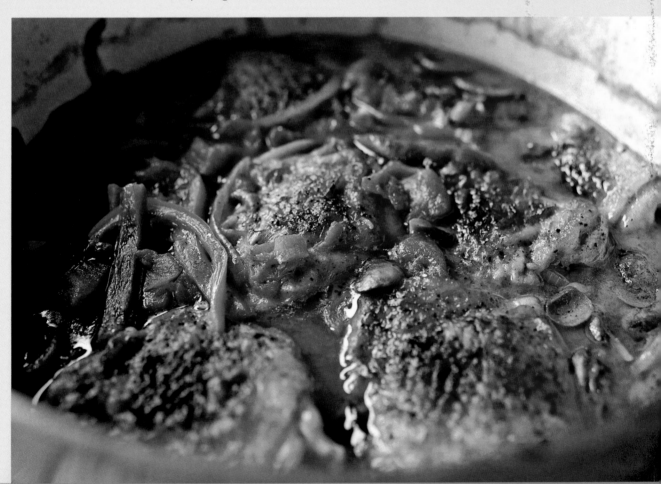

8 skin-on chicken thighs

½ teaspoon kosher salt, more to taste

½ teaspoon black pepper, more to taste

½ cup all-purpose flour

¼ cup olive oil

2 tablespoons butter

1 medium onion, halved and sliced

2 red bell peppers, seeded and thinly sliced

2 green bell peppers, seeded and thinly sliced

5 garlic cloves, minced

12 ounces white button or cremini mushrooms, sliced

½ teaspoon ground thyme

¼ teaspoon ground turmeric

½ teaspoon red pepper flakes

1 cup dry white wine or low-sodium chicken broth

One 28-ounce can diced tomatoes

1 pound wide egg noodles

Minced parsley, for sprinkling

Grated Parmesan cheese, for sprinkling

1. Preheat the oven to 350°F.

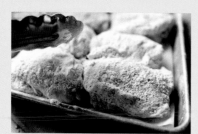

2. Sprinkle both sides of the chicken with salt and black pepper to taste and dredge it in the flour.

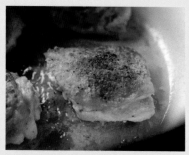

3. Heat the olive oil and butter in a heavy pot (with a lid) over medium-high heat. Working in batches, place the chicken skin side down in the pot. Brown the chicken on both sides, about 2 minutes total, and remove it to a clean plate. Repeat with the remaining chicken. Pour off half the fat from the pot and discard.

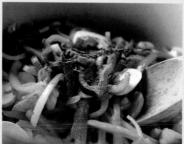

4. Add the onion, bell peppers, garlic, mushrooms, thyme, turmeric, red pepper flakes, and salt and black pepper to taste.

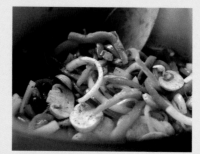

5. Stir and cook the mixture for a few minutes, until the veggies start to soften and turn golden. (The turmeric will also add some gorgeous golden color.)

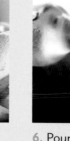

6. Pour in the wine (or broth) . . .

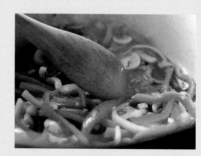

7. Then stir and let the liquid bubble up and reduce for a couple of minutes.

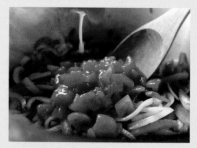

8. Pour in the tomatoes, juice and all . . .

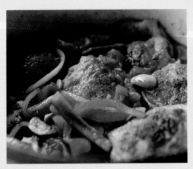

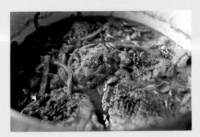

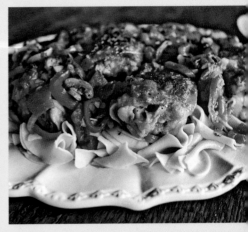

9. Then return the chicken to the pan skin side up, slightly submerging it in the liquid and spooning some of the veggies on top. Place the lid on the pot, put the pot in the oven, and braise the chicken for 45 minutes. Meanwhile, bring a pot of water to a boil and cook the noodles to al dente, then drain.

10. Remove the lid and increase the oven temperature to 375°F. Braise for 15 to 20 minutes more. Remove the chicken from the pot and place it on a plate. Remove the vegetables from the pot and place them on another plate. Set the pot on the stovetop and turn the heat to high. Cook to reduce the sauce for a couple of minutes. Taste and add more salt and pepper if it needs it.

11. Pile the noodles on a large platter, lay on the chicken and veggies, then ladle the sauce all over the top (you probably won't use all of it). Sprinkle on parsley and Parmesan.

M MAKE AHEAD

Cook up to 24 hours in advance. Refrigerate and reheat as described in the Variation below.

V VARIATION

If you have time, remove the chicken and vegetables from the pot after cooking and store them in the fridge separately from the liquid. After several hours, skim off any fat that has risen/solidified on top of the liquid, then return the chicken and veggies to the pan. Warm on the stovetop and serve.

S SERVE WITH

Buttered Parsley Noodles (page 324) instead of the egg noodles

Polenta (page 322) instead of noodles

The Bread (page 336)

Cheese Biscuits (page 332)

Refrigerator Rolls (page 334)

Big, beautiful green salad

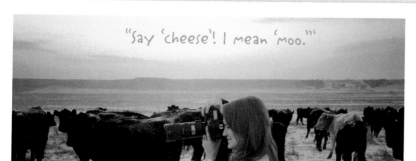

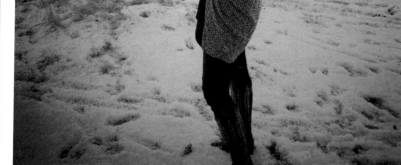

"Say 'cheese'! I mean 'moo.'"

TUNA NOODLE CASSEROLE

MAKES 8 TO 10 SERVINGS

Some people find tuna noodle casserole to be frightening.
That's because they've never had this one. Give it a try sometime soon!

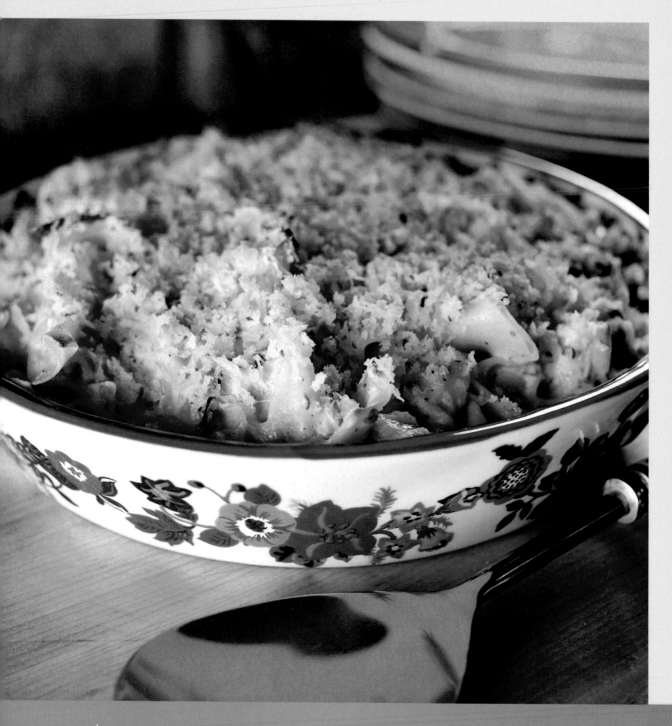

½ cup (1 stick) butter

1 medium onion, diced

6 ounces white button mushrooms, finely chopped

¼ cup all-purpose flour

3 cups whole milk

½ cup dry sherry, more to taste!

Kosher salt and black pepper to taste

Two 6.4-ounce packages white albacore tuna in water, drained

¼ cup finely chopped red bell pepper

2 tablespoons minced parsley

12 ounces wide egg noodles, cooked to al dente and drained

½ cup panko breadcrumbs

1. Preheat the oven to 400°F.

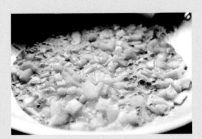

2. Melt 4 tablespoons (½ stick) of the butter in a large skillet over medium heat. Add the onion and cook until it starts to soften, 3 to 4 minutes.

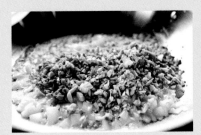

3. Add the mushrooms, stir them around, and cook them for a couple of minutes.

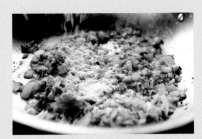

4. Sprinkle the flour evenly over the mixture . . .

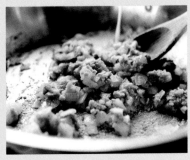

5. And stir so that the flour coats the onions and mushrooms thoroughly. Keep stirring around for another minute.

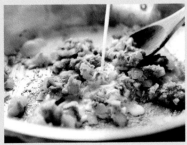

6. Add the milk . . .

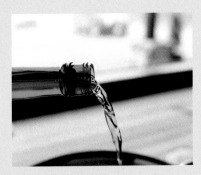

7. And the sherry . . .

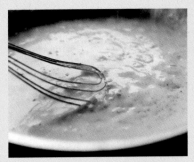

8. And whisk to combine. Cook the sauce until it's nice and thick, 3 to 4 minutes. Sprinkle in salt and black pepper to taste and stir. Adjust the seasonings to make sure the sauce is adequately salted.

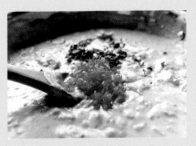

9. Add the tuna and stir it into the sauce . . .

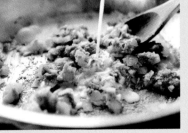

10. Then stir in the bell pepper and 1 tablespoon of the parsley.

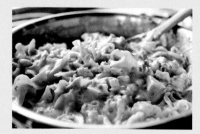

11. Next, stir in the noodles until they're all coated!

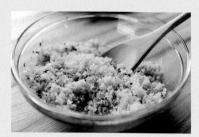

12. Transfer the mixture to a baking dish.

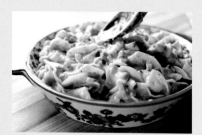

13. Finally, melt the remaining 4 tablespoons of butter in a bowl in the microwave. Stir it around with the breadcrumbs and the remaining 1 tablespoon parsley.

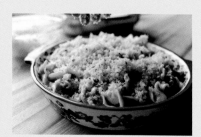

14. Top the casserole with the breadcrumbs . . .

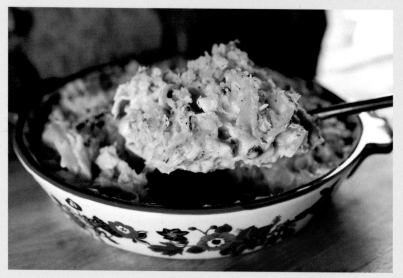

15. And bake it until golden, about 15 minutes. Serve it piping hot!

V VARIATIONS

Use any dry white wine instead of the sherry, or use vegetable or chicken broth.

Substitute low-sodium chicken broth for half or all of the milk for a less creamy sauce.

Add 1 cup frozen peas to the sauce with the red bell pepper and parsley.

Use cooked bite-size chicken chunks instead of tuna!

M MAKE AHEAD

Assemble the casserole and refrigerate it, unbaked, up to 24 hours before baking. Allow an extra 10 to 15 minutes of baking time if you put it in the oven cold.

S SERVE WITH

Green salad

Warm crusty bread

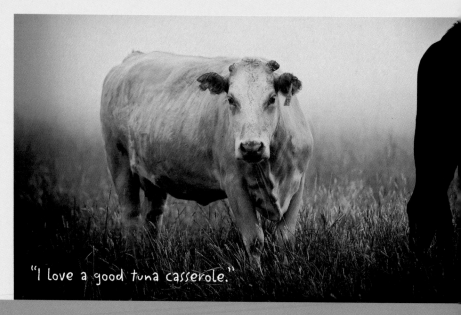

"I love a good tuna casserole."

BEEF STROGANOFF

MAKES 6 TO 8 SERVINGS

Oh, beef Stroganoff . . . how I love thee! This is one of the most classic American comfort foods there is. Never mind that the original Stroganoff came from Russia.

I have a point: Just because a dish doesn't have its origins in this great country of ours doesn't mean we can't occasionally whip up a mean version of the stuff.

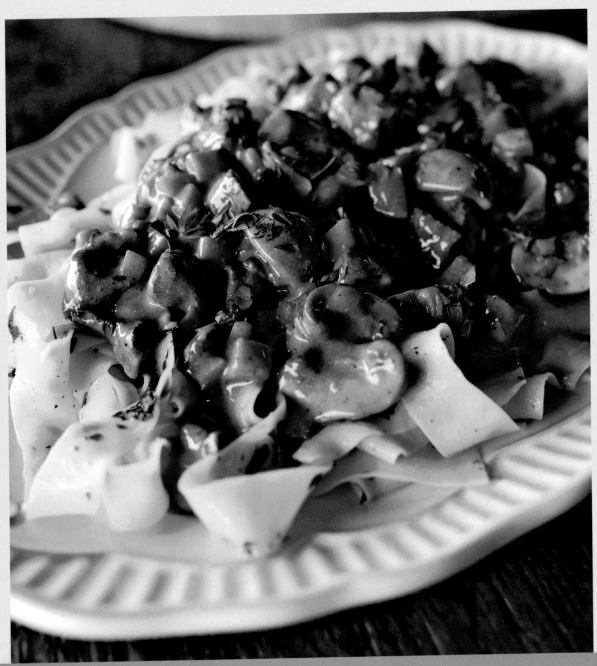

1 pound sirloin steak, cut into small cubes

Kosher salt and black pepper to taste

2 tablespoons olive oil

½ large onion, finely diced

2 carrots, finely diced

8 ounces cremini or white button mushrooms, stemmed and halved

½ cup brandy (or see the next page for alternatives!)

2¼ cups beef stock

2 tablespoons cornstarch

¼ cup sour cream, at room temperature

1 heaping teaspoon Dijon mustard

Buttered Parsley Noodles (page 324), for serving

Minced parsley, for sprinkling

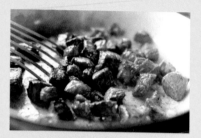

1. Season the steak with salt and pepper, then heat 1 tablespoon of the olive oil in a heavy skillet over medium-high heat. Add half the meat to the pan and brown it quickly, about 2 minutes. Remove the first batch to a bowl and cook the rest of the meat.

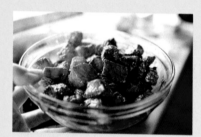

2. Remove and set all the meat aside.

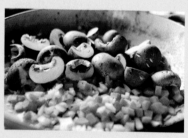

3. Add the remaining 1 table-spoon olive oil to the pan and add the onion, carrots, and mushrooms . . .

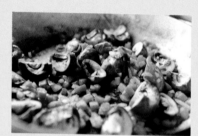

4. And cook until the mixture is deep golden brown, about 5 minutes.

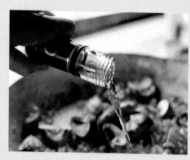

5. Turn off the heat and add the brandy . . .

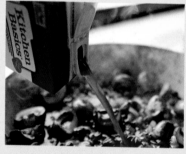

6. And 2 cups of the stock. Stir, scrape the bottom of the pan, and turn the heat to medium-high.

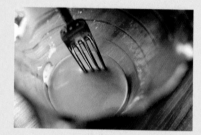

7. Cook to reduce the liquid by about a third, 3 to 4 minutes.

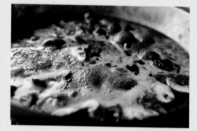

8. In a small pitcher, make a slurry by mixing the remaining ¼ cup stock and the cornstarch with a fork.

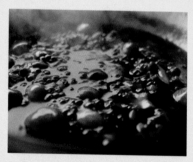

9. Pour the slurry into the skillet and cook until the sauce thickens, 1 to 2 minutes.

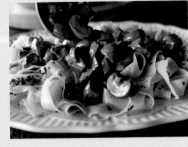

10. Turn off the heat. Stir in the sour cream and Dijon . . .

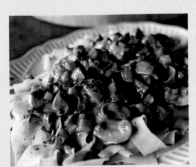

11. Then throw in the beef and stir until the mixture is nice and piping hot. Taste and adjust the seasonings! Yum.

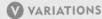

12. Pile the noodles on a platter and spoon the contents of the skillet on top.

13. Sprinkle with parsley at the end. Delicious!

M MAKE AHEAD

Cut up the meat and prepare the vegetables up to 24 hours in advance. Store in separate containers in the fridge until cooking time.

V VARIATIONS

Use cognac, whiskey, or wine in place of the brandy.

Omit the alcohol and just up the amount of stock if preferred.

Use a mix of wild mushrooms instead of creminis or white buttons.

Serve over rice or polenta instead of noodles.

S SERVE WITH

Refrigerator Rolls (page 334)

Cheese Biscuits (page 332)

Roasted Asparagus (page 280)

Lemony Green Beans (page 292)

Roasted Carrots with Vinaigrette (page 300)

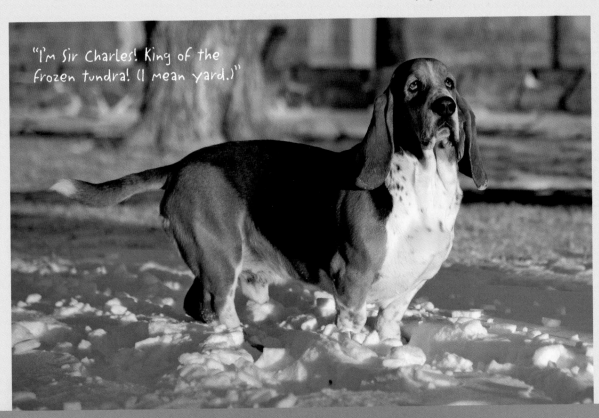

"I'm Sir Charles! King of the frozen tundra! (I mean yard.)"

CLASSIC PULLED PORK

MAKES 12 TO 16 SERVINGS

There are so many different ways to make pulled pork, but you can't beat the good ol' basic barbecue version that's messy and glorious and positively dripping with sauce and should therefore never be eaten on a first date.

Second date? Totally fine. But first date? You just might scare him/her away!

Keep in mind that this pulled pork, while simple, takes a pretty long time to make from start to finish. So just remember to plan ahead!

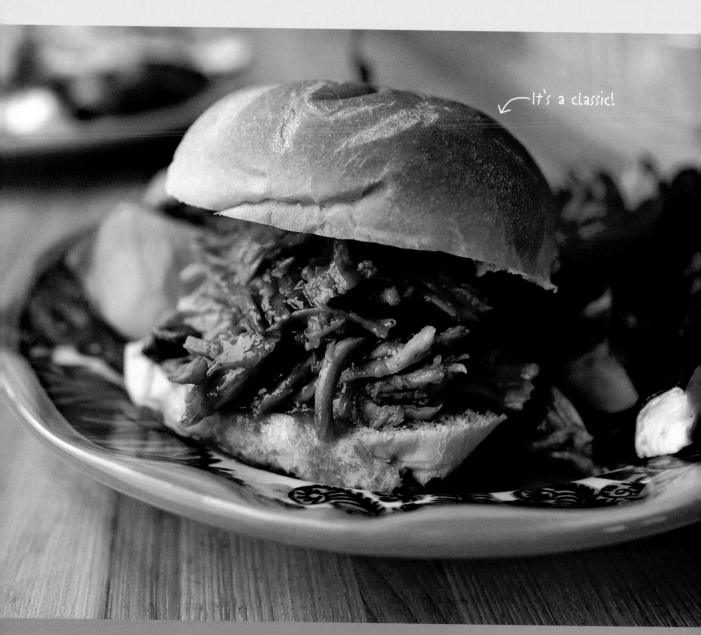

It's a classic!

¼ cup packed brown sugar

1 tablespoon chili powder

1 tablespoon paprika

2 teaspoons garlic powder

2 teaspoons kosher salt

1 teaspoon black pepper

1 teaspoon cayenne pepper

One 7- to 8-pound pork shoulder roast (also called pork butt)

4 onions, quartered

4 cups good-quality barbecue sauce

Good-quality hamburger buns, for serving

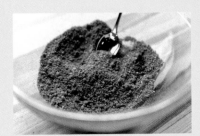

1. In a medium bowl, stir together the brown sugar, chili powder, paprika, garlic powder, salt, black pepper, and cayenne.

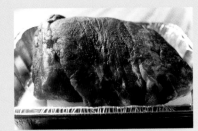

5. Place the quartered onions in the bottom of a large roasting pan (I like to use a disposable foil roasting pan) and place the pork roast right on top.

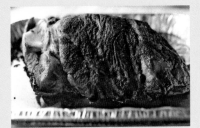

7. And roast until the pork is fork-tender and falling apart, about 7 hours. (Test this by inserting two forks into the pork and pulling them apart; if the meat pulls apart easily, it's done! If you meet with much resistance, cover it and pop it back in the oven for 30 to 45 minutes, then test again. Keep going until it's falling apart.)

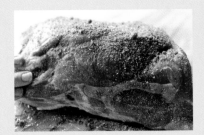

2. Use your hands to rub the mixture all over the pork shoulder . . .

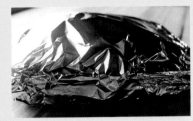

6. Completely cover the pan with heavy foil, put it in the oven . . .

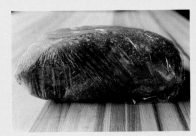

3. Then wrap the pork in plastic wrap and refrigerate for several hours . . . preferably overnight!

4. Preheat the oven to 300°F.

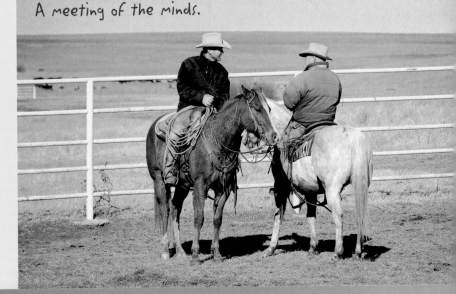

A meeting of the minds.

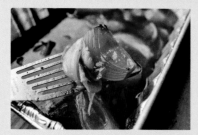

8. Remove the pork from the pan and set it aside on a cutting board or baking sheet. Remove the onions from the pan and set them aside.

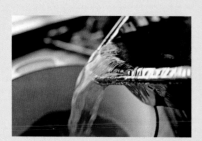

9. Pour 1½ cups of the cooking liquid from the pan into a medium saucepan. Discard the rest of the liquid.

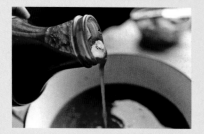

10. Pour in the barbecue sauce . . .

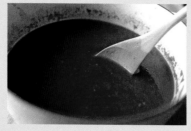

11. And cook the sauce over medium heat for 20 minutes, allowing it to bubble gently, until it thickens slightly.

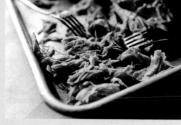

12. Shred the meat with two forks, then put all the meat back into the roasting pan. (Note: You can shred the cooked onions right along with the meat and have them be all mixed in, or you can save the onions to put on top of the meat in a sandwich.)

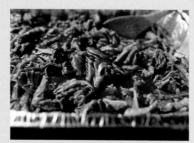

13. Pour the delicious sauce all over the shredded pork, making sure it's all coated. Cover and refrigerate for up to 3 days if you're making it for later, or serve right away. You may also let it cool, then freeze it for up to 6 months!

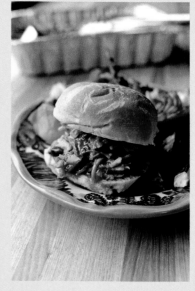

14. Pile the meat on the buns (with the onions, if you've reserved them), making sure you get plenty of sauce on there.

The messier the better!

V VARIATIONS

Up the amount of cayenne to 1 tablespoon for spicier pulled pork.

Add chunks of bell pepper (any color) to the roasting pan with the onions.

S SERVE WITH

Sweet Potato Fries (page 308)

Thin Fries (page 318)

Breakfast Potatoes (page 312)

Colorful Coleslaw (page 294)

S SERVE BUNLESS ON A PLATE WITH

Stovetop Mashed Potatoes (page 310)

Quick Shells and Cheese (page 214)

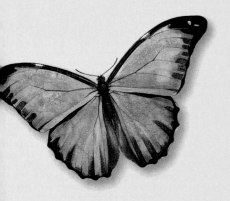

FRENCH DIP SANDWICHES

MAKES 8 TO 10 SANDWICHES

Very few things are more comforting to me than a deliciously drippy French dip sandwich. Fantastically flavorful beef . . . golden toasted rolls . . . dark, beautiful onions . . . and the most delectably savory liquid to dip it in.

Man. That was one delicious daydream just then.

Here's how you can make one in real life.

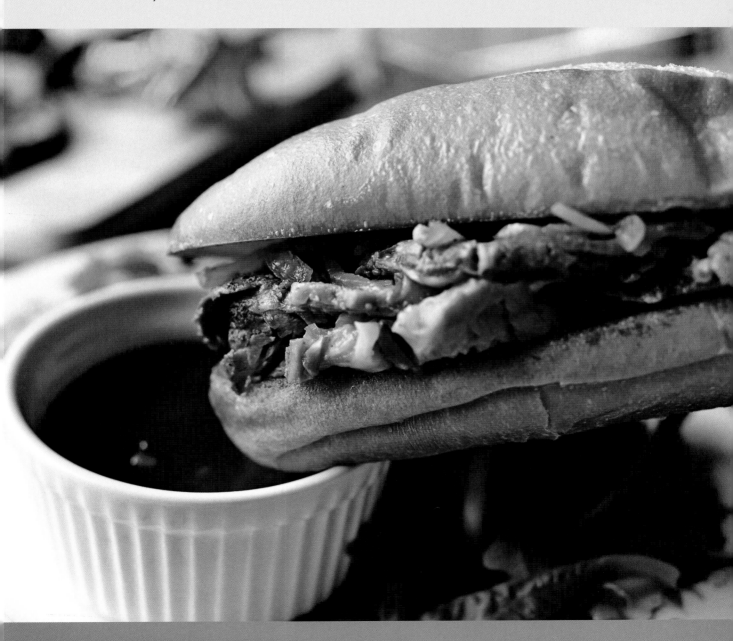

1 tablespoon kosher salt

2 tablespoons black pepper

½ teaspoon ground oregano

½ teaspoon dried thyme

One 4- to 5-pound boneless beef rib loin, tied

2 large onions, halved and thinly sliced

5 garlic cloves, minced

One 2-ounce packet French onion soup mix

One 10.5-ounce can beef consommé

1 cup beef broth

¼ cup dry sherry (or you may use beef broth)

2 tablespoons Worcestershire sauce

1 tablespoon soy sauce

8 to 10 crusty sub rolls, toasted

1. Preheat the oven to 475°F.

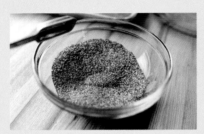

2. In a small bowl. mix together the salt, pepper, oregano, and thyme.

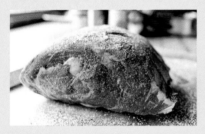

3. Sprinkle the seasoning mix liberally over the beef loin, using your hands to rub it all over the surface.

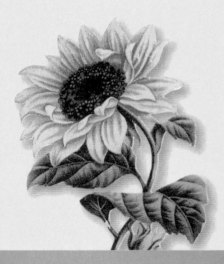

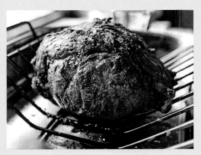

4. Place the meat on a roasting rack in a roasting pan and roast it to medium-rare, about 20 to 25 minutes, until it registers 125°F on a meat thermometer. If you prefer it not as pink, roast it longer.

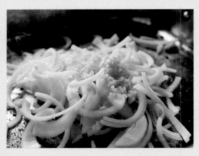

5. Set the meat aside on a cutting board and cover it with foil to keep warm. Place the roasting pan on the stovetop burner over medium-high heat. Add the onions and garlic . . .

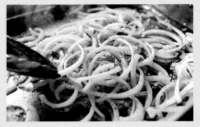

6. And stir them around for 5 minutes, until they get soft and golden.

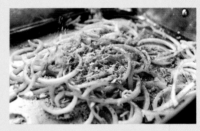

7. Sprinkle in the soup mix . . .

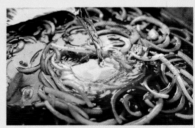

8. Then pour in the consommé, broth, sherry, Worcestershire, soy sauce, and 1 cup water. Bring the mixture to a boil, then turn the heat to low and simmer for 45 minutes, until the flavors are deep and rich.

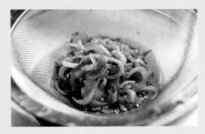

9. Pour through a fine-mesh strainer and reserve both the liquid (*jus*) and the onions for the sandwiches!

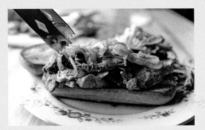

11. Pile beef and onions on each of the bottom halves of the rolls . . .

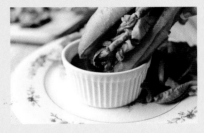

12. And serve the sandwiches with dishes of piping-hot *jus*!

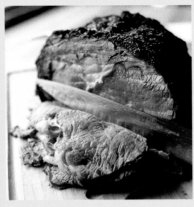

10. Slice the beef very thin with a sharp knife.

ⓥ VARIATIONS

Add 10 ounces sliced white mushrooms to the roasting pan with the onions.

Add 2 sliced bell peppers (any color) to the roasting pan with the onions.

After rubbing the seasoning on the beef, wrap it tightly in plastic wrap and refrigerate overnight to really drive the flavor home.

ⓢ SERVE WITH

Colorful Coleslaw (page 294)

Thin Fries (page 318)

Sweet Potato Fries (page 308)

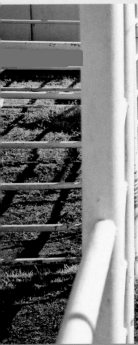
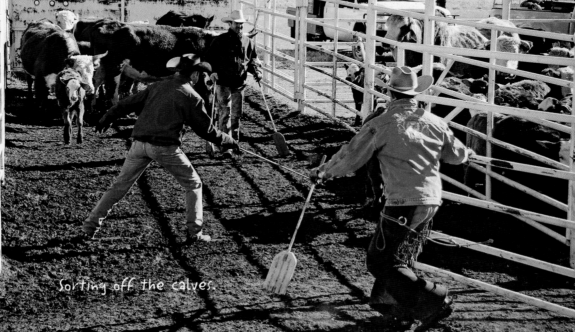

Sorting off the calves.

OVEN-BARBECUED CHICKEN

MAKES 8 TO 12 SERVINGS

This miraculous barbecued chicken is made right in the comfort of your own kitchen. Because you know what? Even though barbecued chicken is delicious when it's made on the grill, that doesn't mean that everyone:

1. Has a grill
2. Is able to grill
3. Wants to grill
4. Believes in grilling
5. Finds joy in grilling
6. Finds fulfillment in sweating, coughing, and singed arm hair.

Friends, I'm here to tell you: This chicken is so darn divine.

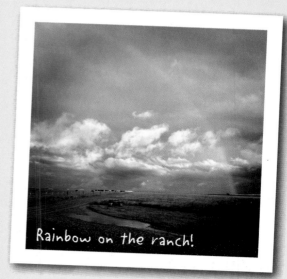

Rainbow on the ranch!

3 cups your favorite barbecue sauce

½ cup peach preserves

1 garlic clove

Olive oil, for drizzling

12 bone-in, skin-on chicken thighs

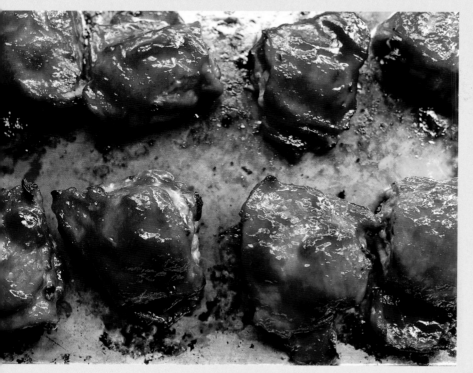

 MAKE AHEAD

Make the sauce ahead of time and store it in the fridge for up to 48 hours. Brush it on the chicken cold.

 VARIATIONS

Use a whole cut-up chicken or chicken legs instead of thighs.

Use apricot, grape, or apple jelly instead of peach.

Add a generous splash of whiskey to the sauce before you heat it up.

 SERVE WITH

Lemony Green Beans (page 292)

Quick Shells and Cheese (page 214)

Stovetop Mashed Potatoes (page 310)

"Slice-Baked" Potatoes (page 314)

Colorful Coleslaw (page 294)

1. Preheat the oven to 400°F.

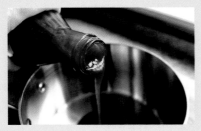

2. Whip up the super-simple sauce: Pour the barbecue sauce into a medium saucepan . . .

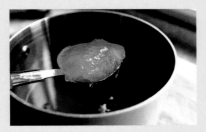

3. Then add the peach preserves . . .

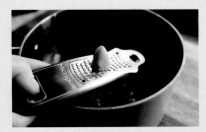

4. And mince or grate in the garlic.

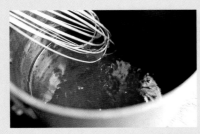

5. Stir the mixture together, then heat it over medium heat until piping hot. Remove it from the heat and set it aside.

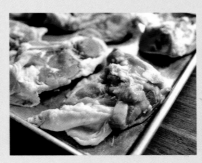

6. Drizzle a large baking sheet (or two) with olive oil and lay out the chicken thighs, skin side down.

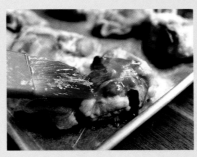

7. Roast the thighs for 25 minutes to start, then pull the pan from the oven and brush the sauce all over the surface of the thighs.

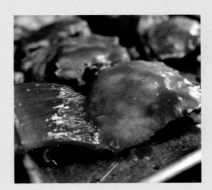

8. Use a spatula to flip the thighs over to the other side, taking care not to tear the skin. Brush the tops with more sauce and roast the thighs for 7 to 8 minutes.

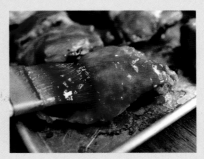

9. Remove the pan from the oven, brush on more sauce, and roast for 7 to 8 minutes more.

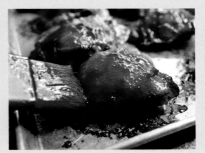

10. Finally, remove the pan from the oven, brush on more sauce, and turn the heat up to 425°F.

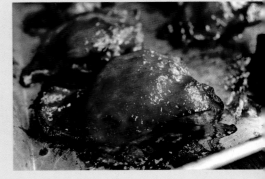

11. Roast for 5 to 7 minutes, or until the thighs are cooked through and the sauce is starting to brown and even blacken a bit around the edges. Remove them from the oven and let them sit for at least 10 minutes before serving. Delicious!

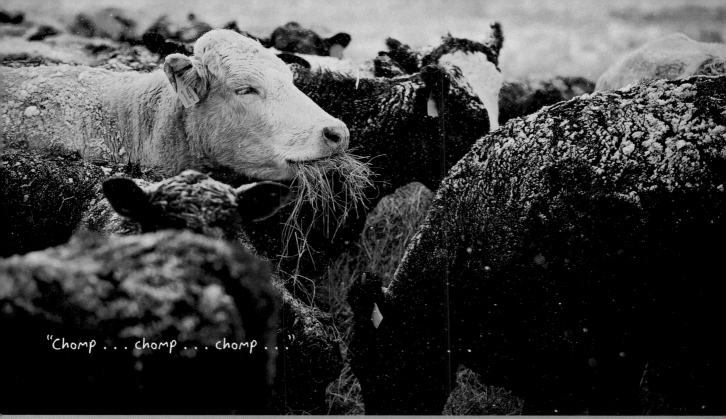

"Chomp . . . chomp . . . chomp . . ."

I LOVE WATCHING COWS EAT HAY IN THE WINTER.

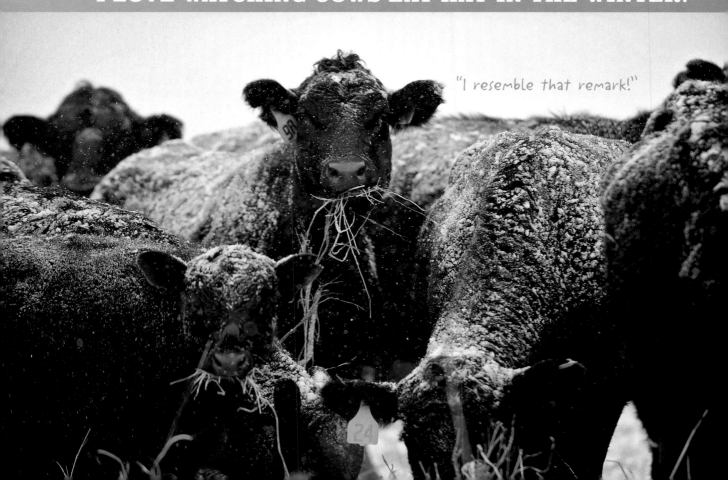

"I resemble that remark!"

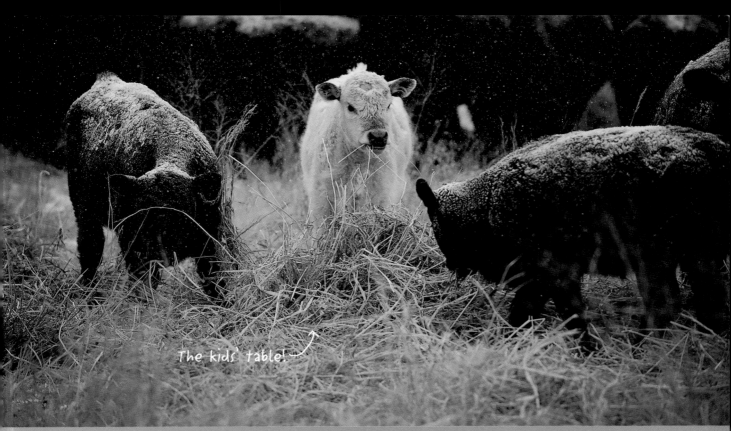

The kids' table! →

THEY AREN'T EXACTLY KNOWN FOR THEIR MANNERS.

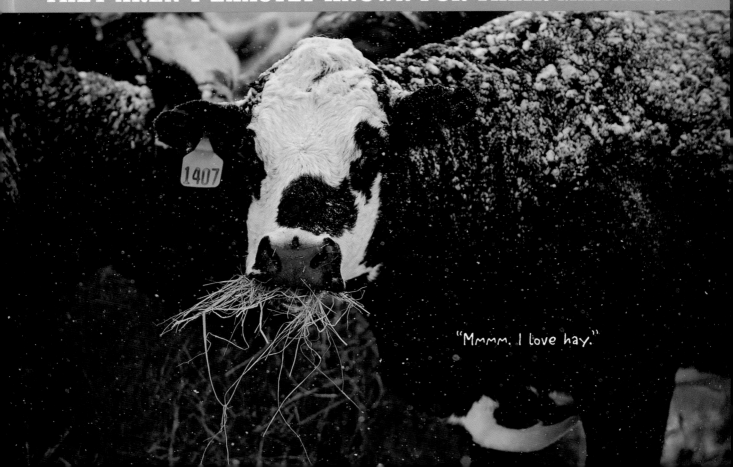

1407

"Mmmm. I love hay."

RED WINE POT ROAST

MAKES 12 SERVINGS

I cracked the pot roast code years and years ago, and I'm so very, very glad I did. Once you master the (very simple but initially elusive) steps to the perfect pot roast, a whole world of comfort and goodness opens up. I have a standby pot roast that has never left my side since I first started making it, and this is its crazy, full-of-life, drunk-on-red-wine first cousin. (A first cousin who brings along a jar of orange marmalade and a bag of root vegetables whenever he visits, by the way. You'll see what I mean here in a second.)

This is a tremendously rich and delightful pot roast, and you'll make it again and again.

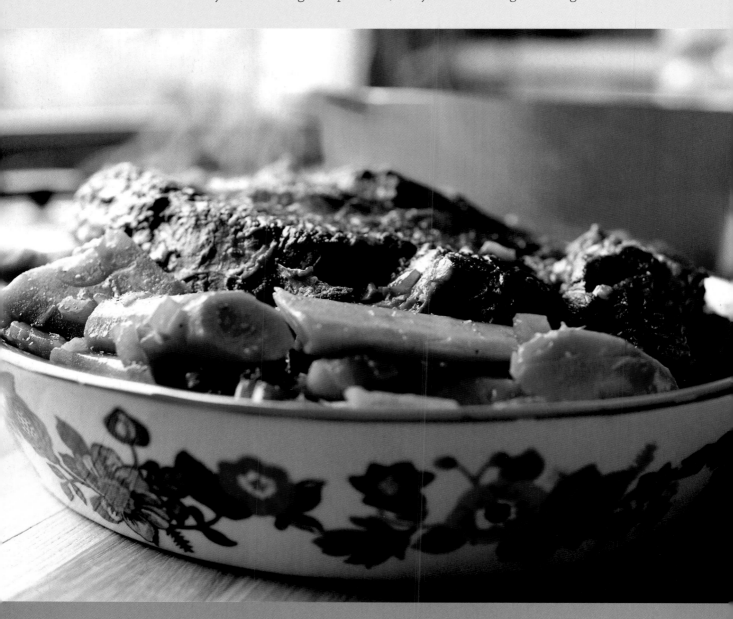

3 tablespoons olive oil

Kosher salt and black pepper to taste

One 4- to 5-pound beef chuck roast

2 onions, diced

3 celery stalks, diced

3 garlic cloves, minced

2 tablespoons tomato paste

2 cups red wine (optional, you can use more beef broth instead)

2 cups beef broth

¼ cup sweet orange marmalade

4 carrots, scrubbed and cut on the diagonal into 1-inch chunks

4 parsnips, peeled and cut on the diagonal into 1-inch chunks

5 large red potatoes, quartered

3 thyme sprigs

3 rosemary sprigs

1. Preheat the oven to 275°F.

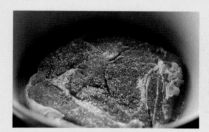

2. Heat the olive oil in a heavy, ovenproof pot (with a lid) over high heat. Salt and pepper both sides of the roast and sear it for about a minute on one side . . .

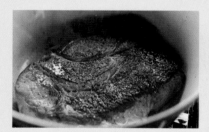

3. And a minute on the other side.

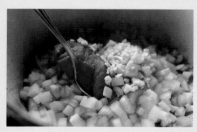

4. Remove the meat to a plate, reduce the heat to medium-high, and add the onions, celery, garlic, and tomato paste.

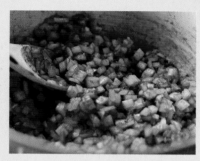

5. Stir it around and cook for 2 to 3 minutes, until the vegetables start to soften and the tomato paste releases its flavor.

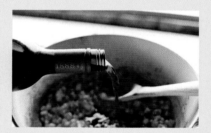

6. Pour in the glorious wine . . .

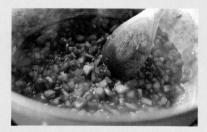

7. Then stir and scrape the pot to get up all the browned bits on the bottom.

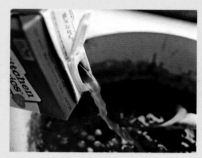

8. Pour in the broth . . .

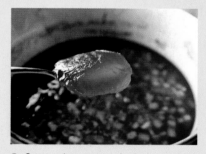

9. Stir in the marmalade . . .

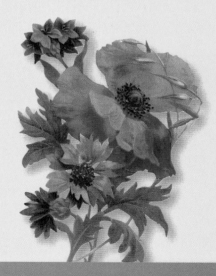

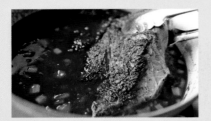

10. Return the meat to the pot . . .

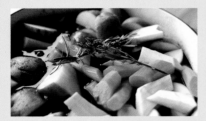

11. And top it all off with the carrots, parsnips, potatoes, thyme, and rosemary. Push the veggies and herbs into the liquid, then put the lid on the pot and roast for 3 to 4 hours, or until the meat is fork-tender. (For a 3-pound roast, plan on 3 hours.)

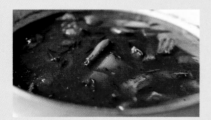

12. Mmm. The liquid becomes something magical!

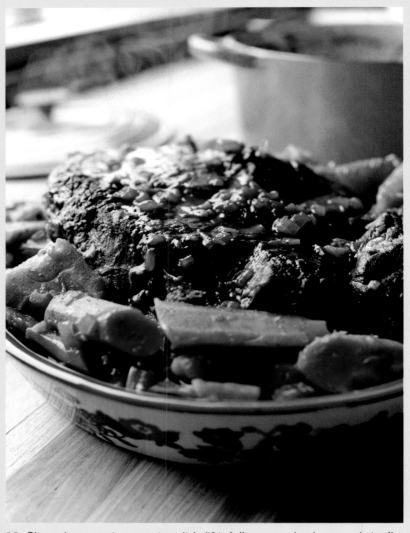

13. Place the roast in a serving dish (if it falls apart, that's a good sign!) and place the vegetables all around it . . . then spoon on as much sauce from the pot as you'd like.

Total, unmistakable comfort food.

Ⅴ VARIATIONS

Increase or decrease the ratio of wine to broth according to your taste.

If you have time, remove the roast and vegetables from the pot after cooking and store them in the fridge separately from the liquid. After several hours, skim off any fat that has solidified on top of the liquid, then return the meat and veggies to the pan. Warm up the roast on the stovetop and serve.

Add 8 ounces halved white button or cremini mushrooms to the pot along with the carrots, parsnips, and potatoes.

Ⓢ SERVE WITH

Lemony Green Beans (page 292)

The Bread (page 336)

Cheese Biscuits (page 332)

Refrigerator Rolls (page 334)

CHICKEN ENCHILADAS

MAKES 8 TO 12 SERVINGS

This is one of those dinners that causes me to sit and stew for hours over what the heck to call it. My title choices were:

Chicken and Green Chile Enchiladas

Green Chile and Chicken Enchiladas

Enchiladas with Chicken and Green Chile

Enchiladas with Green Chile and Chicken

Green Enchiladas (grody!)

Chicken Enchiladas with Caramelized Onions, Green Chiles, and Other Stuff

So I did what I normally do when I feel myself overwhelmed with elaborate recipe title options: I stripped it down to its bare bones and called it Chicken Enchiladas.

I have an unbearable lightness of being all of a sudden. I love it when that happens.

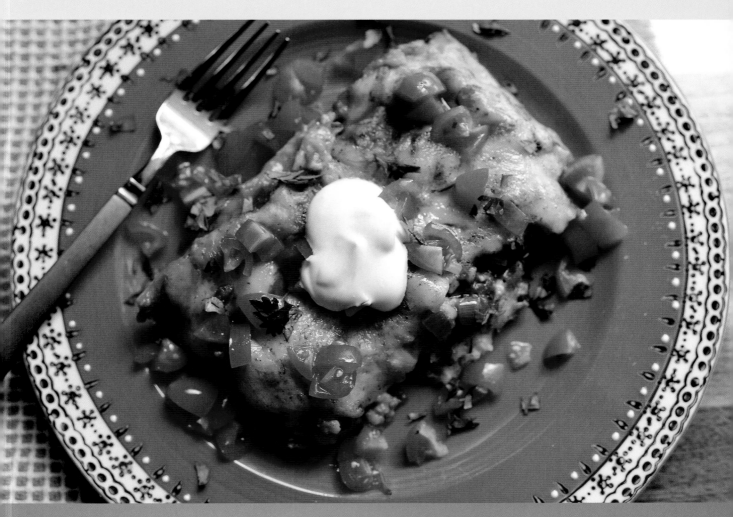

1 teaspoon ground cumin

1 teaspoon chili powder, plus more for sprinkling

½ teaspoon kosher salt

3 boneless, skinless chicken breasts (use 2 if they're very large)

¼ cup vegetable oil

2 onions, diced

Three 15-ounce cans green enchilada sauce

16 corn tortillas

3 cups grated Cheddar-Jack cheese, more as needed

Sour cream, for serving

Diced tomatoes, for serving

Chopped cilantro, for serving

1. Preheat the oven to 350°F.

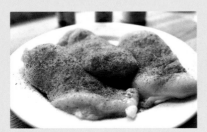

2. Mix together the cumin, chili powder, and salt and sprinkle the mixture on both sides of the chicken.

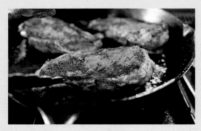

3. Heat the oil in a heavy skillet over medium heat and cook the chicken on both sides until done in the middle, 4 to 5 minutes per side. Remove the chicken to a plate to cool slightly.

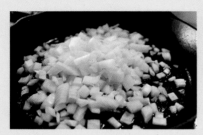

4. Without cleaning the skillet, throw in the onions . . .

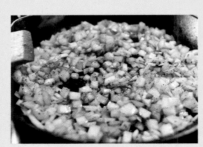

5. Then stir them around and let them cook for 4 to 5 minutes, or until deep golden brown (but be careful not to burn them).

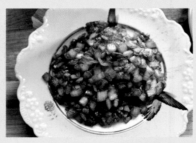

6. Remove the onions to a plate and set aside.

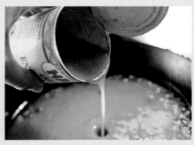

7. Reduce the heat to low and pour the enchilada sauce into the skillet.

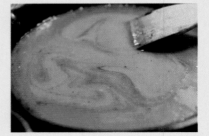

8. Stir it around and let it heat while absorbing all that wonderful chicken and onion flavor!

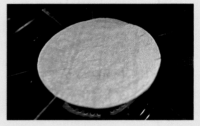

9. Meantime, use tongs to place the tortillas over your stovetop burner (or you can heat them in a small skillet over medium-high heat). Let them brown just slightly, about 30 seconds per side . . .

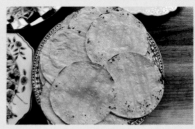

10. Then remove them to a plate and set them aside.

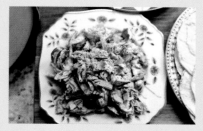

11. Use two forks to shred the chicken completely. Now everything's ready!

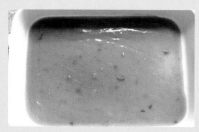

12. Pour 2 cups of the sauce into a 9 x 13-inch casserole dish.

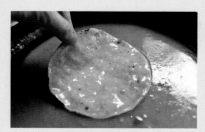

13. Quickly dip a tortilla into the sauce . . .

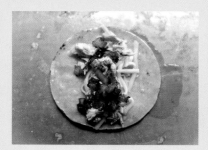

14. Lay it on a baking sheet or plate, and add some shredded chicken, grated cheese, and browned onion.

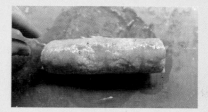

15. Roll it up tightly . . .

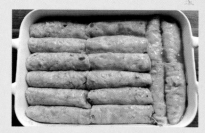

16. Then place it seam side down in the pan! Repeat with the rest of the tortillas and fillings.

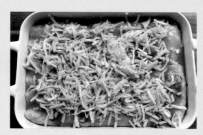

17. Pour on the remaining sauce and top with the remaining cheese (you should have about a cup left) and a light sprinkling of chili powder . . .

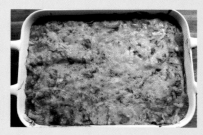

18. Then bake for 30 minutes, until hot and bubbly. Remove it from the oven and let it sit for 10 to 15 minutes to slightly firm up before serving.

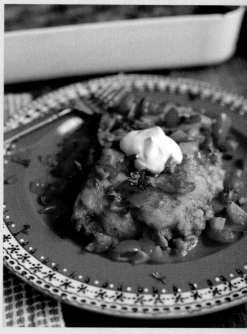

19. Serve with sour cream, diced tomatoes, and cilantro.

Ⓜ MAKE AHEAD

Assemble the casserole and store in the fridge, unbaked, for up to 24 hours. Bake as directed, adding up to 10 minutes more baking time since it will be cold.

Ⓥ VARIATIONS

Use tortillas made from a combination of corn and wheat flour; they hold together nicely!

Use pepper Jack cheese for a slightly different flavor and a little spice.

Use red enchilada sauce instead of green.

Use chopped Beautiful Roasted Vegetables (page 290) instead of chicken for a veggie version.

Use Ready-to-Go Beef Taco Filling (page 124) instead of the chicken for beef enchiladas.

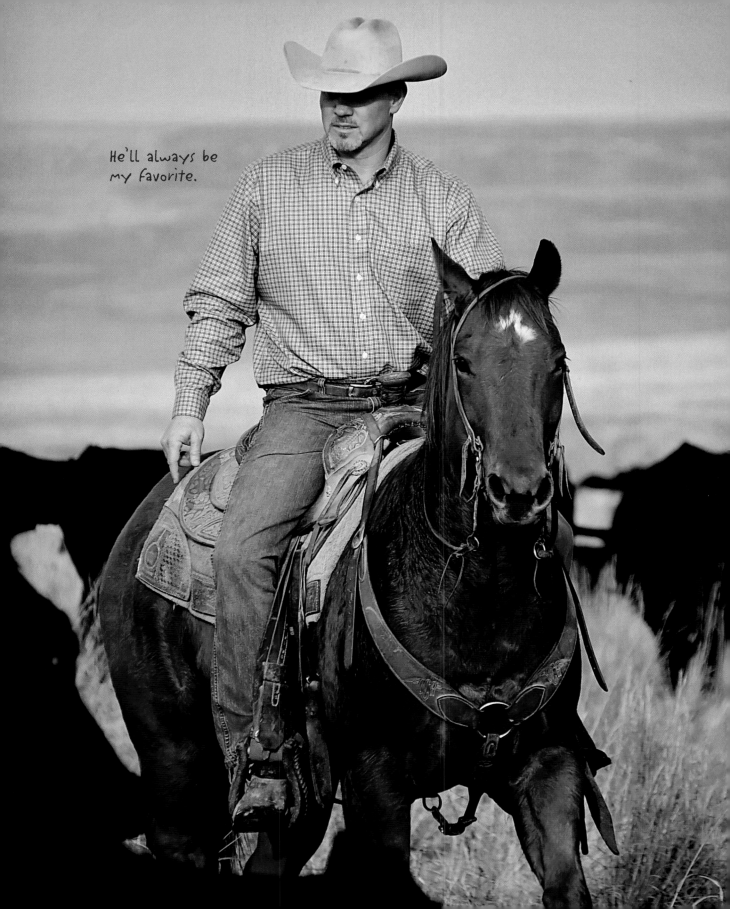

He'll always be
my favorite.

NEW FAVORITES

This is a collection of particularly tasty recipes that aren't necessarily new to Planet Earth but are relatively new favorites of *my* crew. And I don't know about you, but after cooking for a husband and kids for eighteen years, being able to add new recipes to the "Yes" column always represents a major victory for me. In other words, I need to get out more.

PORK CHOPS WITH WINE AND ROASTED GARLIC

MAKES 4 SERVINGS

Pan sauces are everything. Once you figure out the sheer beauty of searing meat in a skillet, then removing it and using the drippings in the pan to make a scrumptious sauce of some sort . . . well, the possibilities are endless.

This pork chop dinner is so divine. Roasted garlic combines with red wine to make the most delectable dish. Perfect for a first date!

(As long as you're not a vampire.)

20 garlic cloves

4 tablespoons olive oil

Kosher salt and black pepper to taste

4 boneless pork chops (medium- to thin-cut)

2 tablespoons butter

1½ cups red wine

1 bay leaf

½ cup beef broth, more as needed

1 tablespoon balsamic vinegar

Chopped chives, for garnish

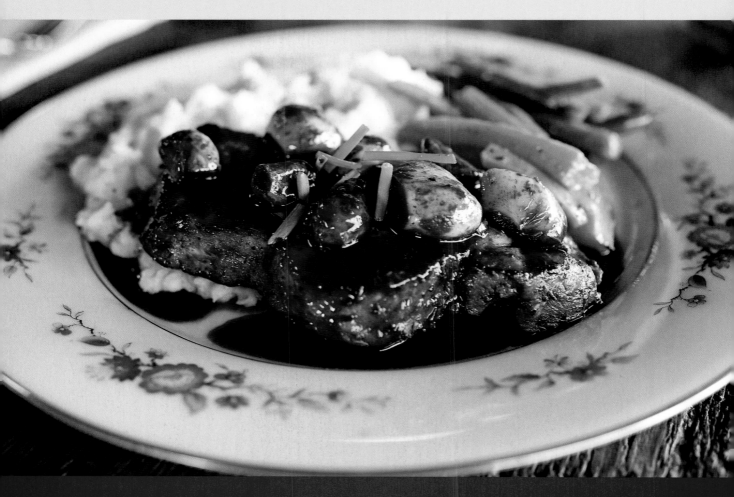

1. Preheat the oven to 350°F.

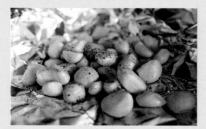

2. Place the garlic cloves on a large sheet of foil. Drizzle in 2 tablespoons of the olive oil, sprinkle with salt and pepper, and fold the edges together to seal.

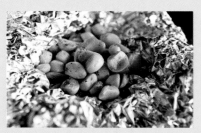

3. Roast the garlic for 1 hour, or until golden and slightly soft but not falling apart. Set aside. (This can be done well in advance!)

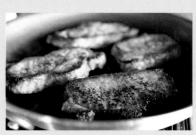

4. Sprinkle the pork chops on both sides with salt and pepper. Heat the remaining 2 tablespoons olive oil and 1 tablespoon of the butter in a large skillet over medium-high heat. Add the pork chops and cook them for a couple of minutes on each side (no need to cook them through at this point; just get great color on the outside).

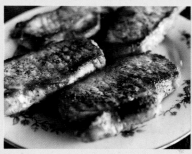

5. Remove the chops to a plate and set them aside.

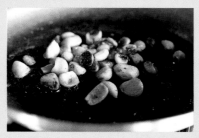

6. Throw the roasted garlic cloves into the same skillet. Stir them around and cook them for a minute or so . . .

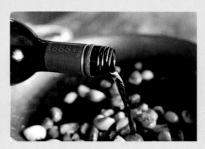

7. Then pour in the wine.

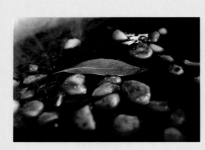

8. Add the bay leaf.

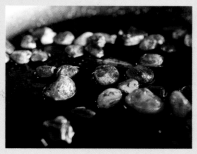

9. And stir, scraping the pan. Cook the mixture for 5 to 7 minutes, or until it has reduced by about two-thirds (raise the heat if necessary).

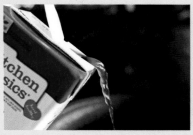

10. Stir in the beef broth and let the liquid come to a bubble . . .

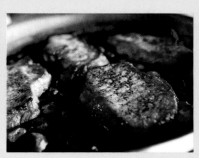

11. Then remove the bay leaf and arrange the chops in the pan so that they're swimming in the sauce. Shake the pan a bit and let the liquid bubble up and reduce while the chops finish cooking through, 3 to 4 minutes.

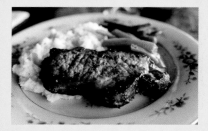

12. Place the chops on serving plates.

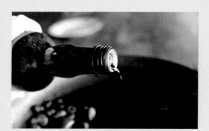

13. Meanwhile, back at the skillet, splash in the balsamic and stir the sauce . . .

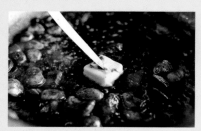

14. Then turn off the heat and swirl in the remaining 1 tablespoon butter.

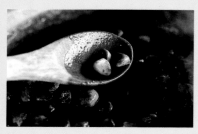

15. Taste and adjust the salt and pepper. Done!

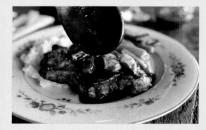

16. Spoon the sauce (including plenty of garlic cloves!) over the chops . . .

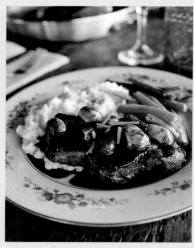

17. And add a few chopped chives on top to make it extra purty.

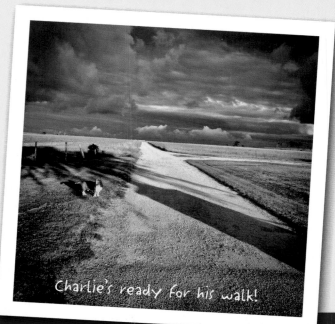

Charlie's ready for his walk!

M MAKE AHEAD

Roast the garlic up to 2 days ahead of time and store in the fridge.

V VARIATIONS

Add 8 ounces halved white mushrooms to the skillet when you add the roasted garlic.

Add 3 tablespoons drained capers to the sauce at the very end.

Use dry white wine instead of red wine for a totally different color and flavor.

Use Marsala wine instead of red or white.

If you prefer a nonalcoholic version, substitute a deep, rich beef stock for the red wine.

S SERVE WITH

Stovetop Mashed Potatoes (page 310)

Lemony Green Beans (page 292)

Roasted Carrots with Vinaigrette (page 300)

Buttered Parsley Noodles (page 324)

Risotto (page 327)

Polenta (page 322)

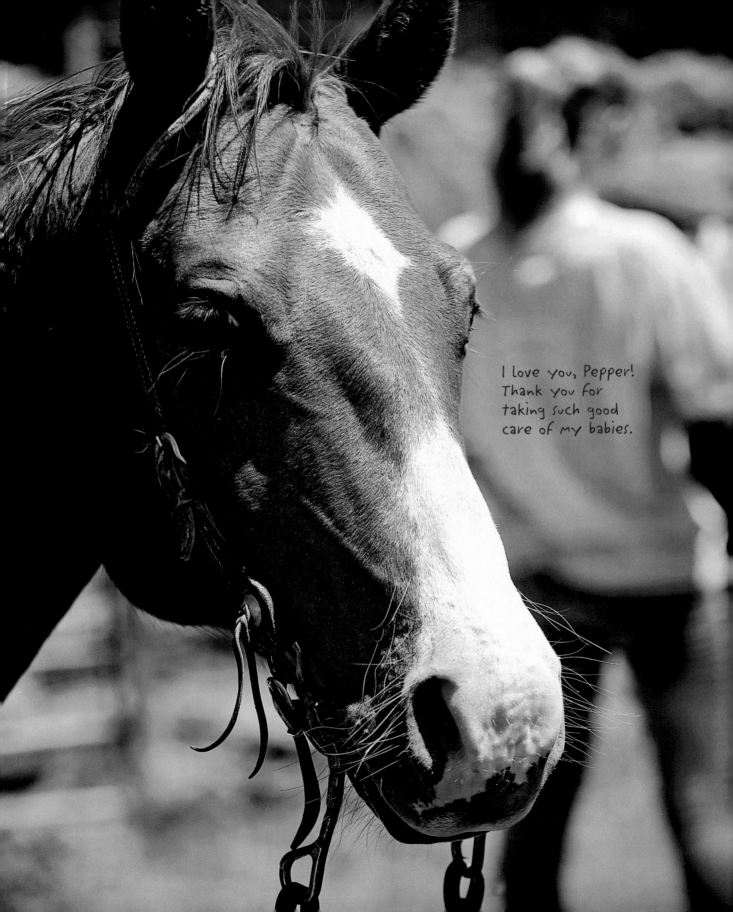

I love you, Pepper!
Thank you for
taking such good
care of my babies.

POLLO ASADO

MAKES 8 SERVINGS

There was an insanely authentic and delicious Mexican food dive in the general vicinity of my college campus. It was basically a hut with a drive-through window—I'm not even sure it had a seating area inside—and it was the perfect fare for my fellow dormmates and me: high on fat and flavor, incredibly cheap, open all night. The two or three people who worked there were friendly and upbeat and made the most incredible quesadillas I've ever eaten—ones I've never been able to duplicate to this day. What was that mysterious cheese? I think it was all a dream. They also sold carne asada and pollo asado tacos and burritos. I didn't eat them because I was a vegetarian in college for reasons I still don't understand. But then again, I still don't understand acid wash. Or neon scrunchies. Or Sun-In.

Pollo asado is marinated Mexican (or Cuban, depending on your perspective) grilled chicken, seasoned in any number of ways. I take a basic citrus approach, but you can add any other ingredients or spices you'd like. But the magic, to me, is not only the flavorful chicken itself, but what you do with it after it's cooked: serve the pieces whole, with warm tortillas and pico de gallo . . . and whatever other scrumptious sides you can manage.

The marinating takes a little time, but just knock it out in the morning, then all you have to do is grill it when it's time for dinner!

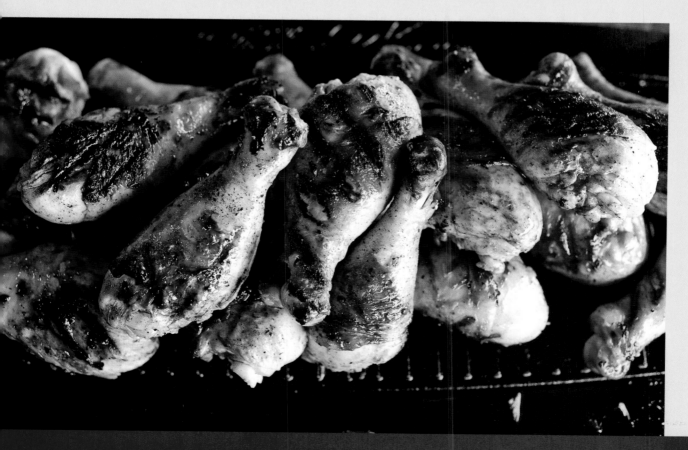

MARINADE

½ cup olive oil

3 large oranges

2 limes

2 lemons

4 garlic cloves, peeled and smashed

1 tablespoon kosher salt

1 teaspoon black pepper

CHICKEN AND FIXINS

16 chicken legs

2 large onions, quartered

Flour or corn tortillas, warmed, for serving

Pico de gallo (see page 23), for serving

Guacamole, for serving

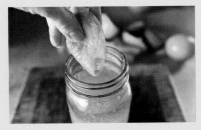

1. To make the marinade, pour the olive oil into a jar. Halve the oranges, limes, and lemons and squeeze in their juice. (Save the squeezed fruit.)

"Yum! Chicken!"

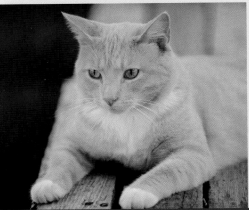

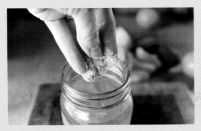

2. Add the garlic, salt, and pepper, then place the lid on the jar and shake it until everything is combined.

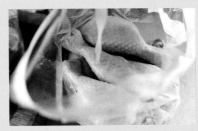

3. Divide the chicken between two large plastic bags and divide the marinade between them.

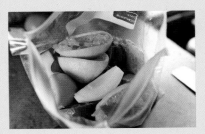

4. Evenly distribute the juiced fruit halves and onions between the two bags.

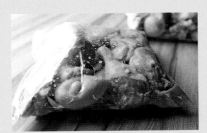

5. Seal the bags and place them in the fridge to marinate for several hours (8 to 12 is ideal, or overnight).

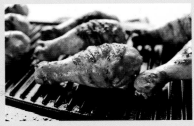

6. Remove the chicken legs from the marinade and grill them on all sides over medium to medium-high heat until the chicken is completely done in the middle, 12 to 15 minutes. (The time will vary depending on the thickness of the chicken legs.)

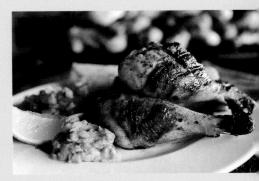

7. Serve with warmed tortillas, pico de gallo, and guacamole!

Ⓥ VARIATIONS

Use any cut of chicken you'd like—chicken thighs, boneless breasts . . .

Add cumin, oregano, or other spices to the marinade.

Add cayenne or red pepper flakes to the marinade to give it a kick.

Double the amount of garlic for a stronger garlic flavor.

Ⓢ SERVE WITH

Black Bean Soup (page 77)

Any cooked beans (pinto, black, and so on)

Colorful Coleslaw (page 294)

CHICKEN MARSALA

MAKES 4 SERVINGS

Chicken Marsala is one of those dishes that sounds fancy and complicated, but it really is one of the easiest dinners to whip up. Marsala is a unique, yummy wine made in Italy, and whether you're using it to make desserts or this classic savory dish, it's a great bottle to keep in your pantry. (Or on your bedside table . . . whichever you prefer.)

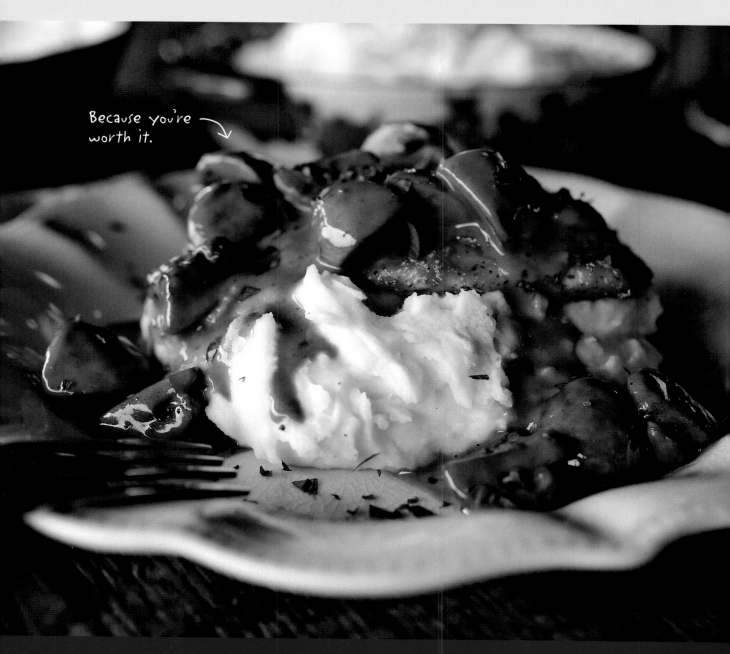

Because you're worth it.

2 boneless, skinless chicken breasts

Kosher salt and black pepper to taste

½ cup all-purpose flour

2 tablespoons olive oil

4 tablespoons (½ stick) butter

12 ounces white button mushrooms, quartered

1 cup Marsala wine

1 cup beef broth

1 teaspoon cornstarch

½ cup heavy cream

Mashed potatoes or cooked noodles, for serving

Chopped parsley, for serving

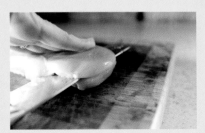

1. Hold one hand on top of one piece of chicken, then use a sharp knife to carefully slice it in half horizontally.

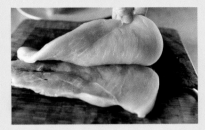

2. Pull the two pieces apart. Repeat with the other chicken breast, to give you four thinner chicken cutlets total.

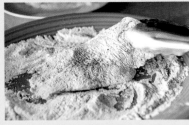

3. Sprinkle the chicken on both sides with salt and pepper, then pour the flour in a dish and dredge the chicken pieces in flour.

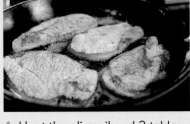

4. Heat the olive oil and 2 tablespoons of the butter in a large skillet (nonstick works well!) over medium-high heat. Add the chicken cutlets and cook for 2 to 3 minutes on the first side, until browned and gorgeous . . .

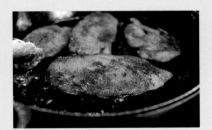

5. Then turn them over and cook them on the other side, 2 to 3 minutes. They should be well browned and cooked through.

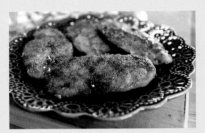

6. Remove them to a plate and set them aside.

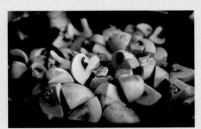

7. In the same skillet, add the mushrooms . . .

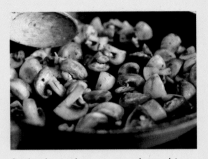

8. And stir them around, cooking them until golden, 5 to 6 minutes.

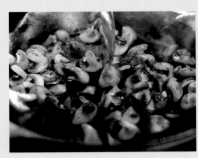

9. Pour in the Marsala and beef broth . . .

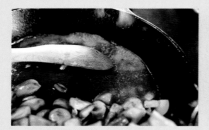

10. Stir to deglaze the pan, scraping up the browned bits . . .

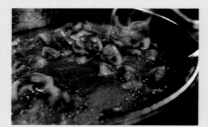

11. And cook for 2 to 3 minutes more, until the liquid reduces by half. (If the liquid reduces too quickly, splash in more broth as needed.)

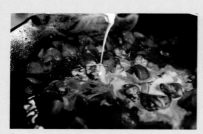

12. Whisk the cornstarch into the cream in a small bowl. When the sauce is dark and rich, pour in the cream mixture . . .

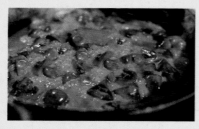

13. And let it bubble up and thicken for another minute. Turn off the heat . . .

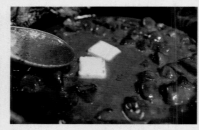

14. And stir in the remaining 2 tablespoons butter.

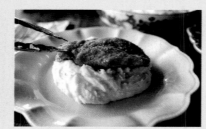

15. To serve, place a piece of chicken on a bed of mashed potatoes or noodles . . .

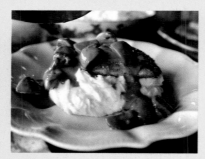

16. Then spoon on some of the sauce . . .

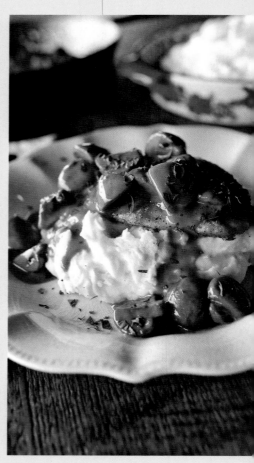

17. And sprinkle on the parsley.

Ⓥ VARIATIONS

Use thin pork chops instead of chicken breasts. Pork marsala!

Use a mix of wild mushrooms instead of white button.

Add ½ cup diced onion and 2 minced garlic cloves with the mushrooms for a pop of flavor.

Use any white wine, whiskey, or bourbon instead of Marsala wine.

Omit the alcohol and use chicken broth instead. (You can still call it Chicken Marsala; I won't tell anyone!)

Omit the cream for a darker, more concentrated sauce.

Ⓢ SERVE WITH

Stovetop Mashed Potatoes (page 310)

Buttered Parsley Noodles (page 324)

Risotto (page 327)

Rice Pilaf (page 320)

Lemony Green Beans (page 292)

Peas and Carrots (page 293)

COCONUT CURRY SHRIMP

MAKES 6 SERVINGS

This is slightly different from the typical stir-fry in that the sauce is creamy and full of unusual curry flavor, and the colors are bright and weird and wonderful.

Let's extract all the adjectives I just rattled off and see what kind of picture it paints: Different, Creamy, Unusual, Bright, Weird, Wonderful.

I'm in!

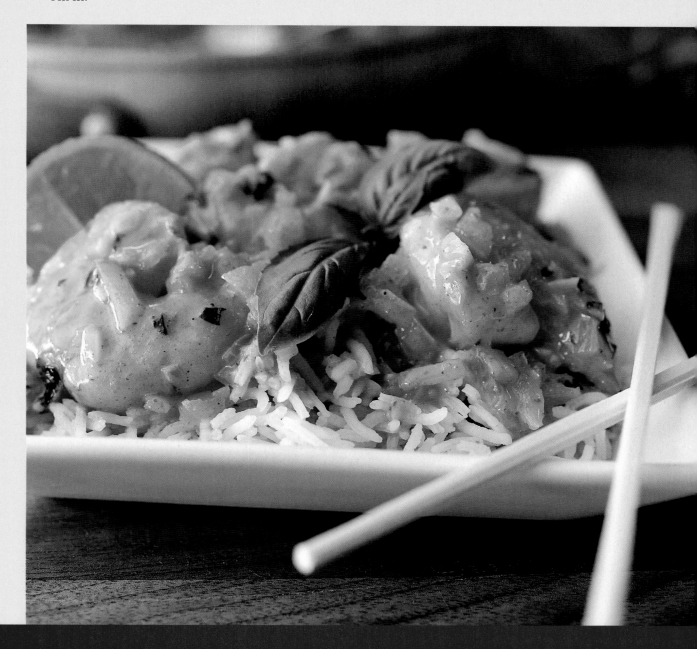

2 tablespoons butter

1½ pounds peeled and deveined shrimp (any size is fine!)

1 medium onion, finely diced

4 garlic cloves, minced

1 tablespoon curry powder (any variety is fine)

One 13.5-ounce can coconut milk

1 large lime

2 tablespoons honey, more to taste

1 tablespoon sriracha, more to taste

¼ teaspoon kosher salt, more to taste

12 basil leaves, chopped, plus more for garnish

2 cups basmati rice, cooked according to the package directions

Lime wedges, for serving

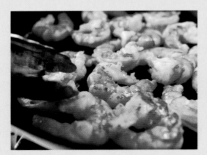

1. Melt the butter in a large skillet (I used nonstick) over medium-high heat. Add the shrimp and cook for 2 to 3 minutes, turning halfway through, until pink, opaque, and fully cooked (the cooking time will depend on the size of the shrimp you use).

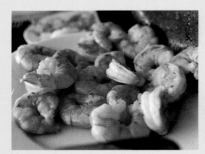

2. Remove them to a plate and set aside.

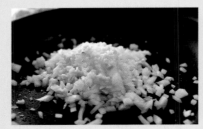

3. Return the skillet to the heat and add the onion and garlic. Stir and cook for 2 minutes to soften a bit . . .

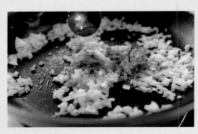

4. Then sprinkle on the curry powder . . .

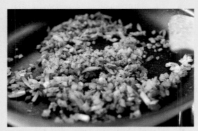

5. And stir it around, cooking the onions and curry for another couple of minutes.

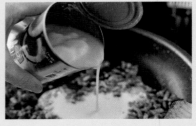

6. Reduce the heat to medium-low and pour in the coconut milk.

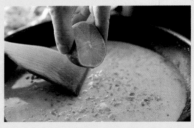

7. Stir the sauce, then add the juice of the lime, honey, sriracha, and salt.

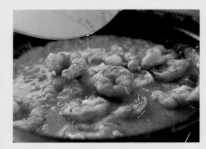

8. Add the shrimp back in and toss it around to coat . . .

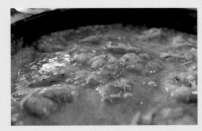

9. Then let the sauce bubble up for a minute or two.

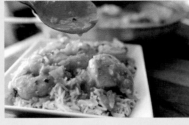

11. Place the rice in bowls and spoon the sauce and shrimp over the top.

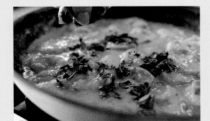

10. Add the basil and toss it around. Taste and adjust the seasonings, adding more of whatever it needs!

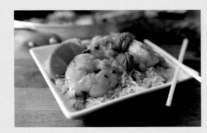

12. Serve with a sprig of basil and a lime wedge.

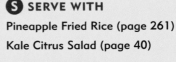

ⓥ VARIATIONS

Add 2 cups diced zucchini, carrots, cauliflower florets, or red bell pepper to the pan with the onions and garlic.

Use Greek yogurt instead of coconut milk.

Add more sriracha for a spicier dish.

Use 4 boneless, skinless chicken thighs cut into bite-size pieces instead of the shrimp.

Ⓢ SERVE WITH

Pineapple Fried Rice (page 261)

Kale Citrus Salad (page 40)

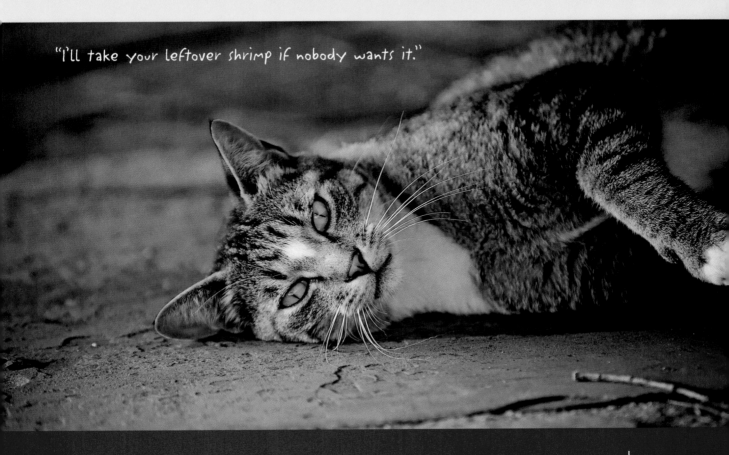

"I'll take your leftover shrimp if nobody wants it."

TOMATO TART

MAKES 8 TO 10 SERVINGS

I love it when my little sister Betsy comes to visit, because we always do our share of cooking and eating. And cooking. And eating. And eating. And eating. Ad infinitum. One evening during her visit at the end of a hot summer, we were trying to figure out how to use a bunch of yellow cherry tomatoes Bets had picked from my garden. They were lusciously ripe and begging to be featured in something special, and after we hemmed and hawed over pasta, frittata, and bruschetta possibilities . . . we wound up deciding to make a tart.

To this day, it's one of the best decisions either of us has ever made.

4 tablespoons (½ stick) butter

2 large onions, halved and thinly sliced

Kosher salt and black pepper to taste

2 rounds store-bought pie dough (or 1 large batch homemade pie dough; see page 140)

1½ cups grated Fontina or Monterey Jack cheese

¼ cup freshly grated Parmesan cheese

¼ cup grated Gruyère or Swiss cheese

3 cups cherry tomatoes (yellow or red, or a mix), more if desired

1 large egg

¼ cup milk

16 basil leaves, more if desired, cut into chiffonade

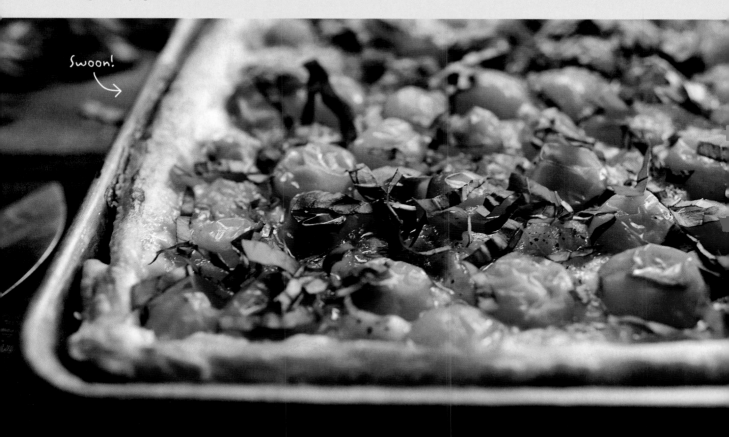

Swoon!

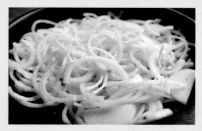

1. Heat a large skillet over medium-low heat. Add the butter, onions, and salt and pepper to taste . . .

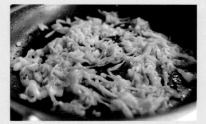

2. And cook, stirring occasionally, until the onions are soft and golden brown, 5 to 7 minutes. Set them aside.

3. Preheat the oven to 450°F.

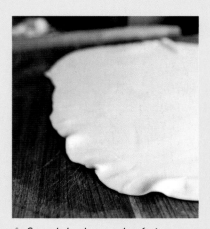

4. Smush both rounds of pie dough into one ball, knead it around a bit to combine them, then roll the ball out into one large, thin rectangle. (You can also keep the dough in separate rounds and use two standard pie pans.)

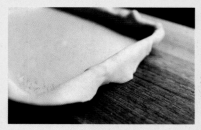

5. Lay the pie dough over a shallow 9 x 13-inch baking sheet, pressing the dough into the edges and allowing a slight overlap.

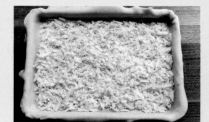

6. Mix the cheeses together and sprinkle them in a single layer over the crust.

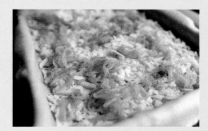

7. Arrange the deliciously golden onions over the cheese . . .

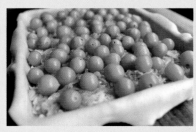

8. Then arrange the tomatoes in a single layer on top.

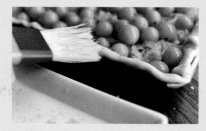

9. Combine the egg and milk in a small bowl and whisk with a fork. Tuck the edges of the crust under themselves, then brush the edge of the crust with the egg mixture.

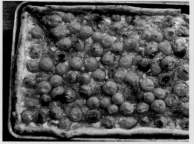

10. Bake the tart for 15 to 18 minutes, watching carefully to make sure the crust doesn't burn. The tomatoes should be starting to burst apart, with some dark and roasted-looking areas on the skin. (Note: When it first comes out of the oven, there will be some liquid surrounding the tomatoes, but it disappears within a few minutes.) Let the tart sit for 5 minutes before serving.

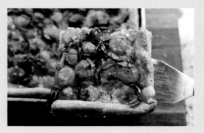

11. Sprinkle on the basil, then cut the tart into large squares and serve it up!

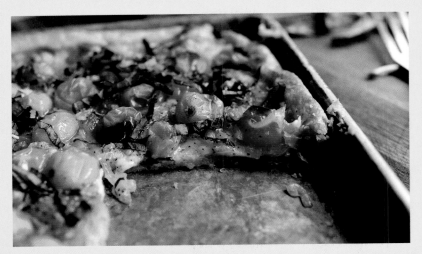

This will disappear before your eyes.

V VARIATIONS

Use Beautiful Roasted Vegetables (page 290) instead of tomatoes.

Top with a mix of chopped herbs: parsley, basil, thyme, and so on.

Spread the crust with a thin layer of prepared pesto before sprinkling on the cheese.

S SERVE WITH

A cold glass of white wine! ☺

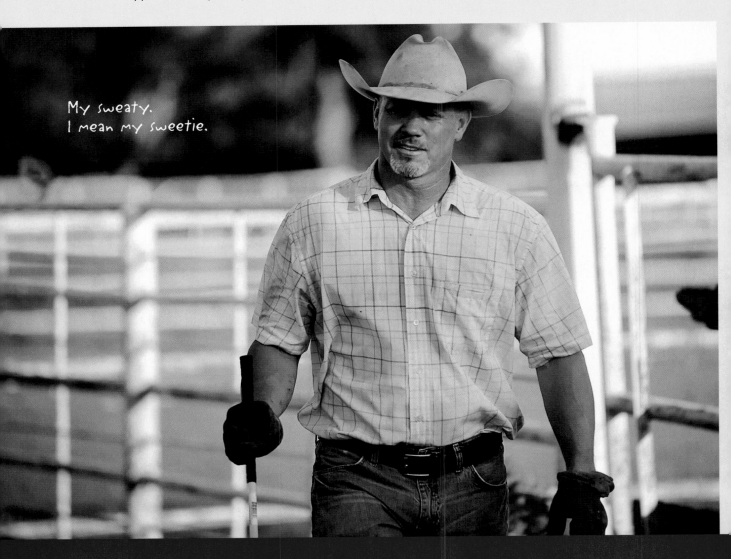

My sweaty.
I mean my sweetie.

PORK CHOPS WITH PINEAPPLE FRIED RICE

MAKES 4 TO 6 SERVINGS

This recipe comes with a bonus: aside from the pork chops and the pineapple, almost everything is a pantry, fridge, or freezer staple . . . and the results are just out-of-this-world delicious. This is one of those dinners that looks way more complicated than it is!

Just note: The ultraflavorful pork chops are a meal in themselves, and you can serve them with salad, noodles, mashed potatoes . . . anything. In that vein, the pineapple fried rice can also be a meal in itself. Many possibilities!

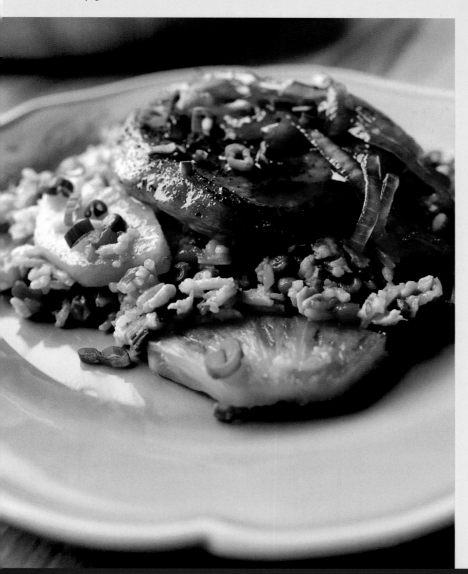

2 tablespoons butter

½ pineapple, peeled, cored, and cut into thin wedges

2 tablespoons peanut or vegetable oil

4 to 6 boneless pork chops (depending on the number you need to serve)

Kosher salt and black pepper to taste

1 large onion, thinly sliced

½ cup low-sodium soy sauce, more as needed

1 tablespoon rice vinegar

2 tablespoons honey

1 tablespoon sriracha or other hot sauce

2 garlic cloves, minced

1 tablespoon minced ginger

3 green onions, thinly sliced

2 large eggs, whisked

1 cup frozen peas

One 4-ounce jar diced pimientos, drained

1½ cups long-grain rice, cooked according to the package directions

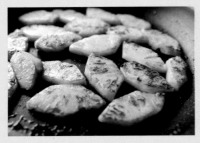

1. Melt the butter in a large skillet over medium-high heat and add the pineapple in a single layer. Cook the pineapple until it's lightly browned on both sides, about 2 minutes per side. Remove and set aside.

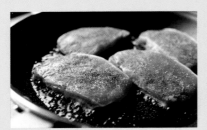

2. In the same skillet, heat 1 tablespoon of the oil over medium-high heat, then season the pork chops with salt and pepper and add them to the pan.

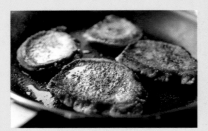

3. Cook the pork chops on both sides until they have a nice deep golden color and are almost cooked through, 4 to 6 minutes total, depending on thickness. Remove them to a plate and set aside.

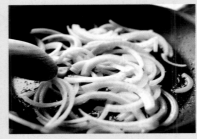

4. Add the onions to the same skillet, still over medium-high heat. Stir and let them cook for a good couple of minutes.

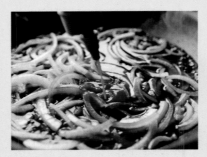

5. When the onions are starting to soften, add 6 tablespoons of the soy sauce, the rice vinegar, honey, and sriracha.

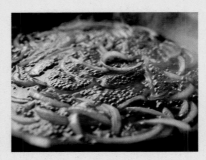

6. Stir and let the liquid cook and bubble up for a good couple of minutes until the sauce starts to reduce. Taste and adjust the seasonings as you wish.

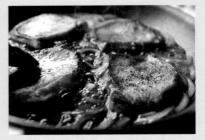

7. Return the pork chops to the pan, reduce the heat to low, and let them simmer while you make the fried rice. Check on the pan occasionally; if the liquid level seems low, splash in ¼ cup water.

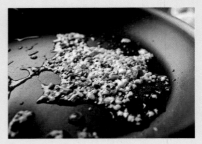

8. Heat the remaining 1 tablespoon oil in a separate large skillet over medium heat. Add the garlic, ginger, and two-thirds of the green onions and sauté for 1 to 2 minutes to release the flavors.

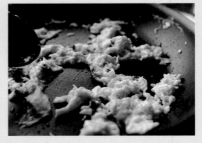

9. Add the eggs to the skillet, stirring to scramble them . . .

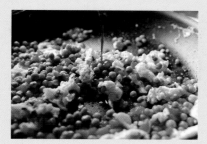

10. Then stir in the peas, pimientos, and remaining 2 tablespoons soy sauce.

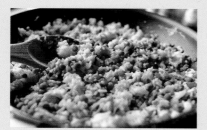

11. Add the rice, turn the heat to high, and stir-fry the rice for 1 to 2 minutes . . .

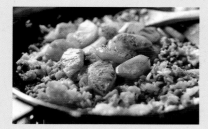

12. Then turn off the heat and stir in the pineapple. Done!

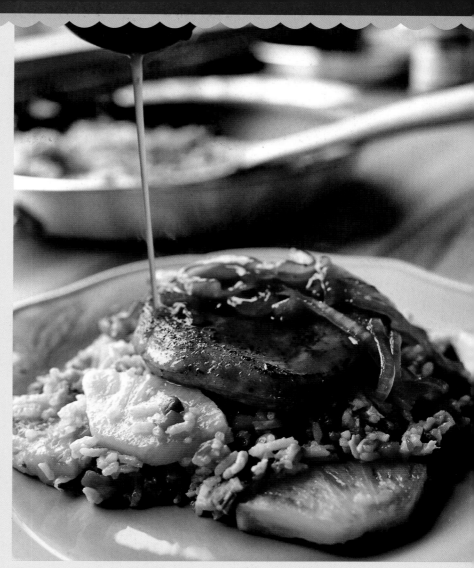

13. To serve, pile the fried rice on a plate and set a pork chop on top. Then spoon on as much sauce (be sure to include onions) as you'd like!

Ⓜ MAKE AHEAD

Have the rice cooked and in the fridge; leftover rice is actually better for fried rice!

Ⓥ VARIATIONS

Use thin boneless chicken cutlets instead of pork chops.

Dice up the pork chops into bite-size pieces before cooking.

Serve the cooked pork chops and sauce with Chow Mein (page 174), Stovetop Mashed Potatoes (page 310), or Polenta (page 322).

Serve the Pineapple Fried Rice as a main dish meal. Add cooked chicken or shrimp if desired.

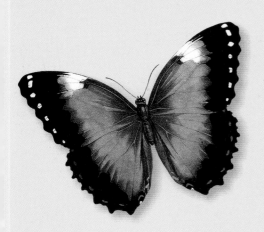

TOFU LETTUCE WRAPS

MAKES 4 TO 6 SERVINGS

The title of this recipe cracks me up, because I picture any self-respecting cowboy reading it and totally running for the hills. It sounds weird, it seems wrong, and it definitely isn't something I'd serve to any human being who works in agriculture—at least not after a long day of work.

But despite all that . . . this dish is a true triumph. A gloriously simple and healthy meatless meal. If you're into that sorta thing. Which cowboys aren't. But that just leaves more for me.

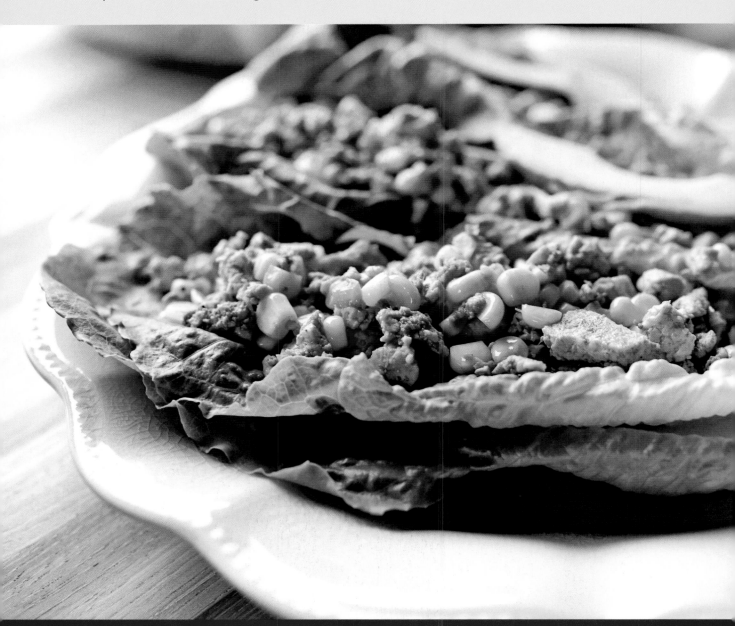

2 teaspoons peanut or olive oil

One 14-ounce package extra-firm tofu, drained

Kernels from 2 ears corn, or 1½ cups frozen corn kernels

¼ teaspoon chili powder, more to taste

¼ cup soy sauce, plus more for drizzling

1 teaspoon balsamic vinegar

2 green onions (green parts only), sliced

Romaine lettuce leaves

2 avocados, peeled, pitted, and sliced

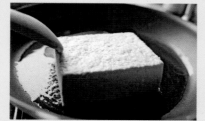

1. Heat the oil in a skillet (nonstick is best) over medium-high heat. Place the tofu in the skillet.

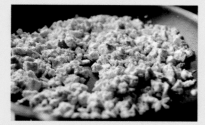

2. Use a spoon to break it into very small pieces as it cooks. Continue cooking the tofu for several minutes, until much of the liquid has cooked off and the tofu starts to turn golden brown.

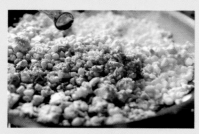

3. Add the corn and stir it around. Cook for 2 to 3 minutes (less time if you're using frozen corn). Stir in the chili powder, soy sauce, and balsamic.

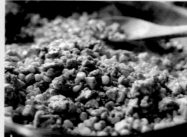

4. Add the green onions and cook the mixture for another couple of minutes!

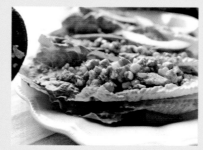

5. To serve, spoon the warm tofu mixture into the lettuce leaves.

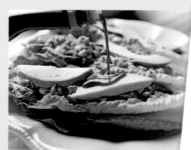

6. To make it extra delicious, lay on some avocado slices and drizzle on more soy sauce. Oh my goodness, you will love this.

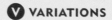 **MAKE AHEAD**

Make the tofu mixture, then pop it in the fridge. Throughout the week, remove the amount you'd like and use for lettuce wraps, burritos, or salads.

V VARIATIONS

Use butter lettuce, iceberg, or any kind of lettuce leaves you like.

Add finely diced carrots along with the corn.

Sprinkle chopped cilantro over each lettuce wrap before serving.

Forgo the veggie approach and use finely chopped chicken or ground beef instead of the tofu.

S SERVE WITH

Chow Mein (page 174)

Pineapple Fried Rice (page 261)

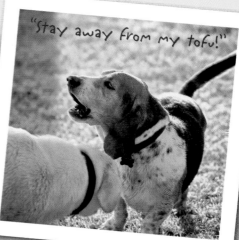

"stay away from my tofu!"

CHICKEN MILANESE

MAKES 4 SERVINGS

First, let's get this out of the way:

Is it Chicken Mee-law-nees?

Or is it Chicken Mi-law-nez?

Or is it Chicken Mi-luh-nees?

Or is it Chicken Mee-luh-nez?

Or is it Chicken Mi-luh-nez?

Oh dear. This could go on for a while. And we don't have time for this! We've got to get dinner on the table! If your household is like mine, your kids are banging their forks and knives on your formerly ding-free table as we speak.

I know I say this a lot . . . but this is one of my absolute favorite things to make for dinner. The chicken is light and crisp, with a buttery golden crust. Topped with greens, lemon, and Parmesan . . . it's pretty much irresistible.

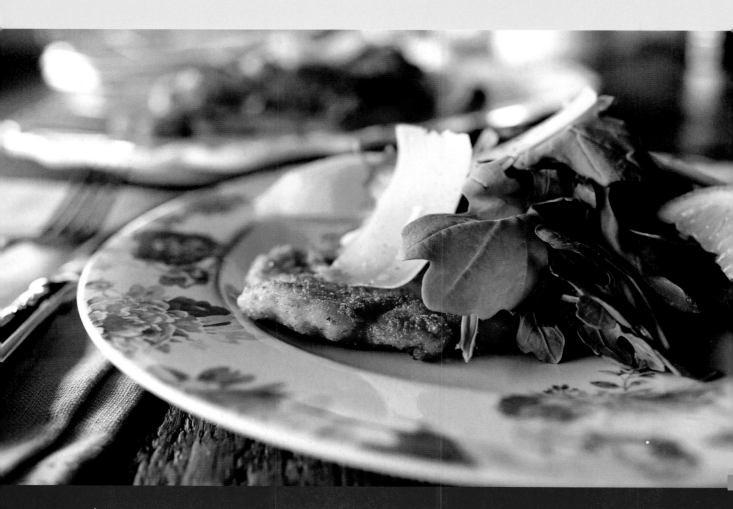

2 boneless, skinless chicken breasts

3 large eggs

¼ cup half-and-half or whole milk

½ cup all-purpose flour

1 cup seasoned breadcrumbs

Kosher salt and black pepper, to taste

4 tablespoons (½ stick) butter

Arugula, baby spinach, or spring greens

½ cup Parmesan shavings

1 lemon, cut into wedges

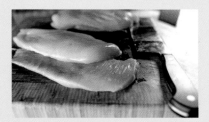

1. Place your palm flat against the top of each chicken breast and carefully slice each piece in half horizontally. You'll be left with 4 thinner chicken breast pieces.

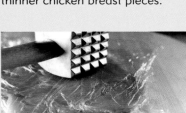

2. Place each chicken cutlet between two sheets of plastic wrap and use the smooth side of a mallet (or a rolling pin) to pound them very thin. If you think they're thin enough . . . pound 'em a few more times! The thinner, the better.

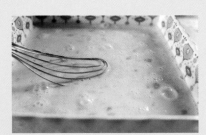

3. In a dish, whisk together the eggs and half-and-half. Place the flour and the breadcrumbs in two separate dishes. Set the three dishes aside for a sec.

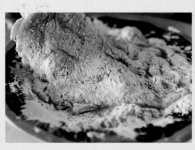

4. Salt and pepper both sides of the chicken pieces, then dredge them one at a time in the flour . . .

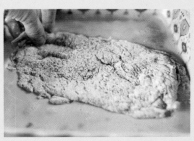

5. Quickly dunk both sides in the egg mixture . . .

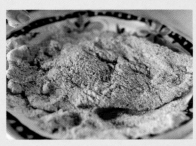

6. Then coat both sides in breadcrumbs. Lay the cutlets on a clean plate as you bread them until you're ready to cook them.

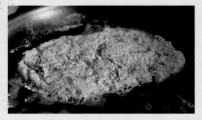

7. Melt 2 tablespoons of the butter in a large skillet over medium-low heat. When it's melted and hot, add two of the breaded chicken cutlets . . .

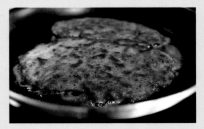

8. And cook them on both sides until the breading is golden brown and the chicken is cooked through, 2 to 3 minutes per side. (Leave them undisturbed in the pan other than to turn them over—you want them to develop a nice, crispy crust!)

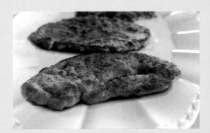

9. Remove the cutlets to a clean plate, then add the remaining 2 tablespoons butter to the skillet and cook the remaining two cutlets.

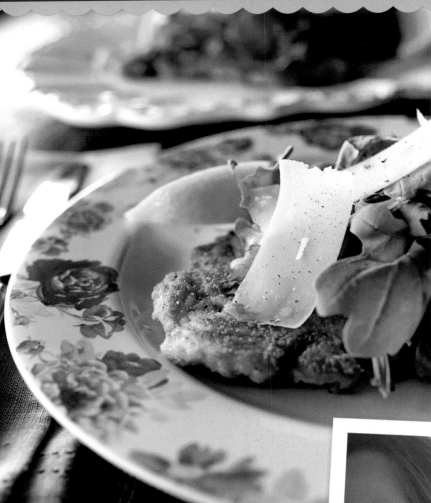

M MAKE AHEAD

Pound the chicken breasts and get your assembly line ingredients ready up to 24 hours in advance. Keep the chicken breasts and egg mixture in the fridge; keep the flour and breadcrumbs in covered bowls on the kitchen counter. Will save you time!

V VARIATIONS

Substitute ½ cup grated Parmesan cheese for half of the breadcrumbs.

Use boneless pork chops instead of chicken breasts.

S SERVE WITH

Buttered Parsley Noodles (page 324)

Lemony Green Beans (page 292)

Roasted Carrots with Vinaigrette (page 300)

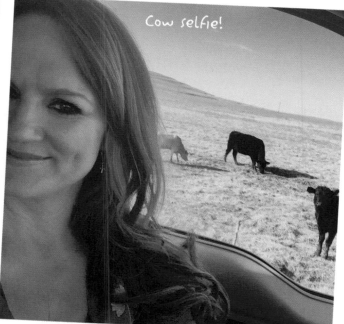

Cow selfie!

10. To serve, place a cutlet on a plate. Top generously with arugula, spinach, or spring greens. Squeeze a little lemon juice over the greens, then sprinkle with a little salt. Finally, sprinkle on Parmesan shavings. Serve with lemon wedges.

PAWHUSKA CHEESESTEAKS

MAKES 6 SERVINGS

I'd like to state for the record that I'm not from Philly. I'm not even from Pennsylvania. I'm not even from the Northeast. I'm not even from the East. I'm not even from. I'm not even. I'm not. I'm!

What I'm saying is, I have about as much authority to make Philly cheesesteaks as I have to make bona fide jambalaya from Louisiana. I get that. So I'm calling these super-easy sandwiches "Pawhuska Cheesesteaks" in order to avoid losing all credibility with residents of Philadelphia.

That's assuming, of course, that I ever had any credibility with them to begin with. Which I most likely did not. So never mind.

8 ounces Velveeta (I used the white "Queso Blanco" version. I'm classy that way.)

½ teaspoon black pepper

¼ teaspoon cayenne pepper

¼ cup milk

6 tablespoons (¾ stick) butter

6 sub rolls, split

2 pounds thinly shaved good-quality deli roast beef

1 yellow onion, cut into thick rings

1 green bell pepper, seeded and cut into thick rings

1 yellow bell pepper, seeded and cut into thick rings

1 red bell pepper, seeded and cut into thick rings

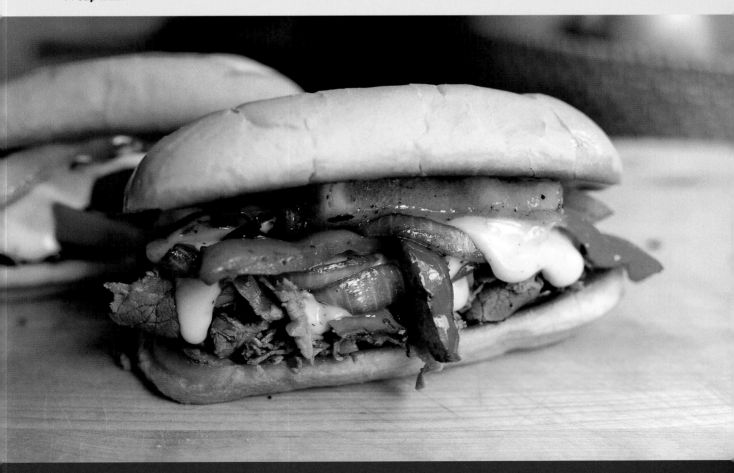

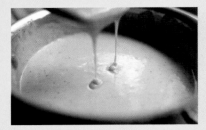

1. In a medium saucepan, combine the Velveeta, black pepper, cayenne, and milk and heat over low heat, stirring occasionally, until totally melted. Set aside and keep warm.

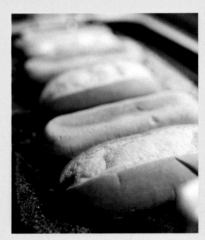

2. Melt 2 tablespoons of the butter on a griddle over medium heat, then place the roll halves on the griddle and toast them until golden brown. Remove them from the griddle and set aside.

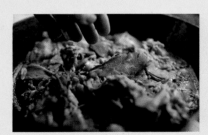

3. Melt 2 tablespoons of the butter in a large skillet over medium-high heat. Throw in the roast beef . . .

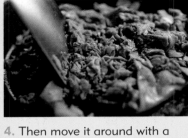

4. Then move it around with a spatula, breaking it up as you go to warm it quickly.

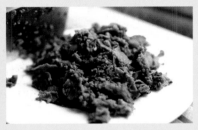

5. After about a minute, remove it to a plate and set it aside.

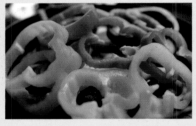

6. Add the remaining 2 tablespoons butter to the skillet and throw in the onion and bell peppers.

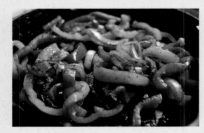

7. Cook until the onions are soft and dark golden and the peppers are soft, 8 to 10 minutes.

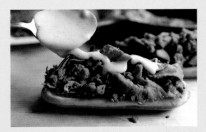

8. To assemble the sandwiches, pile the meat on the bottom halves of the rolls and spoon on a generous amount of the cheese sauce.

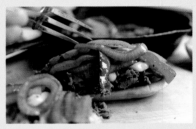

9. Pile on the onions and peppers . . .

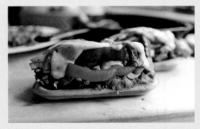

10. Then—why not?—spoon on a little more cheese sauce.

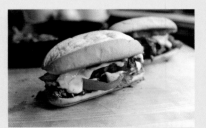

11. Serve them immediately. Hearty appetites are recommended!

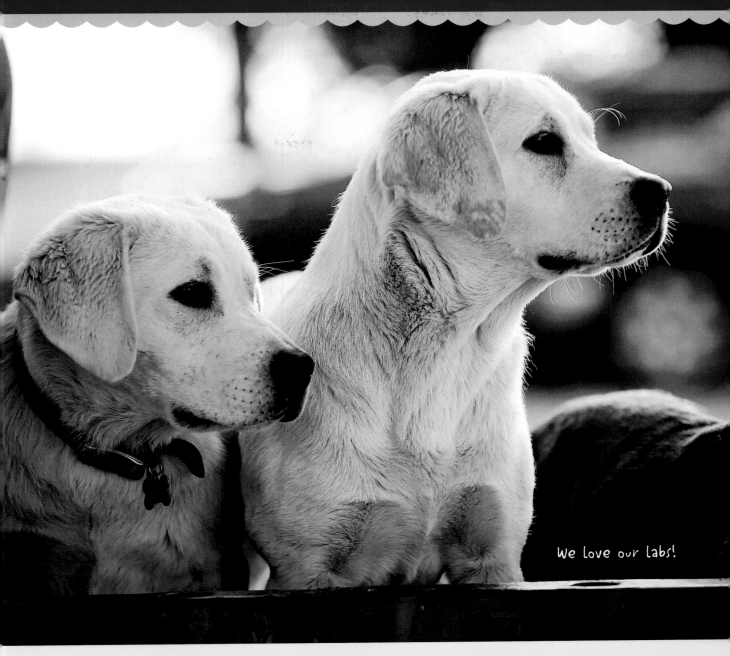

We love our labs!

S SERVE WITH

Thin Fries (page 318)
Sweet Potato Fries (page 308)
"Slice-Baked" Potatoes (page 314)
Colorful Coleslaw (page 294)

V VARIATIONS

Add 8 ounces sliced mushrooms to the onion-pepper mixture while it cooks.

Add a few dashes of Worcestershire or hot sauce to the meat and veggies while cooking.

Spread spicy mustard on the rolls before building the sandwiches.

Make a mixture of mayonnaise and prepared horseradish and spread it on the rolls before building the sandwiches.

Add prepared horseradish to the cheese sauce to give it extra kick.

GREEN CHILE CHICKEN

MAKES 6 SERVINGS

Mmmm . . . roasted green chiles! I love them, and one day when I had a pile of fresh ones, I decided to roast 'em and highlight 'em in a simple grilled chicken dish.

This recipe is ultraversatile! I whipped up my own marinade for the chicken, but you can use store-bought . . . or, if you don't have time for the marinating, you could skip that step and just season the heck out of the chicken before you grill it. And speaking of grilling . . . you don't even have to grill the chicken at all; you can just cook it in a skillet. I served my chicken with rice and beans, but you can serve it with corn tortillas and veggies . . . or you can serve the chicken on a bun and call it a sandwich.

But the most versatility you have with this recipe is this: You can totally change up what you wear whenever you make it. Plaid, polka dots, skirts, shorts, overalls . . . anything goes!

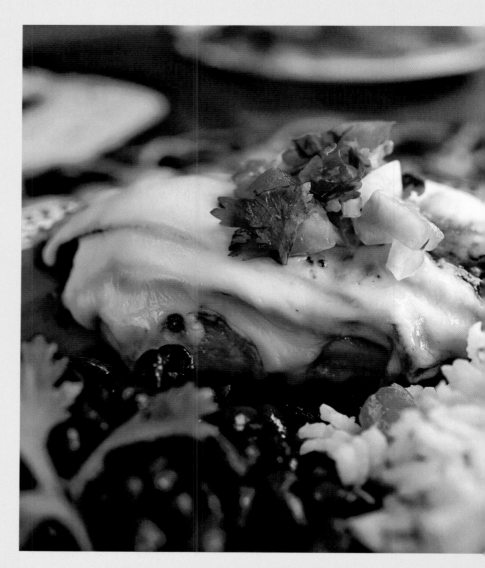

MARINADE

½ cup olive oil

3 tablespoons fresh lime juice

2 chipotle peppers in adobo sauce, more to taste

2 garlic cloves

1 teaspoon ground cumin

1 teaspoon kosher salt

½ teaspoon black pepper

CHICKEN

6 boneless, skinless chicken breasts

6 fresh Hatch, Anaheim, or poblano chiles

Olive oil, for drizzling

½ pound Monterey Jack cheese, cut into thin slices

Pico de gallo (see page 23) or salsa, for serving

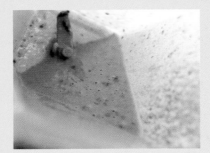

1. To make the marinade, combine the olive oil, lime juice, chipotle peppers, garlic, cumin, salt, and black pepper in a blender and blend until it's totally pureed.

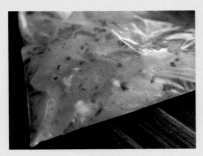

2. Place the chicken breasts in a large plastic bag, pour in the marinade, seal the bag, and marinate in the fridge for at least 6 hours.

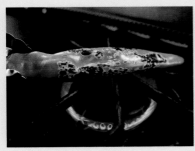

3. Roast the chiles—I use the flame on my stovetop burner, using tongs to hold it over the flame. (You can also do this on an outdoor grill or under the oven's broiler.)

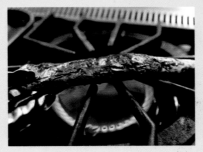

4. Basically, you want to completely blacken the skin until it's hopelessly and deliciously charred.

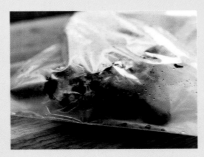

5. Place the charred chiles in a plastic bag and seal it. Let the peppers sit and sweat for a good 20 minutes . . .

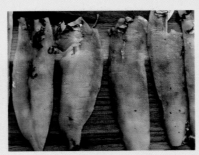

6. Then remove the chiles from the bag, cut off the tops and bottoms, scrape off the skin, scrape out the seeds, and slice them in half. You'll wind up with 12 roasted green chile halves.

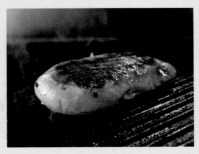

7. When you're ready to cook the chicken, heat a grill, grill pan, or skillet over medium-high heat and drizzle on a little olive oil. Cook the chicken for 4 minutes on the first side, then turn the chicken over and reduce the heat to medium-low.

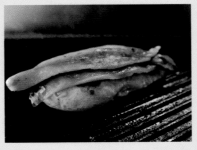

8. Lay two strips of chile on each piece . . .

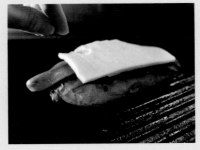

9. Then lay on a slice of cheese . . .

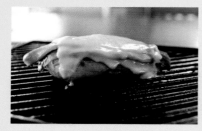

10. And finish cooking the chicken while the cheese totally melts.

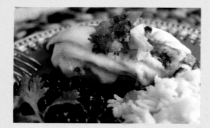

11. Serve it on a plate with a spoonful of pico de gallo or salsa on top. Splendidly yummy!

Ⓜ MAKE AHEAD

Roast and peel the chiles up to 2 days in advance and store in a plastic bag in the fridge.

Ⓥ VARIATIONS

Use canned whole green chiles as a shortcut!

Top with any kind of cheese you'd like: pepper Jack, Cheddar . . .

Omit the cheese for a lighter chicken dish! Just top with pico de gallo.

Ⓢ SERVE WITH

Black Bean Soup (page 77)

Cooked rice or Mexican rice

Warmed corn or flour tortillas

Guacamole, sour cream, queso . . . the works!

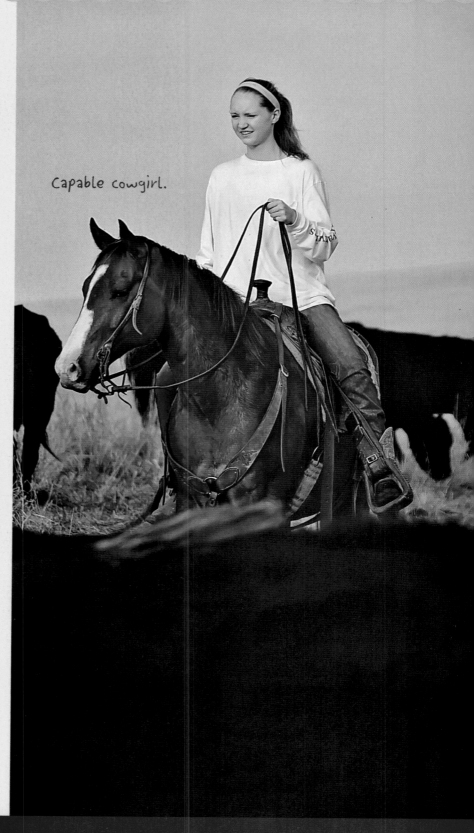

Capable cowgirl.

BURRITO BOWLS

MAKES 8 TO 10 SERVINGS

A burrito bowl is a burrito without the tortilla!

Now, before you turn up your nose and say, "Where's the fun in *that*?" just read the rest of this recipe. You'll be sold by the end! They're fun for company . . . or just dinner with your fam.

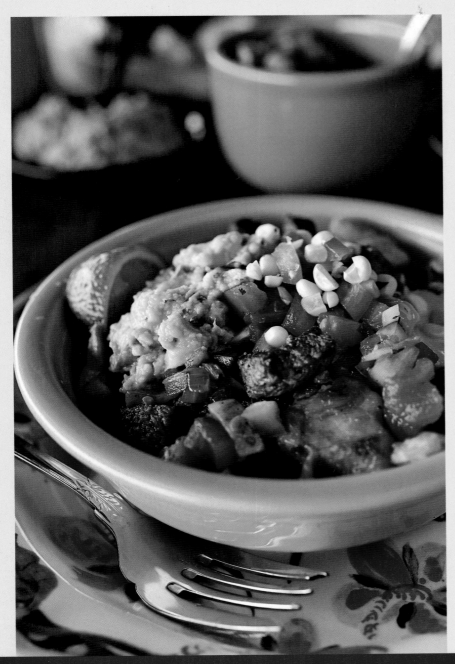

2 cups uncooked long-grain rice

4 cups low-sodium chicken broth

1½ teaspoons kosher salt

1 pound beef sirloin steak, cut into small cubes

1 pound boneless, skinless chicken thighs, cut into bite-size pieces

½ teaspoon black pepper

1 teaspoon ground cumin

1 teaspoon chili powder

4 tablespoons vegetable oil

4 tablespoons (½ stick) butter

1 medium onion, diced

1 zucchini, diced

1 yellow squash, diced

1 red bell pepper, seeded and diced

1 yellow bell pepper, seeded and diced

1 jalapeño, seeded and finely diced

Zest and juice of 2 limes

⅓ cup chopped cilantro

FOR SERVING

Black Bean Soup (page 77), drained, or other canned beans of your choice, heated

Chopped iceberg lettuce

Pico de gallo (see page 23)

Guacamole

Sour cream

Queso (dip made of melted Velveeta and Ro-Tel)

Assorted salsas

Lime wedges

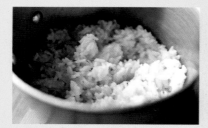

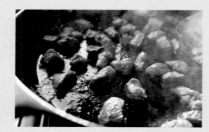

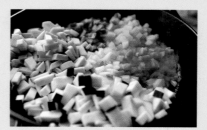

1. Combine the rice, chicken broth, and 1 teaspoon of the salt in a saucepan. Bring it to a boil over medium-high heat, then cover the pan, reduce the heat to low, and simmer for 20 minutes, until light and fluffy. Set aside and keep warm.

4. Heat 2 tablespoons of the oil and 2 tablespoons of the butter in a large skillet over high heat. Throw in the beef in a single layer and leave it in the pan, undisturbed, for a minute to get nice color.

7. Add the remaining 2 tablespoons oil and 2 tablespoons butter to the same skillet and throw in the onion, zucchini, squash, bell peppers, and jalapeño.

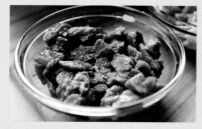

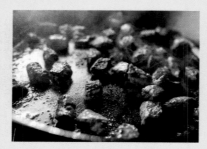

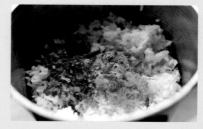

8. Sauté the veggies for a few minutes, until they're deep golden with some dark brown bits.

2. Meanwhile, place the beef and chicken in separate bowls. Mix together the remaining ½ teaspoon salt, the black pepper, cumin, and chili powder, then sprinkle half the mixture over the beef . . .

5. Toss the beef around for 30 to 45 seconds. You want as much color on the outside as possible without completely cooking it through. Remove it to a bowl and keep it warm.

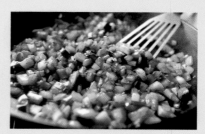

9. Add the lime zest and juice and the cilantro to the rice . . .

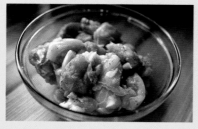

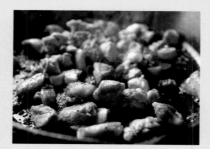

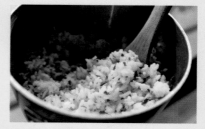

3. And half over the chicken. Toss the beef and chicken to coat.

6. Throw the chicken into the same skillet and cook it for 3 to 4 minutes, until the chicken is completely cooked through. Remove it to a separate bowl and keep it warm.

10. And stir it all together.

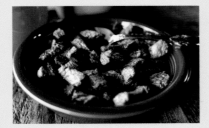

11. To serve the burrito bowls, lay out the beef . . .

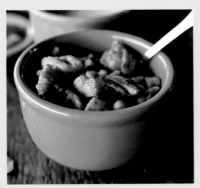

12. And the chicken . . . .

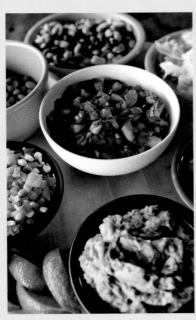

13. Along with the rice, the cooked veggies . . . and whatever fixins you like!

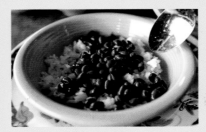

14. Then just let everyone dig in. Let me show you my idea of a good time: Rice in the bowl, then black beans . . .

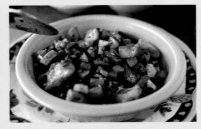

15. Some chicken and some veggies . . .

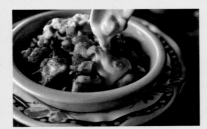

16. And how about some pico, guacamole, and queso? Yes, please!

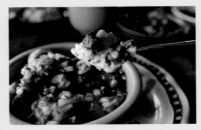

17. Who needs tortillas when you have all this? Not me, that's who.

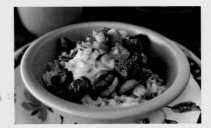

18. My husband's is a little more pared down: Rice, beef, queso, and pico de gallo!

There's no right or wrong way to build a burrito bowl. And that's exactly why I love 'em.

V VARIATION

Cook some deveined shrimp in addition to the beef and chicken.

S SERVE WITH

Good-quality tortilla chips

Margaritas!

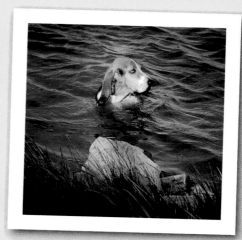

"Nothin' like a cold swim on a hot day."

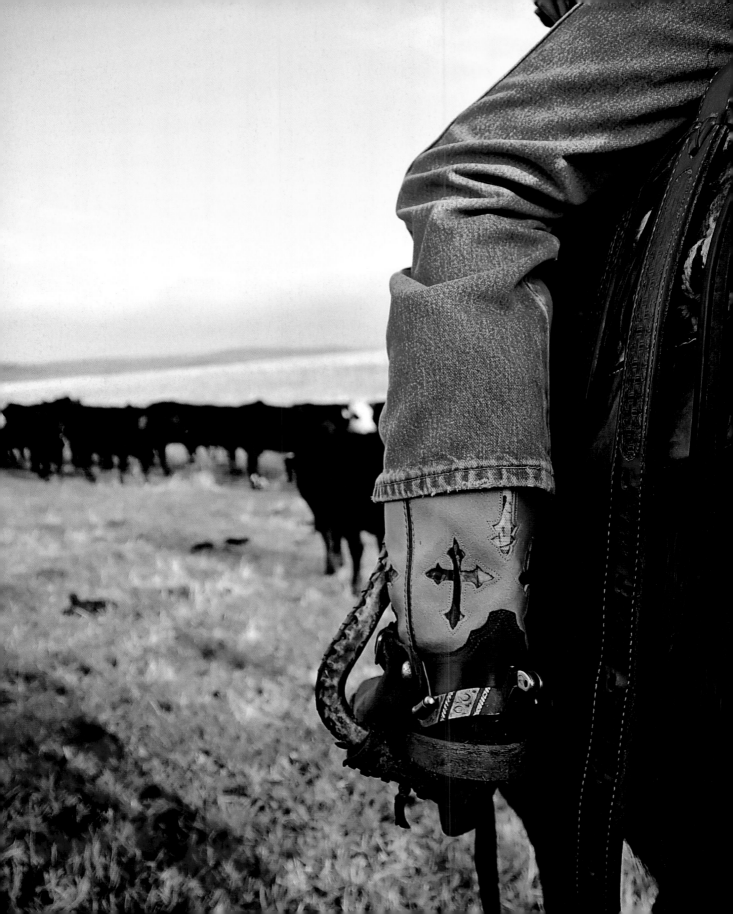

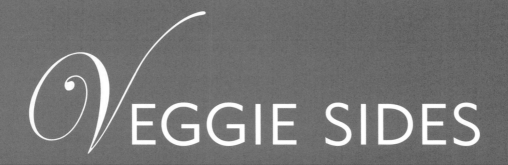

VEGGIE SIDES

Sometimes a pile of pretty vegetables is all a chicken breast or pork chop needs to feel special! From assorted veggies and dip to elegant (but never snobby) roasted asparagus, there's not a main dish anywhere that won't look a little spruced up with one of these sides by its . . . side.

ROASTED ASPARAGUS

MAKES 6 SERVINGS

Now hear this: Roasted asparagus is officially the perfect side dish. It works as part of an elegant meal with company or just a regular weeknight dinner. It can be served piping hot alongside a steak, or chilled in the fridge alongside (or chopped up and put inside!) a pasta salad.

I love the stuff. I think I'll keep it.

2 bunches asparagus, rinsed
½ cup olive oil

Kosher salt and black pepper to taste

1. Preheat the oven to 475°F.

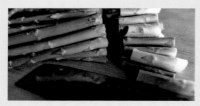

2. First, slice the woody bottom 1½ to 2 inches off the asparagus spears.

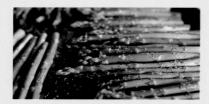

3. Arrange the spears on a large rimmed baking sheet, drizzle on the olive oil, toss them in the oil, and sprinkle on plenty of salt and pepper.

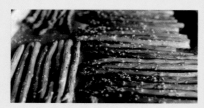

4. Roast for 5 to 7 minutes, or until slightly tender and just starting to brown. (Don't let them go too far or they'll start to turn yellow.)

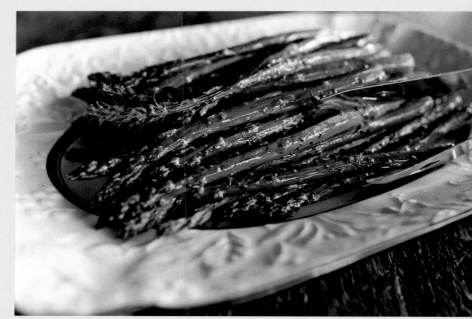

5. Serve immediately!

V VARIATIONS

Add 1 seeded, diced red bell pepper to the asparagus before roasting it.

Just out of the oven, toss the asparagus with ½ cup freshly grated Parmesan cheese.

Just out of the oven, squeeze on the juice of half a lemon.

Chill the asparagus and toss with a simple vinaigrette (see page 300). Serve cold.

S SERVE WITH

Grilled Chicken (page 110)

Quinoa Caprese (page 64)

Mediterranean Orzo Salad (page 62)

Chicken with Mustard Cream Sauce (page 146)

Oven-Barbecued Chicken (page 234)

ROASTED GRAPE TOMATOES

MAKES 6 SERVINGS

This is one of the easiest vegetable side dishes on the planet, as there's hardly any prep at all! And the result is fresh flavor and vibrant color. Perfect with so many things!

2 pints grape or cherry tomatoes (red or yellow or both)

2 garlic cloves

¼ cup olive oil

Kosher salt and black pepper to taste

1. Preheat the oven to 475°F.

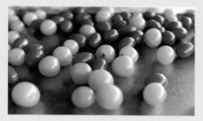

2. Spread the tomatoes on a large rimmed baking sheet.

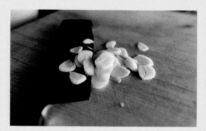

3. Slice the garlic very thin . . .

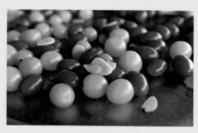

4. Then toss it with the tomatoes.

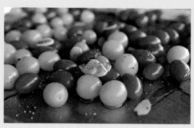

5. Drizzle on the olive oil and sprinkle on salt and pepper to taste . . .

6. Then roast the tomatoes until they're starting to burst, the garlic is golden, and there are some brown bits on the tomatoes. Let the tomatoes sit for 5 to 10 minutes before serving.

V VARIATIONS

Toss in 1 cup Parmesan shavings as soon as the tomatoes come out of the oven.

Stir the roasted tomatoes into cooked pasta or risotto.

Make a delicious appetizer by smearing crostini with goat cheese and topping with roasted tomatoes.

S SERVE WITH

Chicken with Mustard Cream Sauce (page 146)

Tuna Noodle Casserole (page 222)

Chicken Milanese (page 266)

Quick Shells and Cheese (page 214)

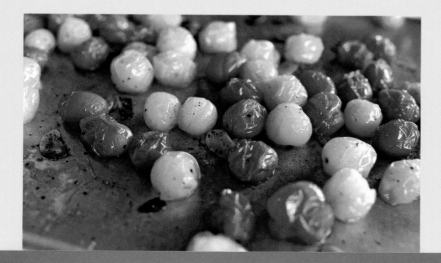

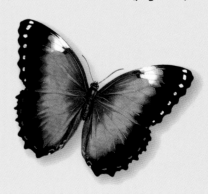

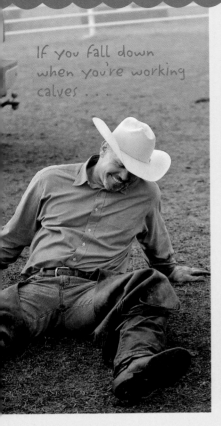

If you fall down when you're working calves . . .

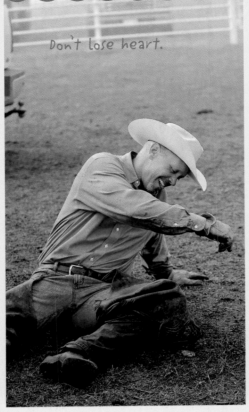

Don't lose heart.

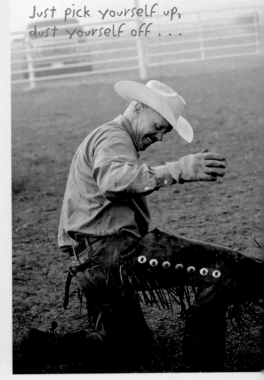

Just pick yourself up, dust yourself off . . .

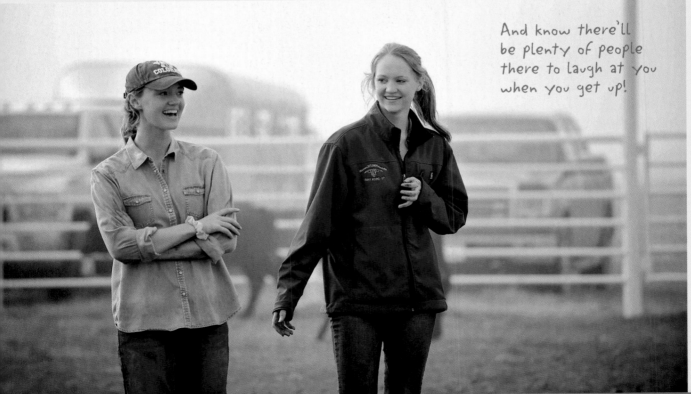

And know there'll be plenty of people there to laugh at you when you get up!

BROCCOLI CAULIFLOWER CASSEROLE

MAKES 4 TO 6 SERVINGS

The most tremendous veggie casserole in the history of veggie casseroles! I started making it around Thanksgiving as an alternative to broccoli-rice casserole, but it has slowly crept into other meals throughout the year. It's irresistible.

1 cauliflower head

1 large broccoli head

½ cup (1 stick) butter

1 medium onion, diced

2 garlic cloves, minced

¼ cup all-purpose flour

2½ cups low-sodium chicken broth

4 ounces cream cheese, at room temperature

¼ teaspoon seasoned salt, more to taste

Kosher salt and black pepper to taste

¼ teaspoon paprika, plus more for sprinkling

⅓ cup seasoned breadcrumbs

1½ cups grated Monterey Jack cheese

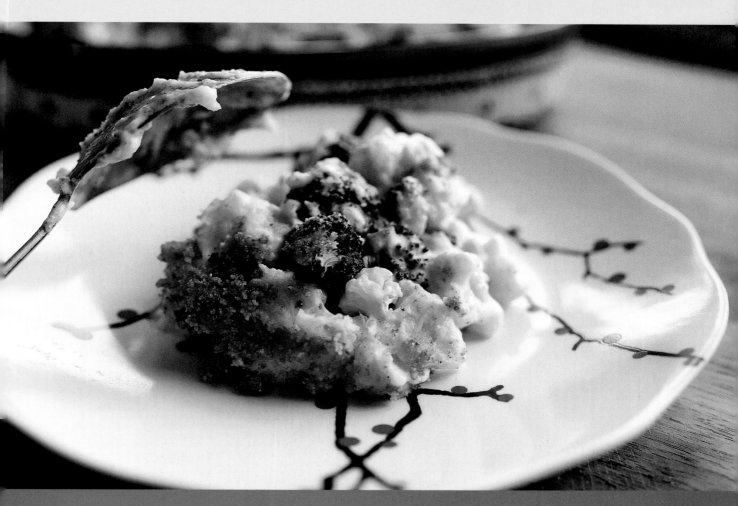

1. Preheat the oven to 375°F.

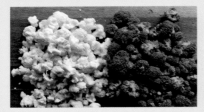

2. Using your hands, break the cauliflower and broccoli into very small florets . . .

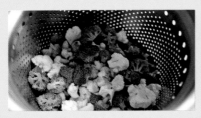

3. Then place them in a steamer and steam them over simmering water until slightly tender, 3 to 4 minutes. Set them aside.

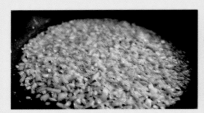

4. Melt 6 tablespoons of the butter in a large skillet over medium heat, then add the onion and garlic and cook until the onion is translucent, 3 to 4 minutes.

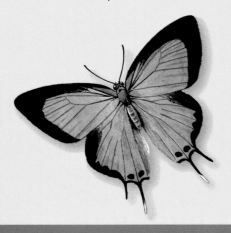

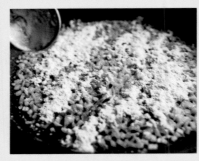

5. Sprinkle in the flour . . .

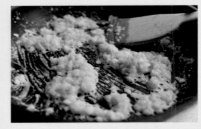

6. Then stir the flour into the onion mixture and cook it for a minute or so.

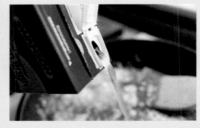

7. Pour in the broth, stirring continuously . . .

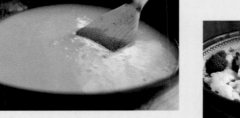

8. And cook the sauce, stirring occasionally, until it begins to thicken, about 3 minutes.

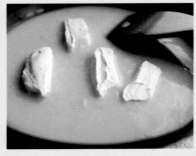

9. Add the cream cheese and stir until it melts completely . . .

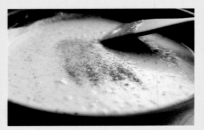

10. Then stir in the seasoned salt, kosher salt, pepper, and paprika. Turn off the heat and set the sauce aside.

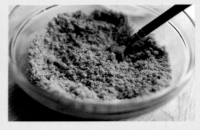

11. In a small bowl, combine the breadcrumbs and the remaining 2 tablespoons melted butter and blend with a fork.

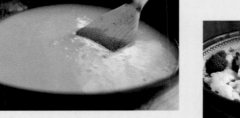

12. To assemble, butter a small (2-quart) casserole and add half the broccoli-cauliflower mixture.

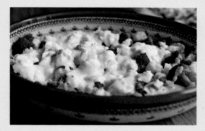

13. Pour on half the sauce . . .

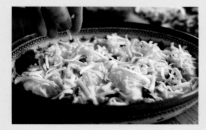

14. Top with half the cheese . . .

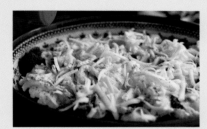

15. And sprinkle on a little paprika.

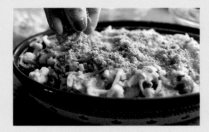

16. Repeat another round of the veggies, sauce, cheese, and paprika . . . then top the casserole with the buttery breadcrumbs.

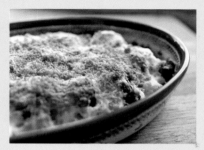

17. Bake the casserole for 25 to 30 minutes, or until the breadcrumbs are golden and the casserole is bubbly around the edges.

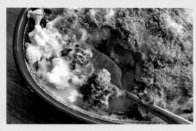

18. Serve it nice and piping hot!

M MAKE AHEAD

The casserole can be assembled and stored in the fridge, unbaked, for up to 24 hours. Allow 10 minutes extra cooking time if baking straight out of the fridge.

V VARIATIONS

This recipe can easily be doubled!

Use all cauliflower or all broccoli, if you prefer.

Use sharp Cheddar cheese instead of Monterey Jack for a slightly different flavor.

Sauté 8 ounces sliced mushrooms with the onions and garlic.

S SERVE WITH

Pan-Fried Pork Chops (page 156)

Salisbury Steak (page 216)

Italian Meatloaf (page 212)

Oven-Barbecued Chicken (page 234)

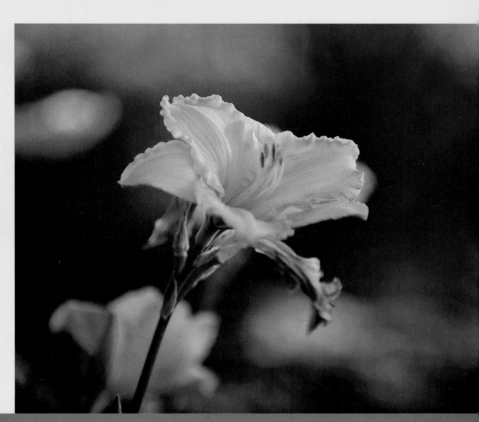

BROCCOLI WITH CHEESE SAUCE

MAKES 6 TO 8 SERVINGS

My boy Bryce loves broccoli with cheese sauce so much that there've been times I've actually feared he would turn into broccoli with cheese sauce. That's a really bizarre old wives' tale, isn't it? That if you eat too much of something, you'll turn into what you're eating? Though sometimes it's definitely fitting: for instance, that time I ate an entire bag of marshmallows when I was eleven? I did actually turn into a marshmallow. It was a very mushy time for me.

Anyway, I stand with B-Man in his love for this perfect combo. It's delicious, and the cheese sauce can be used in any number of different ways. You'll love it!

2 broccoli heads, cut into florets

2 cups whole milk

1 tablespoon butter

1 garlic clove (optional)

12 ounces processed cheese (such as Velveeta)

4 ounces sharp Cheddar cheese

4 ounces Monterey Jack cheese

½ teaspoon seasoned salt

½ teaspoon black pepper

¼ teaspoon kosher salt

¼ teaspoon chili powder, plus more for sprinkling

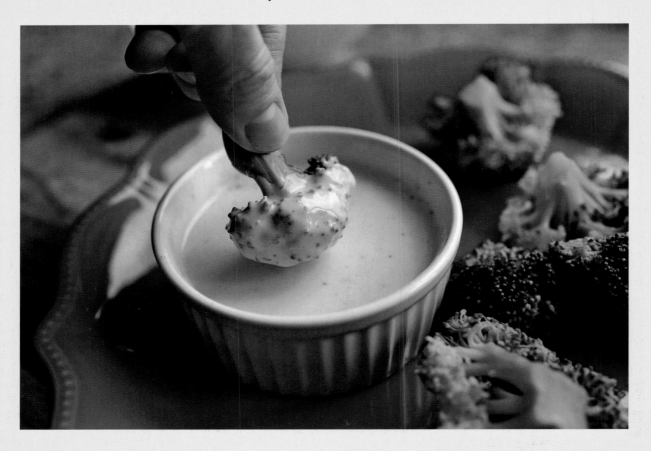

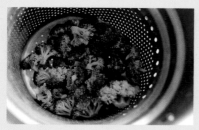

1. Place the broccoli in a steamer over simmering water and steam it for 3 to 4 minutes, until slightly tender but not overly soft.

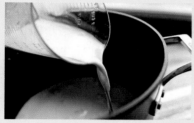

2. Next, pour the milk into a saucepan (nonstick is good) . . .

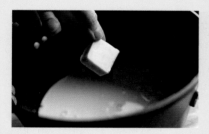

3. Then add the butter.

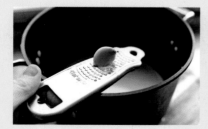

4. If you want to add a nice garlic flavor, grate or press in the garlic. Set the pan over medium-low heat until the butter has melted and the mixture is hot.

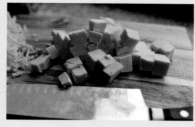

5. Cut the Velveeta into cubes . . .

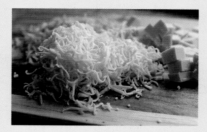

6. And grate the other two cheeses. And now you're ready!

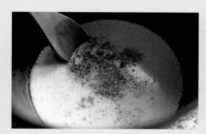

7. Stir in the seasoned salt, pepper, kosher salt, and chili powder . . .

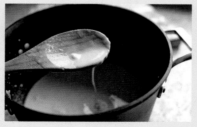

8. Then add the cubed Velveeta and stir until it's melted and silky.

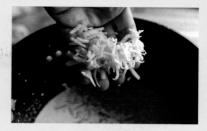

9. Add the Cheddar and Monterey Jack . . .

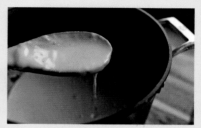

10. And stir the sauce slowly while everything melts together.

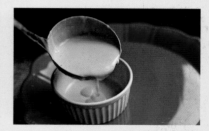

11. While it's nice and hot, ladle the sauce into ramekins . . .

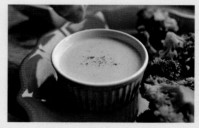

12. Sprinkle a little chili powder on top, just for kicks . . .

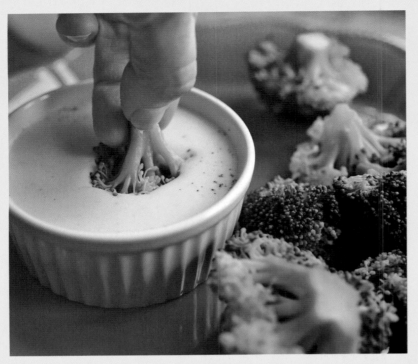

13. And dig right in!

M MAKE AHEAD

The cheese sauce will keep in the fridge for up to 3 days. Just reheat it in the microwave or in a nonstick saucepan as needed.

V VARIATIONS

Use pepper Jack, goat cheese, or any kind of cheese you'd like in place of the Cheddar and/or Monterey Jack.

Stir chopped chives or other herbs into the cheese sauce.

Serve with asparagus or carrots instead of broccoli.

S SERVE WITH

Italian Meatloaf (page 212)
Salisbury Steak (page 216)
Pan-Fried Pork Chops (page 156)

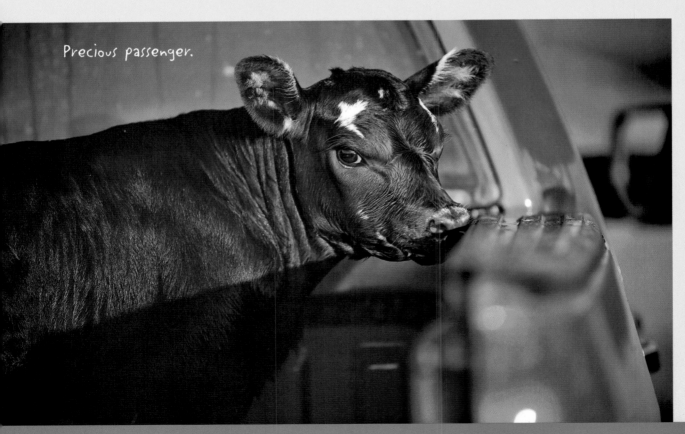

Precious passenger.

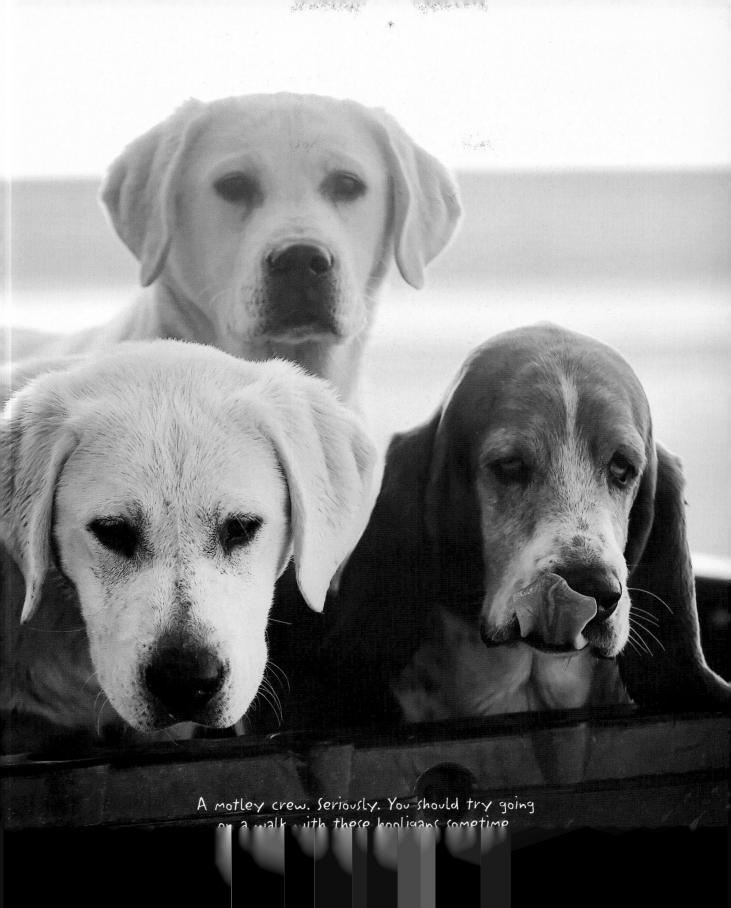

A motley crew. Seriously. You should try going
on a walk with these hooligans sometime.

BEAUTIFUL ROASTED VEGETABLES

MAKES 8 SERVINGS

I think this assortment is so uniquely beautiful, and I love that not all the vegetables come from the same season. Spring vegetables are mixed with fall vegetables, dogs and cats are living together. Mass anarchy!
    And mass deliciousness.

1 bunch asparagus, tough ends removed

1 red onion

1 red bell pepper, seeded

8 ounces mushrooms

1 medium eggplant

½ butternut squash, peeled and seeded

3 garlic cloves, minced

⅓ cup olive oil

Kosher salt and black pepper to taste

1 teaspoon Montreal Steak Seasoning (or any seasoning mix)

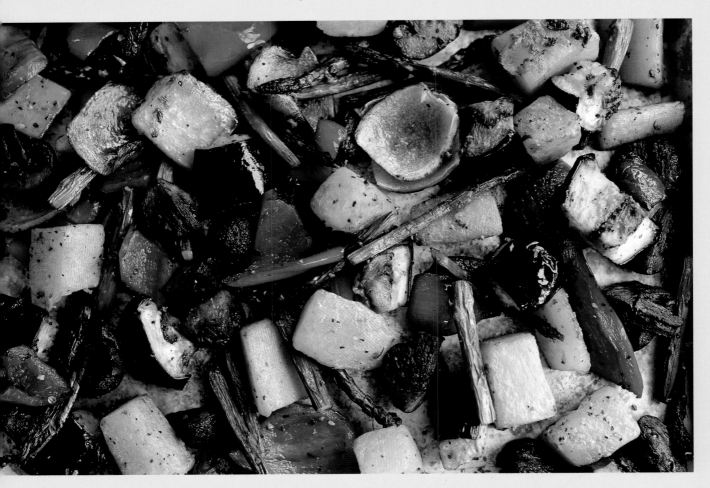

1. Preheat the oven to 450°F.

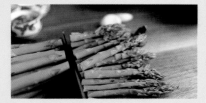

2. Cut the asparagus into 2- to 3-inch pieces . . .

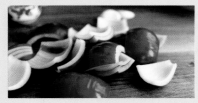

3. Chop the red onion into wedges . . .

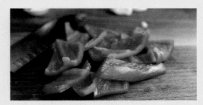

4. Chop the bell pepper into chunks . . .

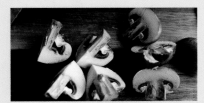

5. And cut the mushrooms into quarters.

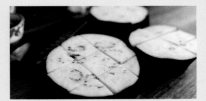

6. Cut the eggplant into thick slices, then cut the slices into chunks . . .

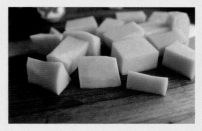

7. And, finally, cut the butternut squash into large pieces.

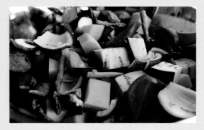

8. Throw all the veggies into a large bowl along with the garlic . . .

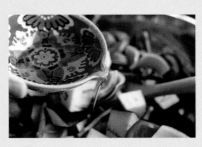

9. Then drizzle in the olive oil . . .

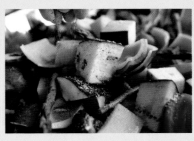

10. Sprinkle on salt and black pepper to taste, and the steak seasoning, and toss it all together.

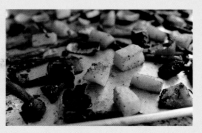

11. Spread the vegetables on two rimmed baking sheets so that they have plenty of breathing room, then roast them for 20 minutes, shaking the pans twice during that time. If needed, roast for 5 to 10 minutes more, until the veggies are nicely browned and tender.

12. Serve them warm or chilled! They're delicious either way.

Ⓜ MAKE AHEAD

The vegetables will keep in the fridge for up to 5 days. Reheat or eat cold!

Ⓥ VARIATIONS

Substitute any vegetables you like: zucchini, yellow squash, parsnips, carrots . . .

Squeeze on some lemon juice when the veggies come out of the oven.

Toss the vegetables with 1 cup freshly grated Parmesan cheese right after they come out of the oven.

Ⓢ SERVE WITH

Quinoa Caprese (page 64), stirred into the salad or served on the side

Panzanella (page 46), stirred into the salad

Chicken with Mustard Cream Sauce (page 146)

Italian Meatloaf (page 212)

LEMONY GREEN BEANS

MAKES 6 SERVINGS

I adore fresh green beans, but I'm sometimes guilty of adding all sorts of naughty/decadent/fattening things to them (Hello, green bean casserole during the holidays!) to make them extra flavorful and delicious. This simple, easy-to-whip-up veggie side dish is the antidote to that: Just add a little butter, lemon juice, salt, and pepper, and simple green beans are totally transformed. They'll disappear quickly!

3 tablespoons butter

1½ pounds fresh green beans, ends snapped or chopped off

1½ lemons, plus a lemon half for garnish

¼ teaspoon kosher salt, more to taste

¼ teaspoon black pepper

Ⓥ VARIATIONS

Use olive oil instead of butter, if you prefer.

Add the zest of the 2 lemons along with the lemon juice for even more citrus flavor.

Sprinkle in a little chili powder with the salt and pepper to give the green beans a kick.

Use frozen green beans straight out of the freezer rather than fresh. You might just need to up the cooking time by 2 to 3 minutes!

Ⓢ SERVE WITH

Italian Meatloaf (page 212)

Chicken with Mustard Cream Sauce (page 146)

Pork Chops with Wine and Roasted Garlic (page 246)

Salisbury Steak (page 216)

Oven-Barbecued Chicken (page 234)

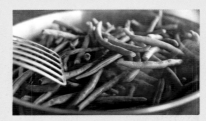

1. Melt the butter in a large skillet over medium-high heat. When the butter sizzles and starts to turn golden, throw in the green beans and sauté them, stirring occasionally, until slightly tender, 3 to 4 minutes.

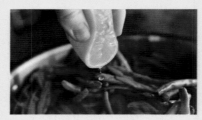

2. Squeeze in the juice of the lemons . . .

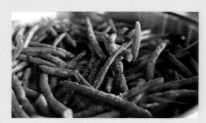

3. Sprinkle in the salt and pepper, then stir to make sure everything is coated and combined. Cook for an additional minute, then turn off the heat.

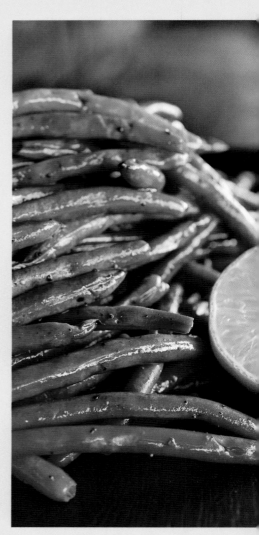

4. Serve them heaped on a platter with a lemon half for squeezing.

PEAS AND CARROTS

MAKES 8 SERVINGS

Peas and carrots go together like . . .
> Like . . .
> Like . . .
> (Warning: I'm going to say it . . .)
> Like peas and carrots.
> There! I said it! (I hope you can forgive me.)

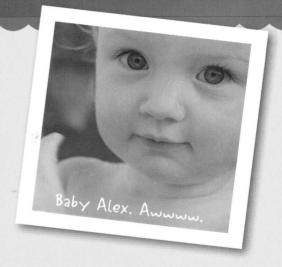
Baby Alex. Awwww.

2 tablespoons butter

4 large carrots, cut into small, uniform dice

1 pound frozen peas

12 basil leaves, cut into chiffonade

Kosher salt and black pepper to taste

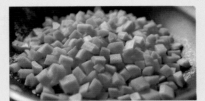

1. Melt the butter in a large skillet over medium heat. Add the carrots . . .

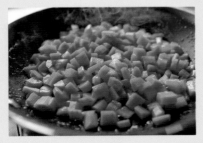

2. And cook until they're tender, 4 to 5 minutes, stirring occasionally.

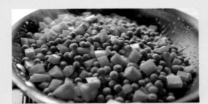

3. Add the peas straight out of the freezer, then toss them around for 2 minutes. (They'll thaw almost instantly!)

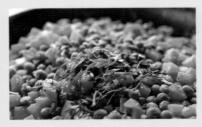

4. Sprinkle in the basil and salt and pepper to taste . . .

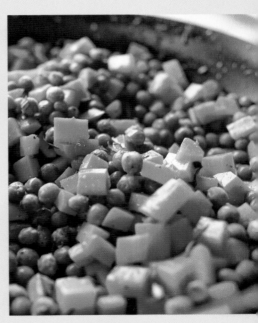

5. And toss to combine. Serve nice and hot!

V VARIATIONS

Squeeze in the juice of half a lemon for a citrusy zip.

Stir in the cheese sauce from page 286 for a cheesy veggie dish.

Add chopped parsley and/or mint for a different herby edge.

S SERVE WITH

Italian Meatloaf (page 212)

Chicken with Mustard Cream Sauce (page 146)

Pork Chops with Wine and Roasted Garlic (page 246)

Salisbury Steak (page 216)

Chicken Milanese (page 266)

COLORFUL COLESLAW

MAKES 12 SERVINGS

Coleslaw has long been relegated mostly to picnics or barbecues, and I would just like to state for the record that I think that is terribly unfair! From now on I shall daily sing the praises of crispy, crunchy coleslaw as a totally legitimate indoor side! Whether it's served with grilled chicken, pork chops, meatloaf, or steak, it always adds color and freshness to your plate.

½ cup mayonnaise

½ cup whole milk

1 teaspoon white vinegar

1 tablespoon sugar

½ teaspoon kosher salt, more to taste

¼ teaspoon black pepper, more to taste

Several dashes of hot sauce

½ head green cabbage, thinly sliced

½ head purple cabbage, thinly sliced

12 mini sweet peppers, seeded and sliced

2 cups julienned carrots

2 cups cilantro leaves

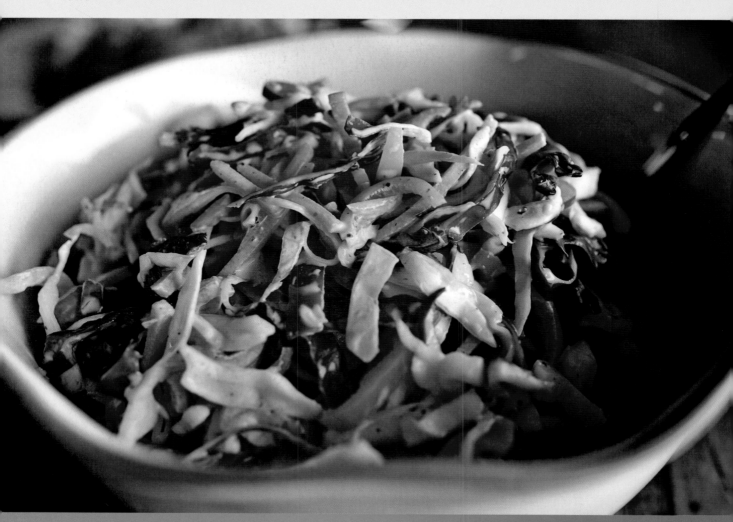

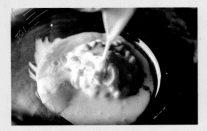

1. Combine the mayonnaise, milk, vinegar, sugar, salt, black pepper, and hot sauce in a medium bowl.

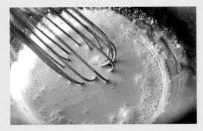

2. Whisk it together until smooth. Taste and adjust the seasonings as desired.

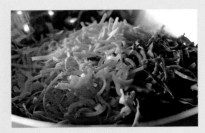

3. Throw the cabbages, sweet peppers, and carrots into a large bowl.

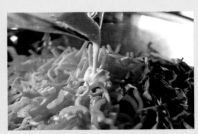

4. Pour on three-quarters of the dressing . . .

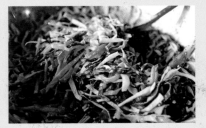

5. And toss everything to coat. If you'd like the coleslaw to have more dressing, add the remaining dressing and toss (just keep in mind that the veggies will give off a little liquid while the slaw is in the fridge). Season the slaw with salt and pepper, if needed.

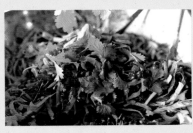

6. Add the cilantro at the very end . . .

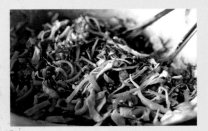

7. Then cover and refrigerate for at least 2 hours to allow the flavors to meld.

Ⓜ MAKE AHEAD

The slaw can be made up to 8 hours before serving and stored in the fridge.

Ⓥ VARIATIONS

Add thinly sliced red or white onion to the cabbage mixture.

Add 6 thinly sliced green onions to the finished slaw.

Add white or black sesame seeds.

Add shelled sunflower seeds for a little nutty crunch!

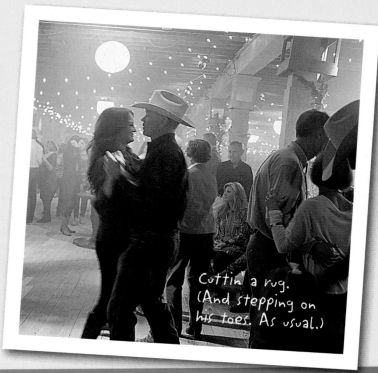

Cuttin a rug. (And stepping on his toes. As usual.)

BUTTERNUT SQUASH AND KALE

MAKES 8 SERVINGS

It doesn't matter how much of this veggie combination I make . . . it disappears before I can say "Butternut Squash and Kale."

See? It's gone again! Now I have to make more.

2 tablespoons butter

½ butternut squash, peeled and diced (as on page 57)

½ teaspoon kosher salt

Black pepper to taste

¼ teaspoon chili powder, more to taste

1 bunch kale, stalks removed, leaves torn into pieces

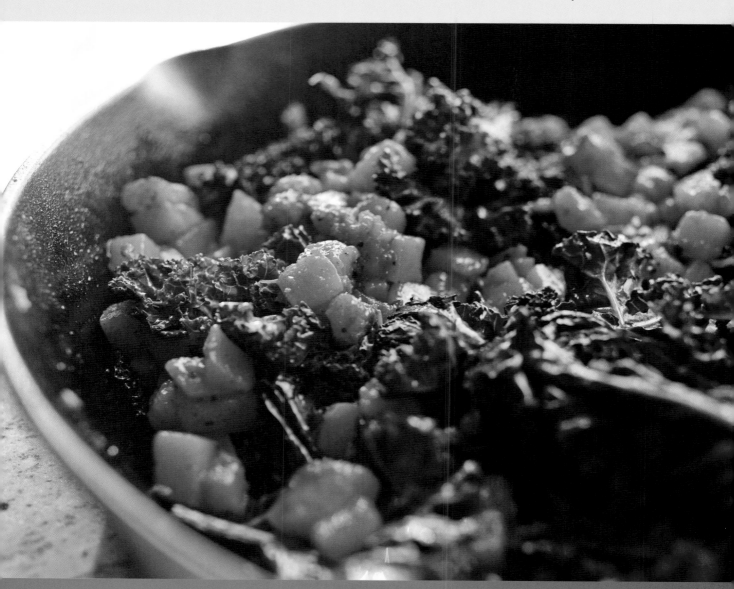

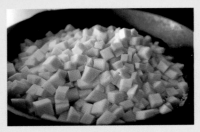

1. Heat 1 tablespoon of the butter in a large skillet over high heat. Throw in the squash and stir it around for a minute to cook . . .

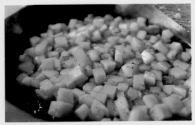

2. Then add the salt, pepper to taste, and the chili powder . . .

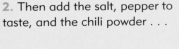

3. And continue cooking for several minutes, until the squash is tender but not falling apart.

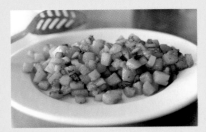

4. Remove it from the pan and set it aside.

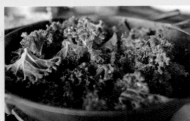

5. Melt the remaining 1 table-spoon butter in the skillet, lower the heat to medium, and add the kale. Sauté it for 2 to 3 minutes, until it begins to wilt . . .

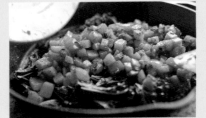

6. Then add the squash and toss it to combine. Serve warm. This is scrumptious!

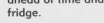 MAKE AHEAD

The butternut squash can be cubed and the kale torn up to 24 hours ahead of time and stored in the fridge.

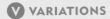 VARIATIONS

Toss in 1 cup Parmesan shavings when you add the squash to the kale.

Mix this veggie mixture into Risotto (page 327) or buttered noodles.

Use the veggie mixture in quesadillas or panini.

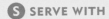 SERVE WITH

Italian Meatloaf (page 212)

Chicken with Mustard Cream Sauce (page 146)

Pork Chops with Wine and Roasted Garlic (page 246)

Salisbury Steak (page 216)

Chicken Milanese (page 266)

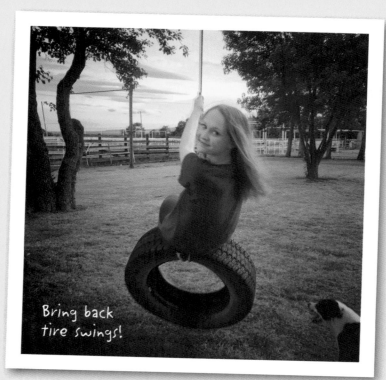

Bring back tire swings!

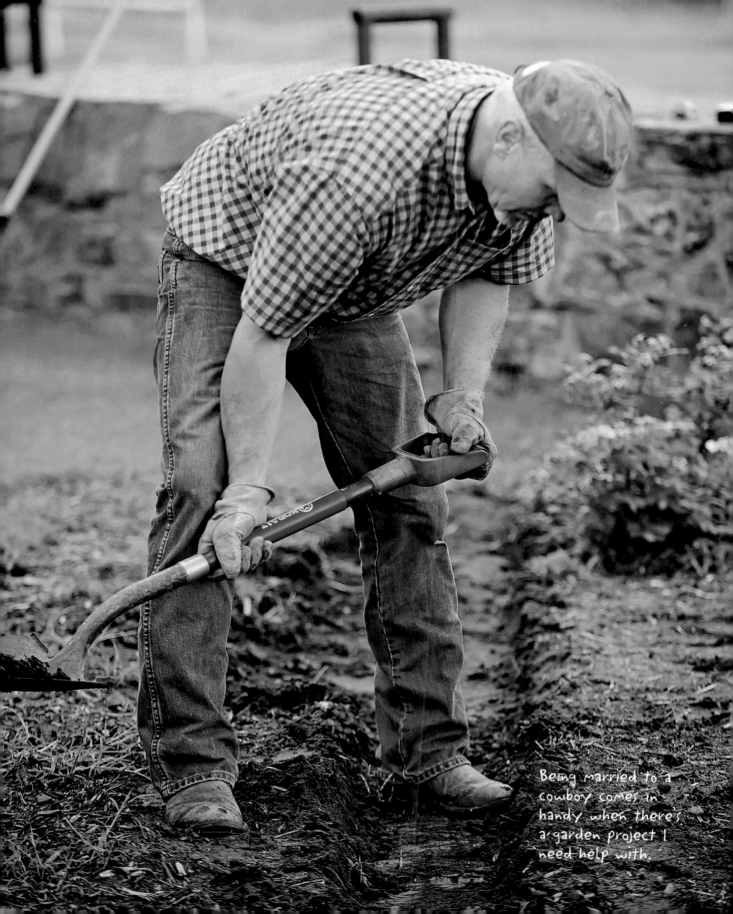

Being married to a cowboy comes in handy when there's a garden project I need help with.

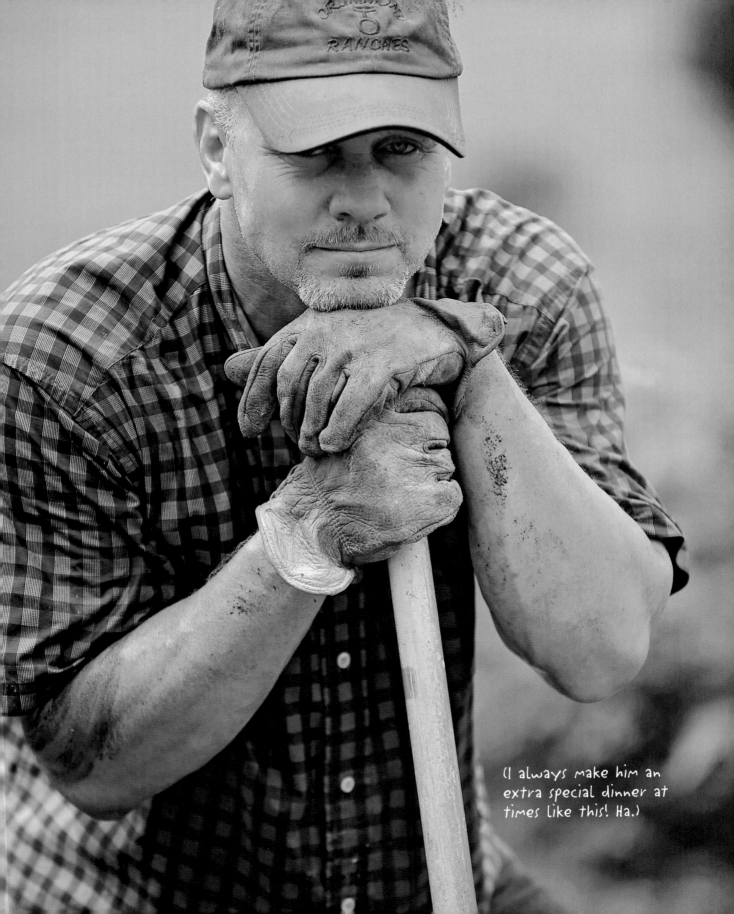

(I always make him an
extra special dinner at
times like this! Ha.)

ROASTED CARROTS WITH VINAIGRETTE

MAKES 8 TO 10 SERVINGS

Roasted vegetables are served in Heaven, no two ways about it. Something happens when the high heat of the oven hits the natural sugars in the vegetables . . . Wait, what's that called again? . . . It's on the tip of my tongue . . .

Oh! I just remembered. *Bliss.* Bliss is what happens.

I love these beautiful roasted carrots straight out of the oven, but when they're drizzled with a simple, herbalicious vinaigrette? Well, they're pretty much too tasty to take.

¼ cup plus 2 tablespoons olive oil

2 tablespoons white wine vinegar

1 tablespoon Dijon mustard

1 tablespoon chopped garlic

Leaves from 3 thyme sprigs, minced

Leaves from 1 rosemary sprig, minced

Kosher salt and black pepper to taste

5 pounds carrots

1. Preheat the oven to 475°F.

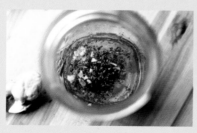

2. Make a simple vinaigrette by combining ¼ cup of the olive oil, the vinegar, Dijon, garlic, thyme, rosemary, and salt and pepper to taste in a jar. Shake it vigorously for 30 seconds or so to emulsify it, then set it aside.

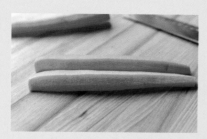

3. Slice the carrots in half . . .

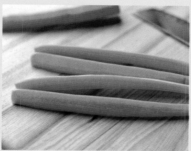

4. Then in quarters lengthwise.

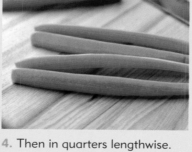

5. Next, cut them into 2- to 2½-inch pieces.

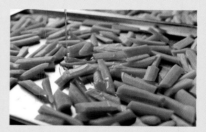

6. Arrange them on two rimmed baking sheets and drizzle them with the remaining 2 tablespoons olive oil . . .

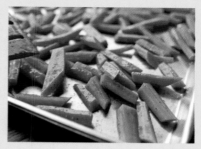

7. Then sprinkle them with salt and pepper.

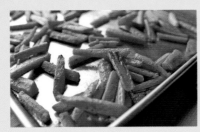

8. Roast the carrots for 10 to 12 minutes, shaking the pan twice during roasting to toss them, until the carrots are tender and brown along the edges.

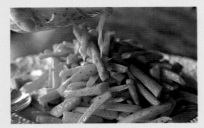

9. Pile the carrots onto a serving plate and drizzle on the vinaigrette. (You might not want to use all the vinaigrette; store the extra in the fridge for a future salad!)

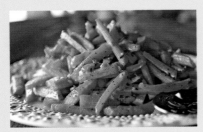

10. Serve these delectable carrots hot, warm, or at room temperature. They're lovely!

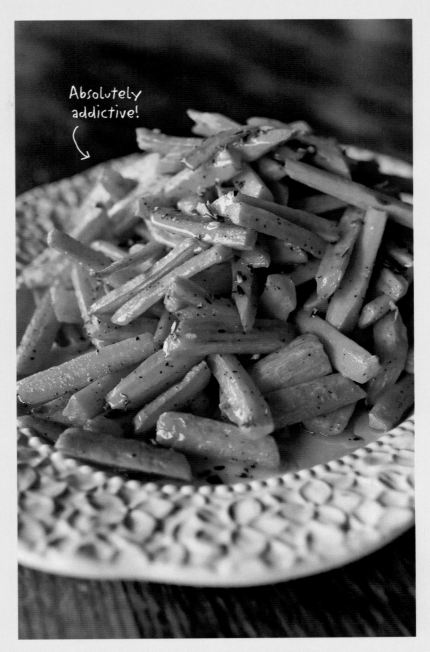

Absolutely addictive!

🄢 SERVE WITH

Italian Meatloaf (page 212)

Chicken with Mustard Cream Sauce (page 146)

Pork Chops with Wine and Roasted Garlic (page 246)

🄥 VARIATIONS

Just out of the oven, toss the carrots with ½ cup freshly grated Parmesan cheese.

Use lemon juice in the vinaigrette instead of vinegar.

Chill the finished carrots in the fridge and serve as a cold salad.

Boil or steam the carrots instead of roasting, if you prefer!

VEGGIES AND THREE DIPS

EACH DIP MAKES 2 CUPS

There's no more versatile veggie dish in the world than a bunch of fresh raw veggies with a bowl of your favorite dip. It can be a snack, an appetizer, or a side dish, and it will satisfy your need to eat something crunchy along with your need to stare at the natural beauty of the fruits of the earth.

I mean the vegetables of the earth.

Here are three of my favorite dips!

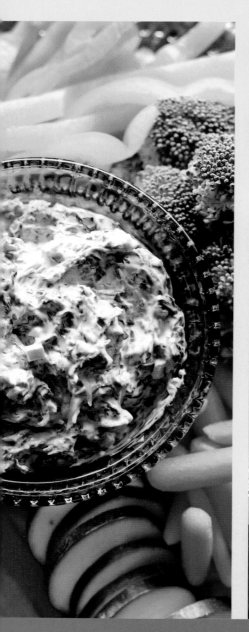
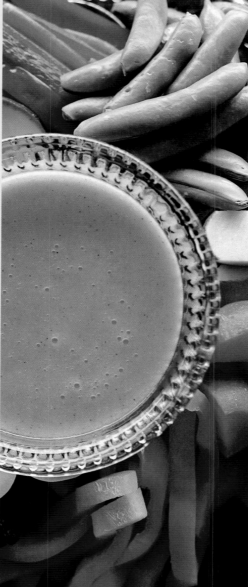
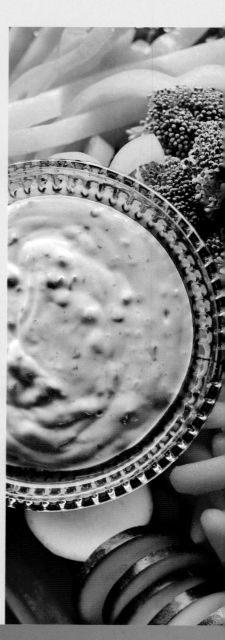

RAW VEGGIES

Cucumber slices

Baby carrots

Sugar snap peas

Bell peppers, seeded and cut into strips

Radishes, halved

SPINACH DIP

Crisp carrots, beautiful spinach . . . this lovely dip tastes like spring!

½ cup mayonnaise

1 cup sour cream

1 garlic clove, pressed

One 10-ounce package frozen spinach, thawed and squeezed between paper towels to remove excess moisture

1 carrot, finely diced

3 green onions, chopped

Juice of ½ lemon

Kosher salt and black pepper to taste

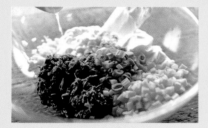

1. Combine all the ingredients in a bowl.

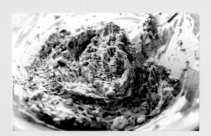

2. Mix everything together, then cover the bowl and refrigerate for 2 hours to allow the flavors to meld.

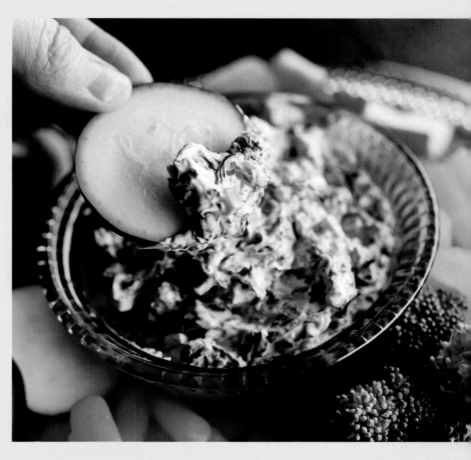

HONEY MUSTARD DIP

Tangy and irresistible, this beautifully golden dip is as delicious with veggies as it is with fries.

½ cup mayonnaise

½ cup honey

⅓ cup mustard
(yellow, Dijon, country)

1 teaspoon paprika

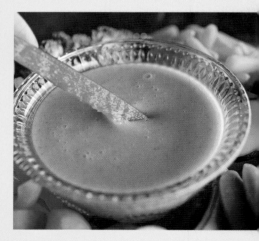

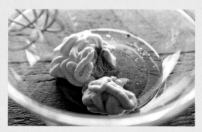

1. Combine all the ingredients in a bowl . . .

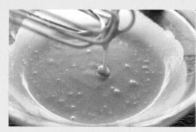

2. And whisk them together until smooth.

CREAMY CHIPOTLE DIP

When I'm in the mood for a veggie dip with a nice kick, I take about 90 seconds out of my day and whip up this spicy wonder.

2 cups mayonnaise (or 1 cup mayo plus 1 cup sour cream)

2 to 3 chipotle peppers in adobo sauce, minced

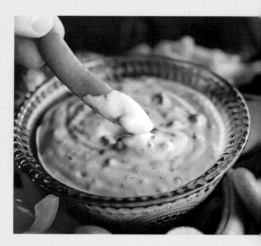

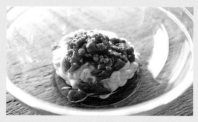

1. Place the mayo and chipotle in a bowl . . .

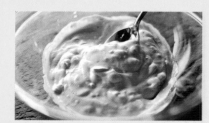

2. And stir until smooth. Add a little more adobo sauce from the chipotle can if you'd like more spice.

Ⓥ VARIATIONS

You may substitute plain nonfat Greek yogurt for the mayonnaise and/or sour cream in the dips.

Use any of the dips as a sandwich or panini spread.

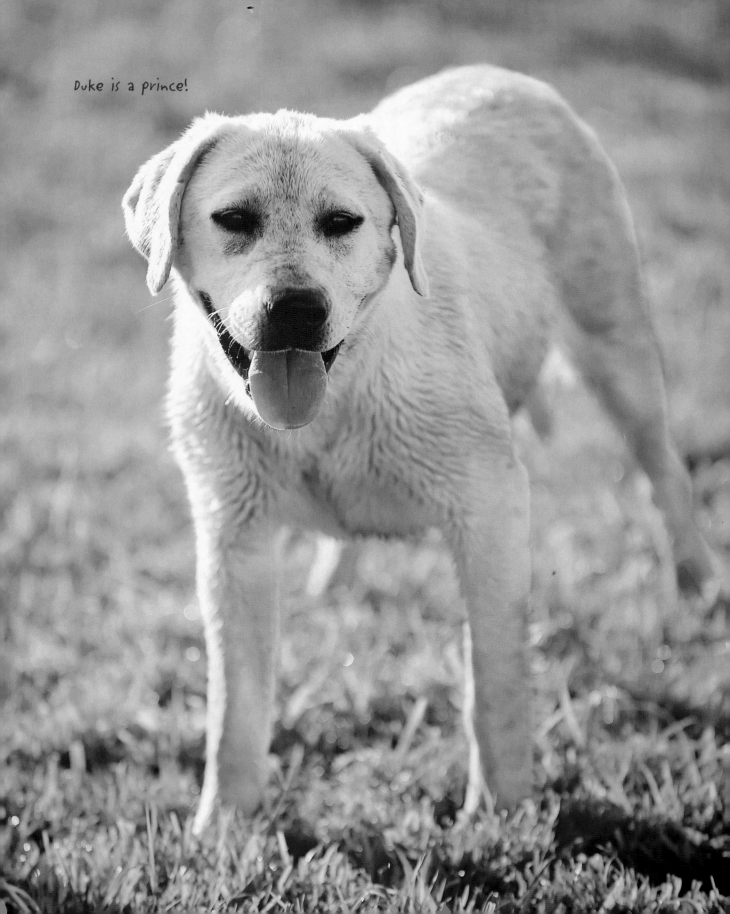

Duke is a prince!

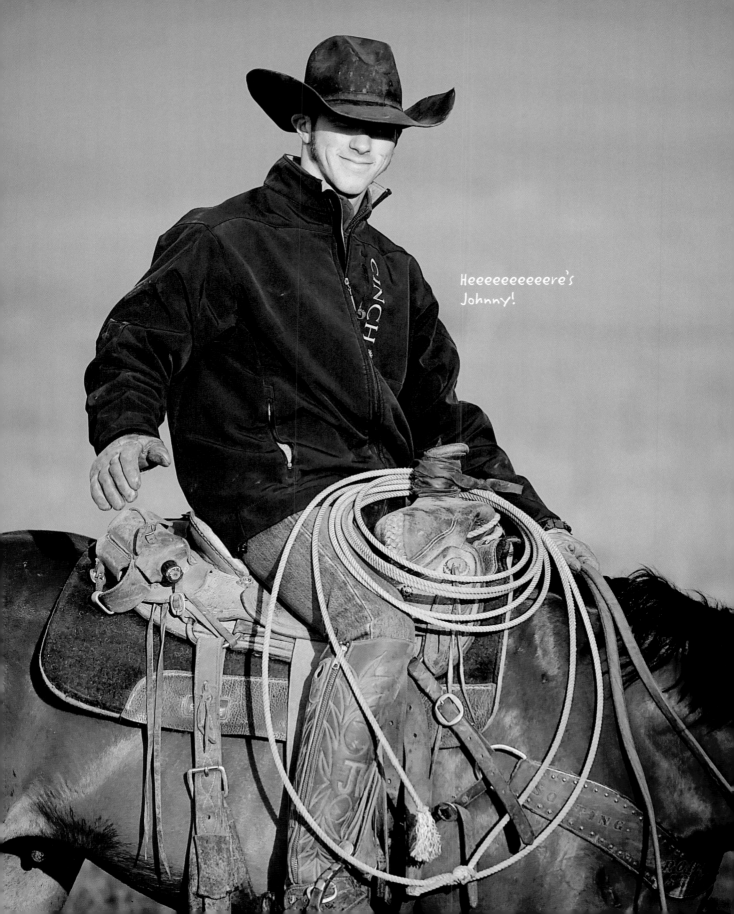

Heeeeeeeeeere's
Johnny!

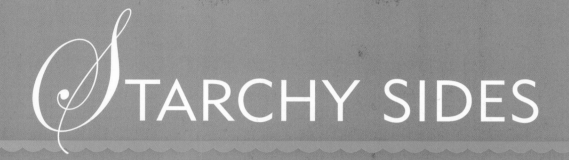

$\mathcal{S}$TARCHY SIDES

In the meat-and-potatoes world in which I (happily, I should state) reside, a mere baked potato won't always do. The more standby potato recipes I can have at the ready, the better, and in this section, you'll find some seriously good ones. But the fun doesn't stop there: I also include soul-satisfying rice, noodle, and bread recipes—all guaranteed to make you stop, close your eyes, and go "yesssssssss."

SWEET POTATO FRIES

MAKES 6 TO 8 SERVINGS

Sweet potato fries are both naughty and nice, and if you bake them in the oven, they're easy, too!

Naughty, nice, and easy.

Never mind! I'm not going to go there. (See? I can be mature sometimes.)

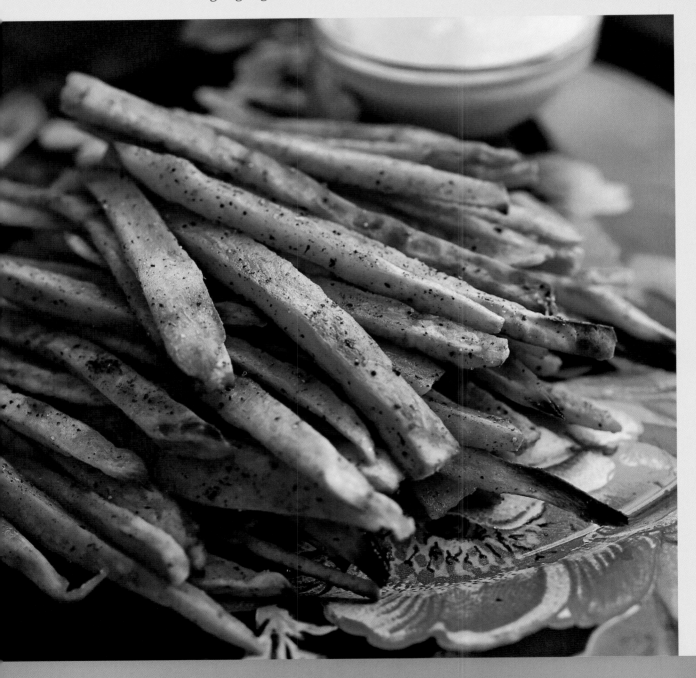

6 large sweet potatoes

½ cup (1 stick) butter

2 garlic cloves, pressed or minced

**1 teaspoon seasoned salt
or kosher salt**

1 teaspoon chili powder

½ teaspoon black pepper

½ cup mayonnaise

2 tablespoons sriracha or ketchup

Kosher salt, for sprinkling

1. Preheat the oven to 450°F.

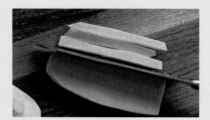

2. Peel the sweet potatoes, then slice them into wide strips. Stack the strips and slice them into thin sticks.

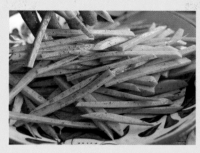

5. Pour the butter mixture over the sweet potatoes and use your hands to toss them to coat.

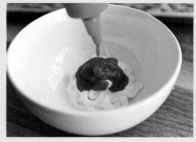

8. To make a quick dipping sauce, combine the mayonnaise and sriracha (or ketchup) and stir to combine.

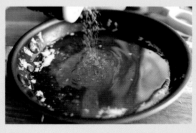

3. Place all the potatoes in a large bowl.

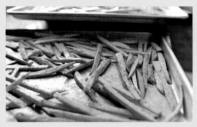

6. Place them on two rimmed baking sheets to avoid crowding . . .

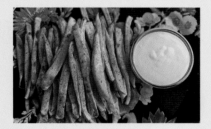

9. Pile the fries on a plate next to the sauce and go for it!

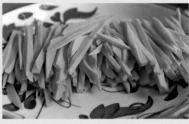

4. Melt the butter in a small skillet or saucepan over medium-low heat, then use a spoon to skim off the foam. Add the garlic, seasoned salt, chili powder, and pepper and stir it all together.

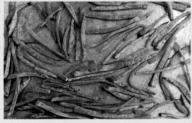

7. And bake them for 15 to 17 minutes, shaking the pans a couple of times during baking. Let them rest on the baking sheets for 5 minutes before serving.

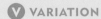 **MAKE AHEAD**

Prepare the potatoes and toss them in the butter-seasoning mixture up to 3 hours before baking. Store them in the fridge until you're ready to put them in the oven. Allow for 10 more minutes of baking time if the potatoes are cold.

V VARIATION

Toss the uncooked fries in 2 tablespoons cornstarch for slightly crisper fries.

STOVETOP MASHED POTATOES

MAKES 6 TO 8 SERVINGS

Making mashed potatoes doesn't have to be a big production! Just boil some potatoes, then drain them. While they're sitting in the colander, make a creamy, buttery concoction in the same pan, throw the potatoes back in, and mash away! Peel the potatoes or don't peel them, wear high heels or don't . . . it's all up to you!

3 pounds Yukon gold potatoes, peeled or unpeeled and scrubbed clean (your preference!)

1 cup whole milk

½ cup (1 stick) butter

¼ cup heavy cream, more to taste

Kosher salt and black pepper to taste

4 ounces cream cheese

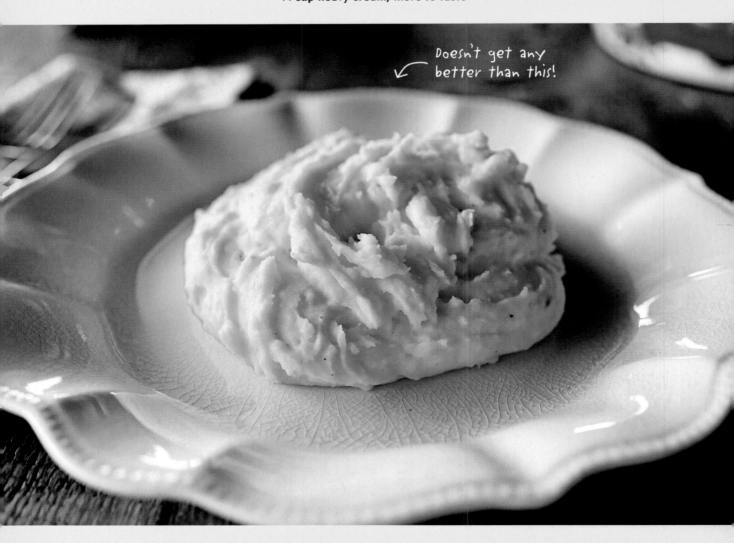

Doesn't get any better than this!

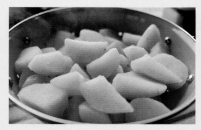

1. Cut the potatoes into wedges. In a pot or large saucepan, boil them in water over medium-high heat until fork-tender, about 25 minutes. Pour them into a colander to drain them, then set aside.

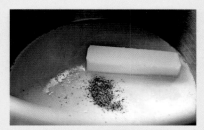

2. Return the same pot to the stovetop over medium heat and add the milk, butter, cream, and salt and pepper to taste.

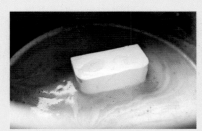

3. Stir to heat the milk mixture and melt the butter, then add the cream cheese and stir as it melts.

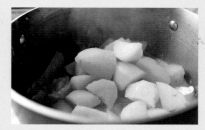

4. When the mixture is melted and creamy, throw in the potatoes and turn off the heat . . .

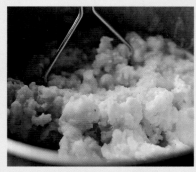

5. And use a potato masher . . .

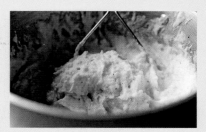

6. To mash them until they're totally smooth. (You can also use a potato ricer!) Put the lid on the pan and keep warm, splashing in a couple tablespoons of cream if you need to reheat them.

S SERVE WITH

Salisbury Steak (page 216)

Chicken Cacciatore (page 219)

Pan-Fried Pork Chops (page 156)

BBQ Meatballs (page 108)

Chicken with Mustard Cream Sauce (page 146)

Italian Meatloaf (page 212)

Oven-Barbecued Chicken (page 234)

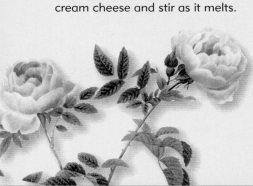

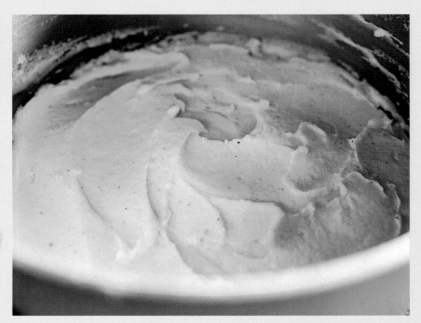

BREAKFAST POTATOES

MAKES 8 SERVINGS

I call these "Breakfast Potatoes," but they make a really nice potato side dish whether it's morning, noon, or night. Serve them next to grilled steak, grilled chicken, or (if you wanna be really wacky) rolled up inside a breakfast burrito with scrambled eggs and cheese! They're versatile and very, very good. A definite staple in our household.

5 pounds red potatoes

1 large onion, cut into chunks

2 green bell peppers, seeded and coarsely chopped

2 red bell peppers, seeded and coarsely chopped

4 garlic cloves, minced

¼ cup olive oil

4 tablespoons (½ stick) butter, melted

1 teaspoon seasoned salt

½ teaspoon cayenne pepper

Kosher salt and black pepper to taste

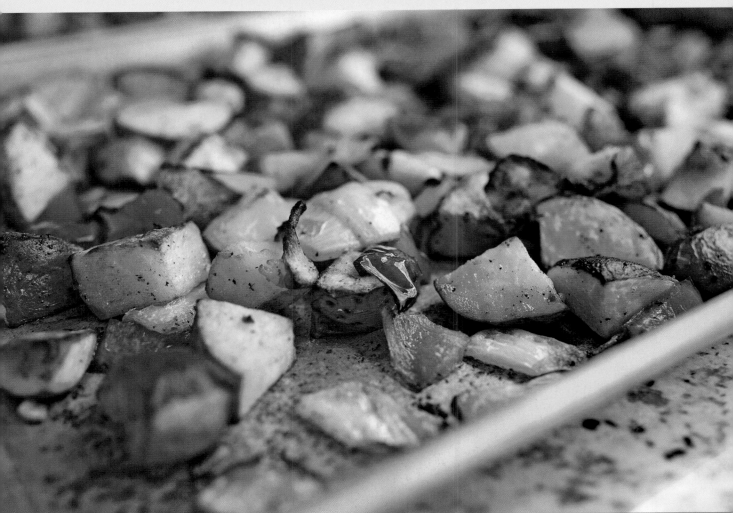

1. Preheat the oven to 425°F.

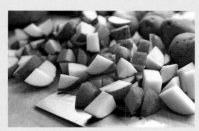

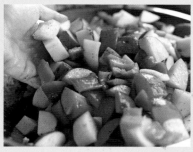

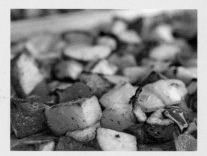

2. Scrub the potatoes clean, then chop them into large chunks or wedges.

6. Use your hands to mix everything together . . .

9. And roast for 15 to 20 minutes more, tossing twice again. Sprinkle with a little more kosher salt and black pepper before serving.

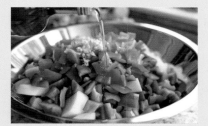

3. Pile the potatoes in a large bowl with the onion, bell peppers, and garlic, then drizzle in the olive oil . . .

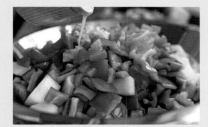

4. And the melted butter.

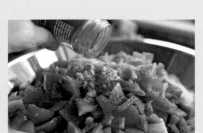

5. Sprinkle on the seasoned salt, cayenne, and kosher salt and black pepper to taste.

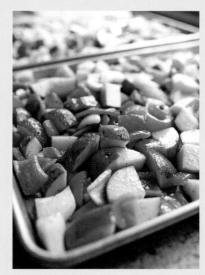

7. Then spread the mixture in an even layer on two rimmed baking sheets.

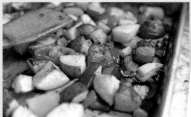

8. Roast the veggies for 20 minutes, shaking the pan to toss them twice during roasting. Raise the oven temperature to 475°F . . .

V VARIATIONS

Do a pared-down batch with only potatoes and onions.

Use 1 to 2 packets of taco seasoning in place of the other seasonings. Taco Potatoes!

Add several dashes of hot sauce to the bowl with the potato mixture.

S SERVE WITH

Ready-to-Go Grilled Chicken (page 110)

Burgers or steaks

Pan-Fried Pork Chops (page 156)

Classic Pulled Pork (page 228)

French Dip Sandwiches (page 231)

Oven-Barbecued Chicken (page 234)

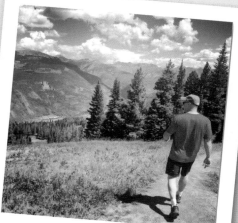

What a view! (The mountains are really nice, too.)

"SLICE-BAKED" POTATOES

MAKES 8 SERVINGS

One night, when my family and I were on a trip to Colorado, we ordered twice-baked potatoes from room service. But instead of the traditional twice-baked potatoes our souls were used to—the hollowed-out potato *halves* stuffed with luscious filling and baked—they brought a plate of curious potato *rounds,* each with a layer of melted cheese on top. We all looked at one another with panicked expressions. What were these unusually diminutive discs? Who would mess with the simple beauty of a traditional twice-baked potato? *What has happened here in Colorado,* we thought? When did everything go so horribly wrong?

(I suggested under my breath that it was all the marywanna. But Ladd and the kids didn't hear me.)

After closer examination—i.e., after we all got over our initial trauma and took our first bites—we discovered that they were simply reconstructed little twice-baked potatoes; but instead of potato halves, they used potato slices. A simple and clever twist on the twice-baked theme!

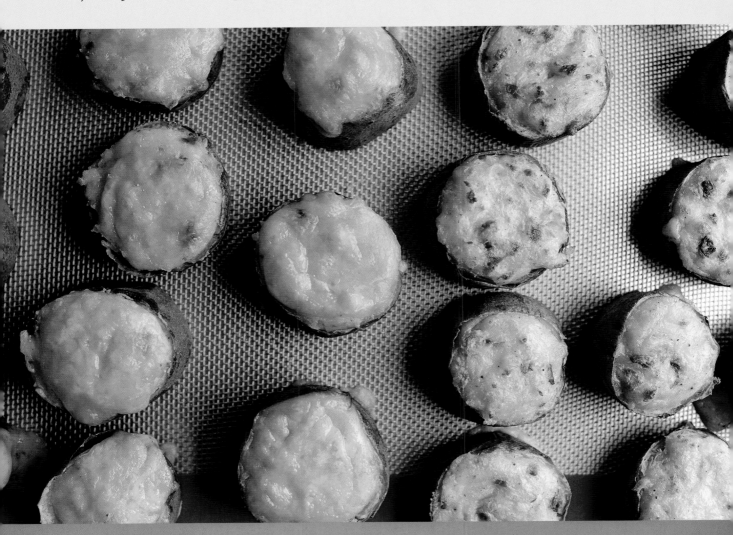

8 medium russet potatoes, scrubbed clean

½ cup (1 stick) butter, softened

¾ cup sour cream

¼ cup milk

6 thin slices bacon, fried crisp and chopped

1 teaspoon seasoned salt

Kosher salt and black pepper to taste

¾ cup grated Cheddar-Jack cheese, plus more for topping

1. Preheat the oven to 375°F.

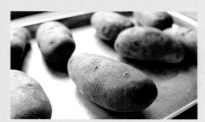

2. Place the potatoes on a baking sheet and bake them for 45 to 50 minutes, until the potatoes are tender and the skins are slightly crisp. Remove them from the oven and let them cool slightly.

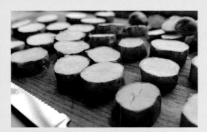

3. Cut off the very ends of the potatoes, then cut the potatoes crosswise into 3 or 4 equal slices.

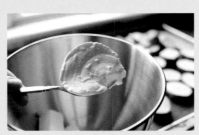

4. Place the butter and sour cream in the bowl of an electric mixer. Set aside.

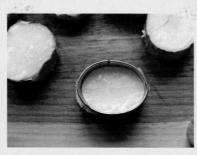

5. Grab a round biscuit cutter slightly smaller than the potato rounds (you might have to use two different sizes) and use it to cut out the center of each round . . .

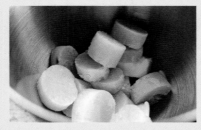

6. And as you go, drop the center potato pieces into the mixer bowl with the butter and sour cream.

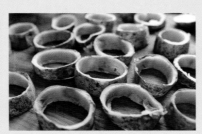

7. Keep going until you've cut them all out! Set the cut-out skins aside.

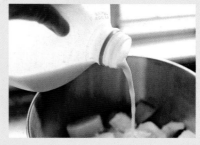

8. Pour the milk into the mixer bowl . . .

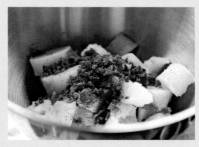

9. Add the bacon, seasoned salt, kosher salt, and pepper . . .

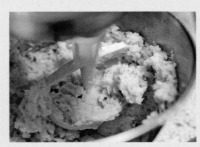

10. And mix on low using the paddle attachment until the mixture is mostly smooth (small lumps are fine). You can also do this by hand using a potato masher; just keep going until it's smooth.

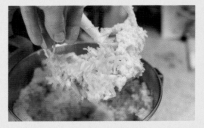

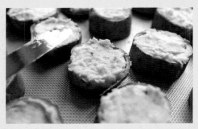

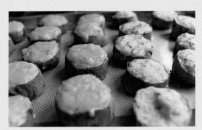

11. Finally, add ½ cup of the cheese and mix it in gently.

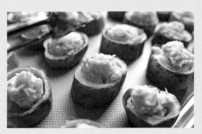

12. Place the cut-out skins on two baking sheets lined with baking mats or parchment paper. Use a scoop or spoon to fill each skin with the potato mixture . . .

13. Then use a knife or spatula to smooth the tops. (You can slightly overfill the skins; they'll shrink a little bit as they bake.)

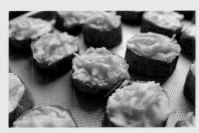

14. Top some with extra cheese and leave some plain, according to your taste . . .

15. And bake them for 8 minutes, or until the cheese has melted. Turn on the broiler and broil the slices for 2 to 3 minutes, or until the cheese is bubbling, watching carefully so they don't burn. Remove them from the oven and let them sit on the baking sheet for 10 minutes, then remove them with a spatula and serve. (Note: The filling will be soft.)

Ⓜ MAKE AHEAD

Make these well in advance, then flash freeze on a baking sheet and transfer to large zipper bags. Remove from the freezer, preheat the oven to 375°F, and bake for 20 to 25 minutes, or until hot.

Ⓥ VARIATIONS

Do a pared-down version with just potato, butter, and seasoning in the potato mixture.

Ⓢ SERVE WITH

Ready-to-Go Grilled Chicken (page 110)

Burgers or steaks

Pan-Fried Pork Chops (page 156)

Classic Pulled Pork (page 228)

French Dip Sandwiches (page 231)

Oven-Barbecued Chicken (page 234)

Green salad and a glass of wine!

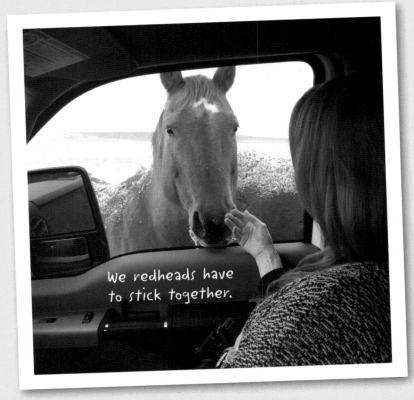

We redheads have to stick together.

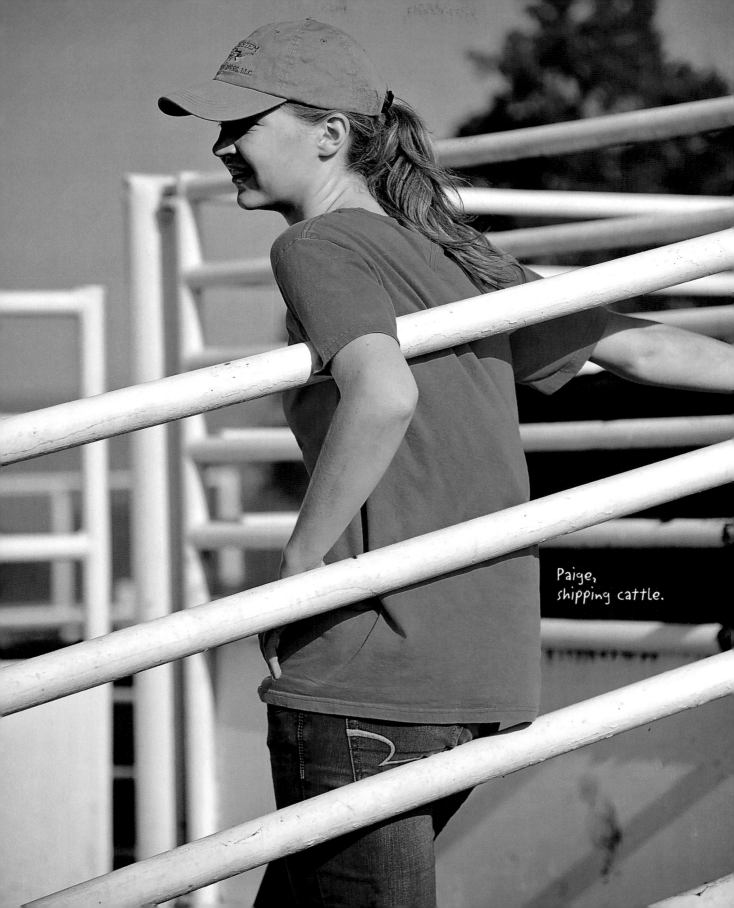

Paige,
shipping cattle.

THIN FRIES

MAKES 6 TO 8 SERVINGS

My entire family is addicted to these super-thin fries, and I don't remember an instance in which a single fry was left. And usually when I plan on making them, I try not to let the word get out until the last batch is being fried—otherwise they disappear sooner than I can get them on the table!

Important: Please be careful when frying with hot oil. Keep the pot on the back burner so little kiddos won't get hurt.

6 large russet potatoes
Vegetable or peanut oil for frying
Sea salt

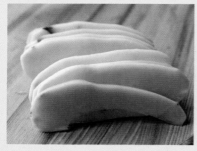

1. Peel and rinse the potatoes, then cut them into sticks by carefully slicing the potato into 5 or 6 thin slabs . . .

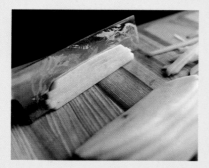

2. Then stacking a few pieces at a time and slicing them into thin sticks.

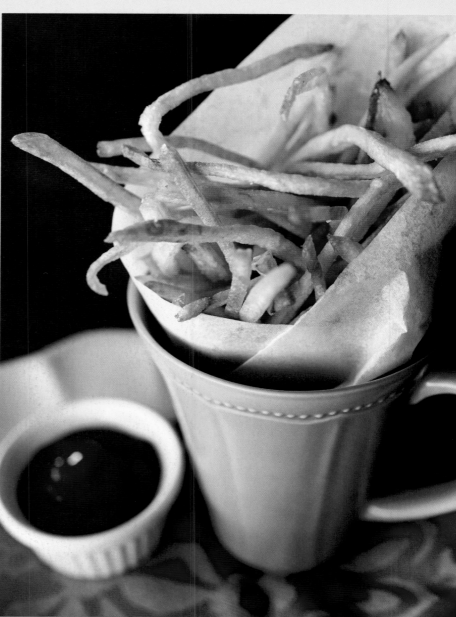

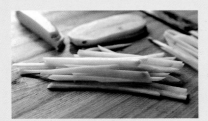

3. Take your time to get them nice and thin!

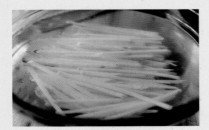

4. Place the fries in a large bowl and cover them with cold water. Swish them around to remove the extra starch, then pour off the starchy water and replace it with fresh. Do this once more, covering with fresh water and setting them aside to soak for 2 to 3 hours. (You can also stick them in the fridge, covered with plastic wrap, and let them soak for up to 3 days.)

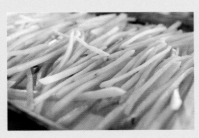

5. When you're ready to make the fries, drain off the water and lay them on baking sheets lined with paper towels. Blot them with more paper towels to dry them as much as you can. Any water left on them will make the hot oil splatter!

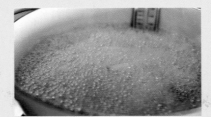

6. Heat a few inches of oil in a heavy pot to 300°F (use a deep-fry thermometer to make sure the temperature is accurate). In three or four batches, use tongs to place a small number of fries into the oil. Fry until the potatoes are soft but not at all starting to brown, about 2 minutes per batch.

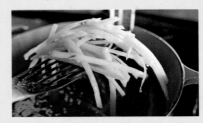

7. Remove each batch . . .

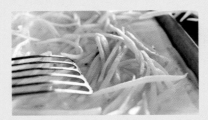

8. And drain them on new/dry paper towels.

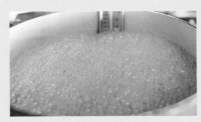

9. When all the potatoes have had their initial frying, turn up the heat until the oil reaches 400°F. When the oil's hot, start frying the potatoes in batches again . . .

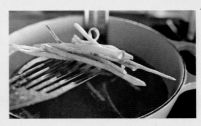

10. This time cooking them until they're golden and slightly crisp.

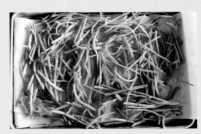

11. Remove them from the oil and drain them on new paper towels.

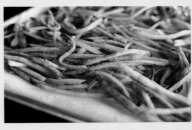

12. Sprinkle them generously with sea salt and dive in!

Ⓥ VARIATIONS

Top with grated Parmesan and minced parsley for a super-decadent treat.

Ⓢ SERVE WITH

Supreme Pizza Burgers (page 154)

Hawaiian Burgers (page 152)

Black Bean Burgers (page 149)

French Dip Sandwiches (page 231)

Pawhuska Cheesesteaks (page 269)

Any salad in the Salad for Dinner chapter (hee hee)

RICE PILAF

MAKES 8 TO 10 SERVINGS

The classic rice side dish that's perfect for any occasion.

2 tablespoons butter

1 medium onion, finely diced

2 celery stalks, finely diced

2 carrots, finely diced

½ cup dry white wine (or substitute chicken or vegetable broth)

1 bay leaf

2 cups uncooked long-grain white rice

4 cups low-sodium chicken or vegetable broth

Kosher salt and black pepper to taste

Minced fresh parsley, for garnish

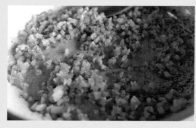

1. Melt the butter in a large skillet over medium heat. Add the onion, celery, and carrots and sauté until they start to soften, about 4 minutes.

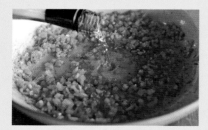

2. Pour in the wine . . .

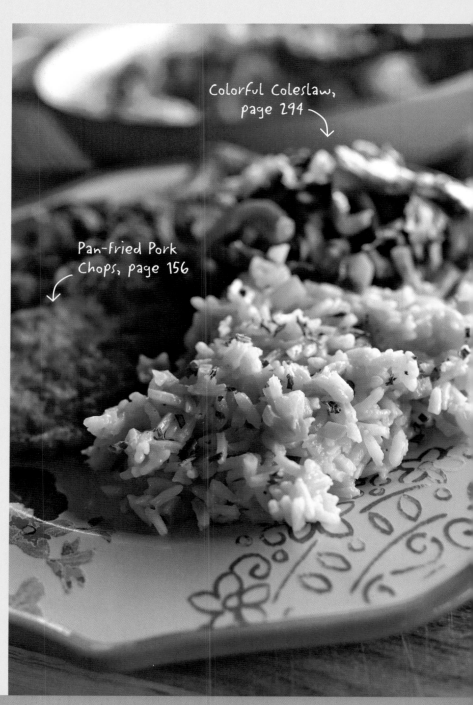

Colorful Coleslaw, page 294

Pan-fried Pork Chops, page 156

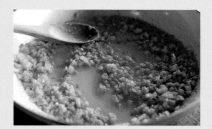

3. And stir and cook until the liquid has reduced by about half.

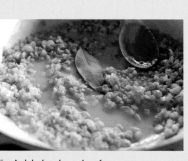

4. Add the bay leaf . . .

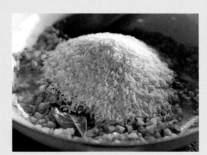

5. Along with the rice . . .

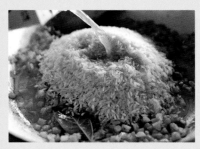

6. And the broth and salt and pepper to taste.

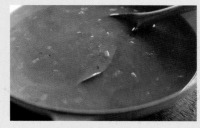

7. Reduce the heat to low, cover the pot, and let the rice simmer for 18 to 20 minutes . . .

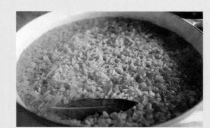

8. Until the liquid has been absorbed and the rice is perfectly cooked! Turn off the heat . . .

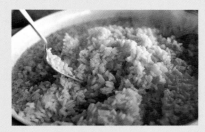

9. And use a fork to lightly fluff the rice. Remove the bay leaf.

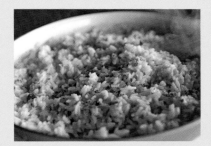

10. Sprinkle with parsley . . .

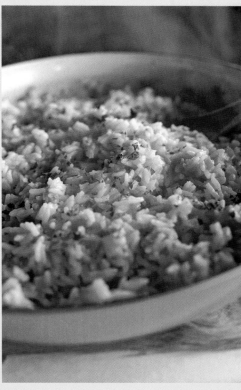

11. And serve!

Ⓥ VARIATIONS

Add any finely chopped or diced veggies to the skillet with the onion. Mushrooms are a favorite of mine!

Add finely chopped pecans or walnuts to the finished pilaf.

Stir in any chopped fresh herbs.

Ⓢ SERVE WITH

Ready-to-Go Grilled Chicken (page 110)

Italian Meatloaf (page 212)

Salisbury Steak (page 216)

Red Wine Pot Roast (page 238)

Pan-Fried Pork Chops (page 156)

Chicken with Mustard Cream Sauce (page 146)

Pork Chops with Wine and Roasted Garlic (page 246)

POLENTA

MAKES 8 TO 10 SERVINGS

Polenta is a lovely side dish, and is very similar to grits, its Southern first cousin. While grits are made from boiling ground hominy, polenta is made from boiling cornmeal. The result in both cases is grainy and naturally creamy, with the beautiful flavor of corn—and it takes on the flavor of whatever else you add to it!

Here's the basic polenta recipe I use. Hope you fall in love with this super-simple side.

6 cups no-salt chicken broth

2 cups polenta or yellow cornmeal

½ teaspoon kosher salt, more to taste

Black pepper to taste

2 tablespoons salted butter

¾ cup heavy cream, more to taste

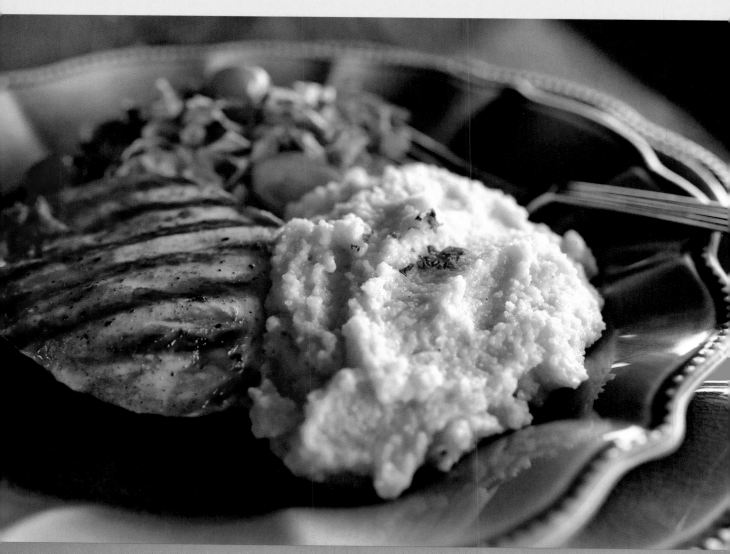

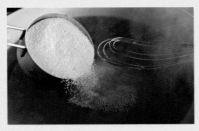

1. Bring the broth to a gentle boil in a high-sided skillet or saucepan over medium heat. Pour the polenta into the pan, whisking as you go.

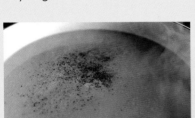

2. Add salt and pepper . . .

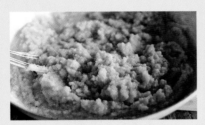

3. Then whisk the polenta slowly as it begins to absorb the liquid. Depending on whether you're using fine-ground or regular polenta, this will take anywhere from 2 to 15 minutes.

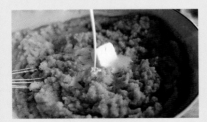

4. When three-quarters of the liquid has been absorbed, add the butter and cream . . .

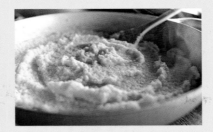

5. And stir while it finishes cooking. Taste and adjust the seasonings, and add a little more cream if you like your polenta nice and creamy. Which I do, of course.

6. Serve it with your favorite dinner recipes!

V VARIATIONS

Stir in 1 to 2 cups grated Cheddar, Fontina, or Monterey Jack cheese. (Just watch the salt content, as cheese adds a lot.)

Stir in 6 crumbled cooked bacon slices.

Stir in caramelized sliced onions or shallots. Yum!

Spread the polenta on a rimmed baking sheet and chill it for 1 hour. Cut the set polenta into squares (or circles), then panfry them in a skillet with a little olive oil over medium-high heat. Yum!

S SERVE WITH

Ready-to-Go Grilled Chicken (page 110)

Italian Meatloaf (page 212)

Pan-Fried Pork Chops (page 156)

Salisbury Steak (page 216)

Red Wine Pot Roast (page 238)

Beautiful Roasted Vegetables (page 290)

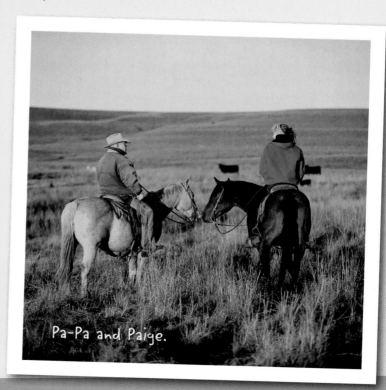

Pa-Pa and Paige.

BUTTERED PARSLEY NOODLES

MAKES 6 TO 8 SERVINGS

Any time a recipe you encounter calls for you to serve it with buttered egg noodles, do yourself a favor: Serve them with these instead. Wide, beautiful noodles are tossed with a butter-lemon-garlic-parsley mixture, and the result is just absolute perfection.

2 tablespoons butter

1 tablespoon olive oil

1 teaspoon chopped garlic

3 tablespoons minced parsley

Zest of 1 lemon

12 ounces pappardelle or other wide noodle, cooked to al dente

¼ teaspoon kosher salt, more as needed

¼ teaspoon black pepper

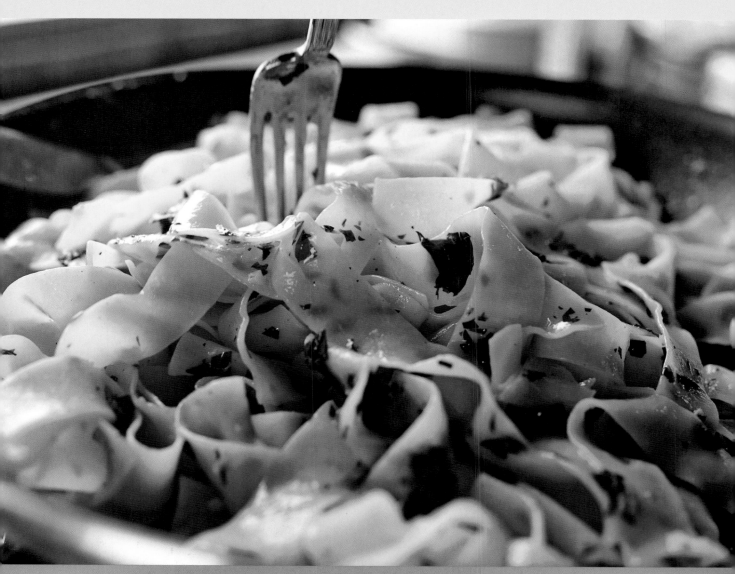

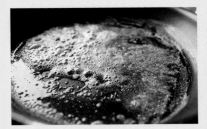

1. Heat the butter and olive oil in a large nonstick skillet over medium heat. When hot, add the garlic and stir to cook for 30 seconds, taking care not to burn it.

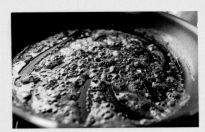

2. Add the parsley and stir it in . . .

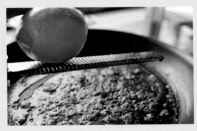

3. Then grate in the zest of the lemon and stir.

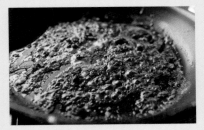

4. Cook the mixture for 1 minute more.

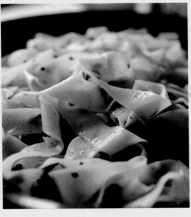

5. Throw in the pasta, sprinkle with the salt and pepper, and toss to coat the noodles. Divine!

V VARIATIONS

Use a mix of herbs along with the parsley: basil, thyme, sage, and so on.

Stir in 1 cup Parmesan shavings at the end.

Splash in a little heavy cream to make the noodle dish delicious!

S SERVE WITH

Chicken with Mustard Cream Sauce (page 146)

Pork Chops with Wine and Roasted Garlic (page 246)

Swedish Meatballs (page 106)

Salisbury Steak (page 216)

Italian Meatloaf (page 212)

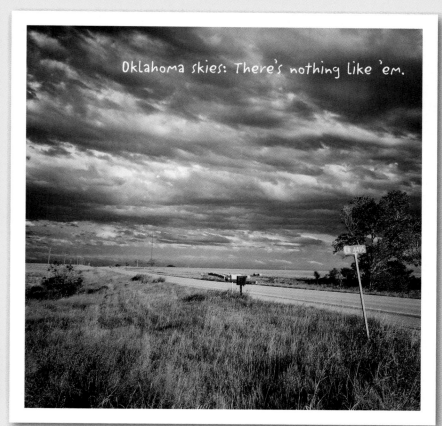

Oklahoma skies: There's nothing like 'em.

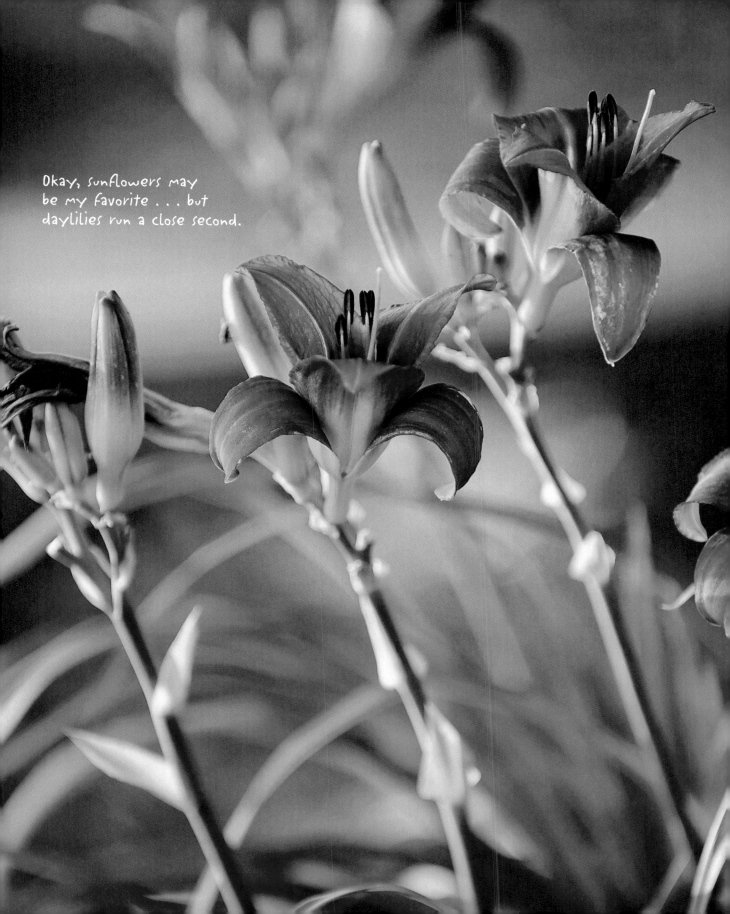

Okay, sunflowers may
be my favorite . . . but
daylilies run a close second.

RISOTTO

MAKES 8 TO 10 SERVINGS

The only downside to risotto—well, besides the fact that it can, if you eat it too regularly, establish permanent residence on your bottom—is that it takes at least thirty minutes to make, and that thirty minutes is spent over a hot stove, slowly adding liquid in increments and stirring continuously until the risotto reaches just the right level of doneness. And because risotto is best served immediately, you'll want to make sure other components of your meal are pretty much ready to go beforehand, because the risotto will take up most of your time and focus.

Oh, believe me . . . it's worth it. But risotto does require a little effort, so just make sure you plan for that. I happen to think that's part of the joy of risotto, though—the organic process of cooking and stirring and cooking and stirring . . . plus it burns an extra twelve calories, so you can have an extra grain or two!

This is how my twisted mind works.

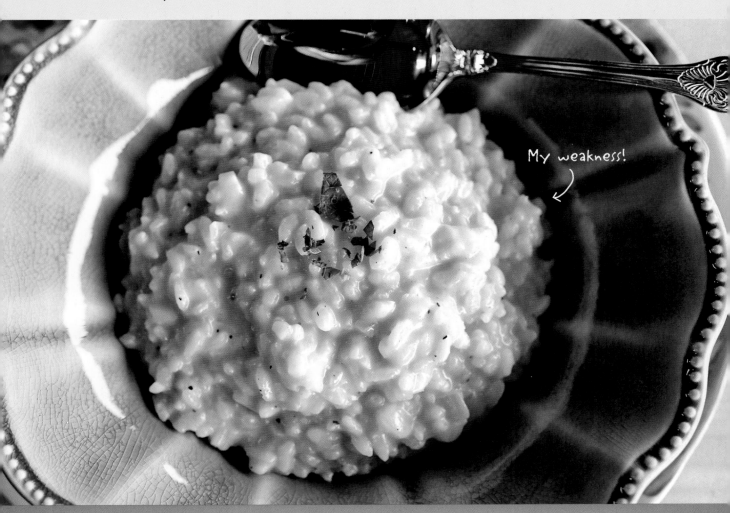

My weakness!

1 tablespoon olive oil

1 tablespoon butter

1 medium onion, diced

3 garlic cloves, minced

2 cups Arborio rice

6 cups no-salt or low-sodium chicken broth, more as needed

Kosher salt and black pepper to taste

⅓ cup heavy cream (optional)

1 cup grated Parmesan

1 tablespoon minced parsley, for garnish

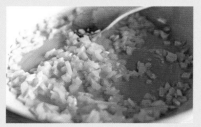

1. Heat a large skillet over medium heat and add the olive oil and butter. Add the onion and garlic and sauté for a few minutes, until the onion is translucent.

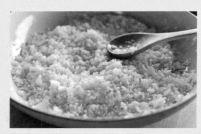

3. And stir to mix it all together.

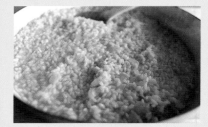

7. And again, stir the rice until it has completely absorbed the broth.

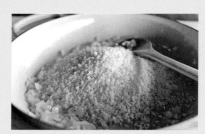

2. Add the rice . . .

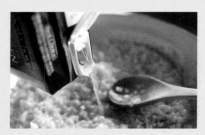

4. Add 1 cup of the broth . . .

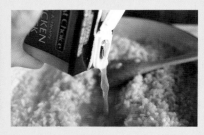

8. Continue this process of adding broth . . .

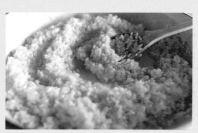

5. And stir, letting the rice absorb the broth completely.

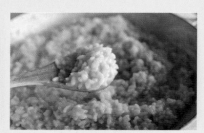

9. And stirring while the rice absorbs it until the rice is perfectly cooked and creamy. It should have a tiny bit of a bite to it but be mostly tender (if you feel it needs one or two more additions of broth to achieve the right consistency, go ahead and add extra). Add salt and pepper to taste at this stage.

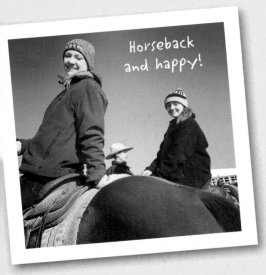

Horseback and happy!

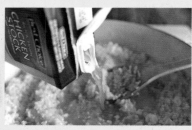

6. Repeat with another cup of broth . . .

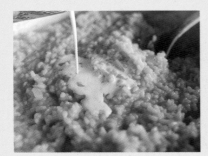

10. Now, you can leave it as is, but I like to add a little cream. It's the kind of gal I am.

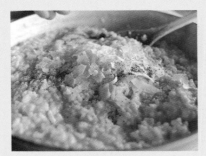

11. Add the Parmesan and a little extra pepper . . .

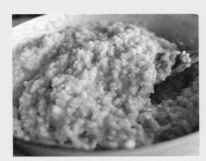

12. And stir it in.

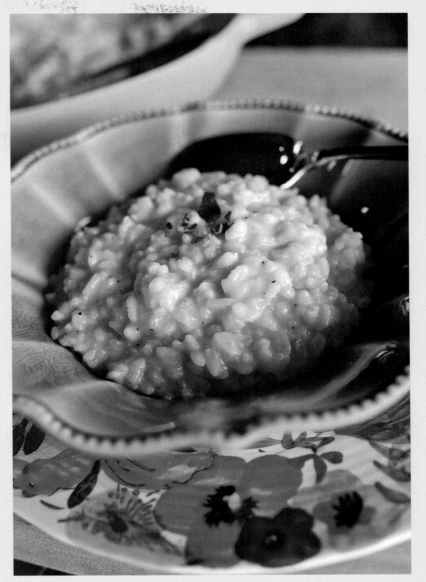

13. And add a little garnish of parsley. It's magical. Wonderful. Gorgeous. Perfect.

I'll love it till the day I croak.

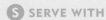

Ⓢ SERVE WITH

Ready-to-Go Grilled Chicken (page 110)

Italian Meatloaf (page 212)

Salisbury Steak (page 216)

Red Wine Pot Roast (page 238)

Ⓥ VARIATIONS

Stir in any ingredients you want to make a more elaborate side dish or a main dish risotto: sautéed mushrooms, caramelized onions, roasted veggies, sautéed shrimp, fresh herbs, prepared pesto, lemon zest, and so on.

Save leftover risotto in the fridge. Form the cold risotto into balls, then bread and deep-fry them. Delicious!

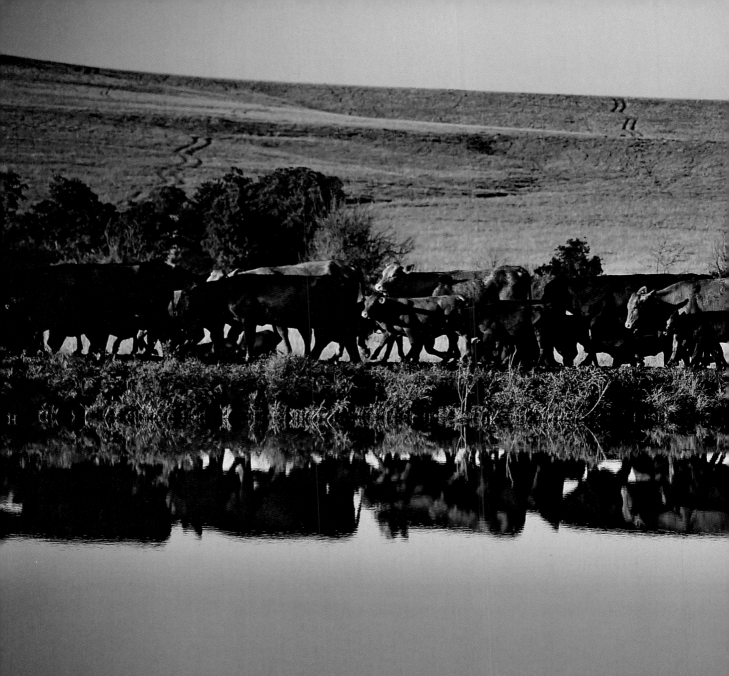

Paige, driving the cattle
across the pond dam.

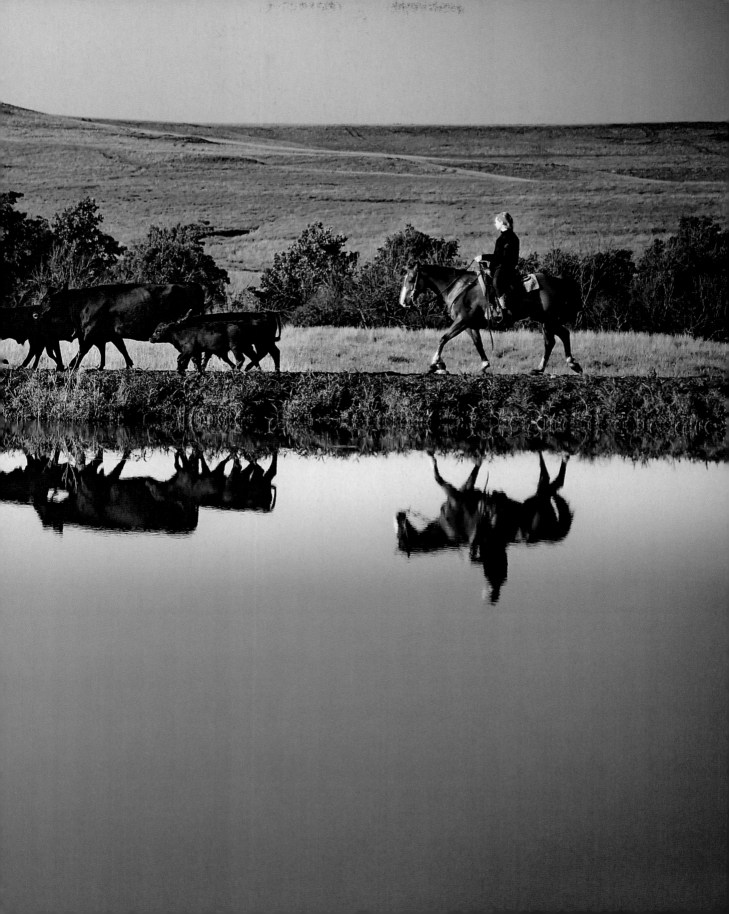

CHEESE BISCUITS

MAKES 24 BISCUITS

These cheesy, irresistible biscuits go with absolutely everything—and absolutely nothing! They're as delicious next to a bowl of chili as they are as a super-tasty afternoon snack.

I love 'em. Big time.

4 cups all-purpose flour

1 heaping tablespoon baking powder

1½ teaspoons kosher salt

½ cup (1 stick) cold unsalted butter, plus more for greasing the pans and serving

1½ cups whole milk

½ cup vegetable oil

2 large eggs

2½ cups grated Cheddar-Jack cheese

1. Preheat the oven to 375°F. Spray 24 muffin cups with baking spray.

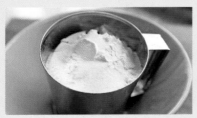

2. Place the flour, baking powder, and salt in a sifter or fine-mesh strainer . . .

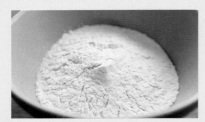

3. And sift them into a large bowl.

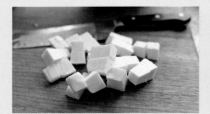

4. Cut the butter into cubes . . .

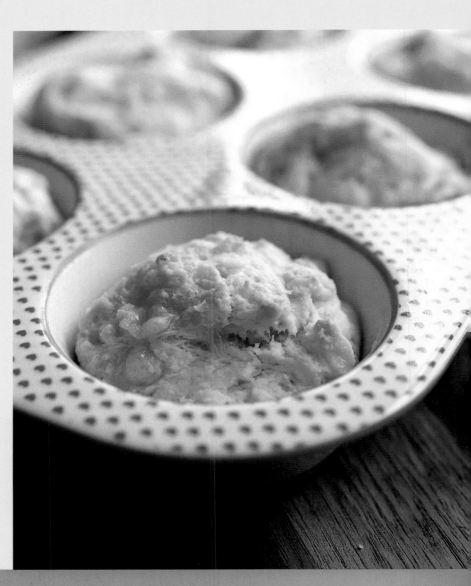

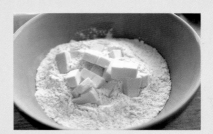

5. Add it to the bowl . . .

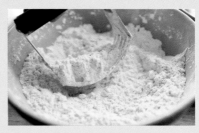

6. And use a pastry cutter to cut the butter into the dry ingredients until the mixture resembles coarse crumbs.

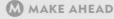

7. In a separate bowl, whisk together the milk, oil, and eggs.

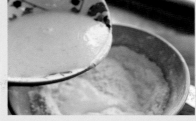

8. Pour the wet mixture into the butter-flour mixture and stir until it just comes together.

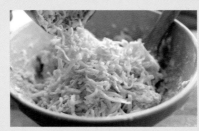

9. Add the grated cheese . . .

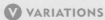
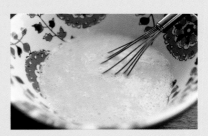

10. And stir until everything's mixed together. The mixture will be a little on the thick side.

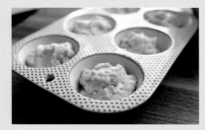

11. Drop a scant ¼ cup helping into each cup . . .

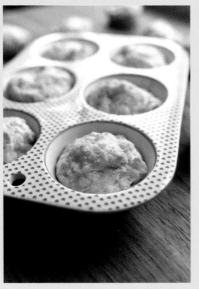
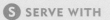

12. And bake the biscuits for 20 to 22 minutes, or until they're golden brown on top. Serve them nice and warm with a little softened butter.

Ⓜ MAKE AHEAD

Make the dough up to 3 hours in advance and store in the fridge. Allow 2 to 3 extra minutes of baking time if the dough is cold.

Ⓥ VARIATIONS

Add ½ cup diced green chiles to the wet mixture.

Add 1 diced, caramelized onion.

Add 1 teaspoon of any of the following for different flavors and heat levels: garlic powder, cayenne pepper, or black pepper.

Ⓢ SERVE WITH

Veggie Chili (page 96)

Ready-to-Go Chili Packets (page 115)

Tomato Soup (page 68)

Hamburger Soup (page 71)

Buffalo Chicken Salad (page 59)

Cobb Salad (page 50)

REFRIGERATOR ROLLS

MAKES 24 ROLLS

This age-old dinner roll recipe will completely transform the way you look at dinner rolls. The gist of it is, you whip up the dough, keep it in the fridge, then scoop out as many helpings as you need at a time and bake them. Gone are the days of making a full batch of rolls and either (a) feeling psychologically pressured to eat them all or (b) seeing them go to waste. A cowboy's wife I knew years ago used to whip up a batch of this dough at the beginning of every week, and she'd just bake two rolls at a time, every single night, until the dough was gone.

I remember that cowboy being a particularly happy man, too.

2½ teaspoons yeast
1 cup (2 sticks) butter

½ cup vegetable shortening
¼ cup sugar
1 large egg

4 cups self-rising flour (must be self-rising, not all-purpose)
1 teaspoon kosher salt

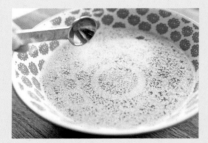

1. Fill a bowl with 2 cups very warm water and sprinkle the yeast over the surface. Let the yeast sit for 5 minutes, until totally dissolved.

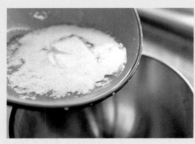

3. Pour it into the bowl of an electric mixer . . .

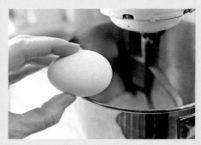

5. Crack in the egg and mix it in until combined . . .

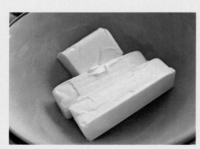

2. Combine the butter and shortening in a separate bowl and melt it in the microwave.

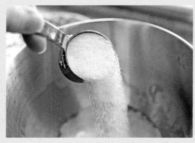

4. Along with the sugar. Mix using the paddle attachment on medium speed until smooth.

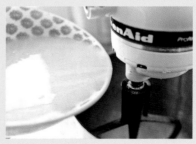

6. Then pour in the yeast-water mixture and mix until smooth.

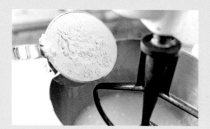

7. With the mixer on low, sprinkle in the flour . . .

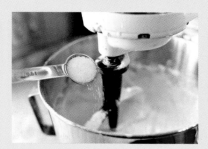

8. And the salt.

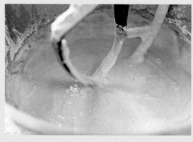

9. Mix everything together until very smooth—it will resemble a batter more than a dough at this point.

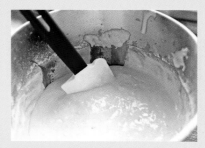

10. Scrape down the bowl and make sure it's all combined . . .

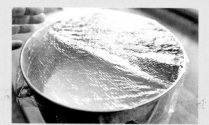

11. Then cover the bowl with plastic wrap and pop it in the fridge! (You can also transfer it to another bowl if you want to free up your mixer bowl.) Refrigerate it for at least 8 hours or up to 5 days.

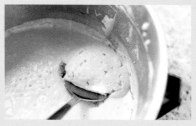

12. When you're ready for warm rolls, preheat the oven to 350°F. Scoop out batter for however many rolls you'd like . . .

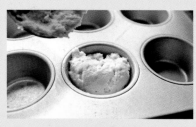

13. And drop it into greased muffin cups.

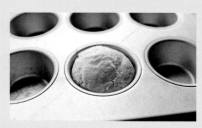

14. The rolls need to bake for 20 to 22 minutes, until golden. Bake one at a time . . .

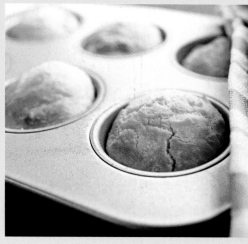

15. Or bake the whole batch!

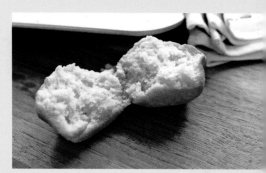

16. Light, fluffy, melt-in-your-mouth deliciousness!

M MAKE AHEAD

Whip up the dough at the beginning of the week and keep it in the fridge. You'll have hot rolls all week!

V VARIATION

Drop the dough into greased mini-muffin pans instead of standard and bake for 13 to 15 minutes.

S SERVE WITH

Any dinner recipe!

THE BREAD

MAKES 12 SERVINGS

Whenever I have a friend or family member over for dinner, they often ask the following question:

"*Are you making The Bread?*"

And I always smile and say:

"*Yes. I am making The Bread.*"

I smile because it's a foregone conclusion that I will be making The Bread.

I smile because The Bread is so darn delicious and no one who tastes it can believe it contains only two ingredients.

I smile because it's probably the easiest, simplest, most effortless thing I make.

I smile. Because butter is involved.

1 loaf French or Italian bread, any variety

1 cup (2 sticks) butter, softened

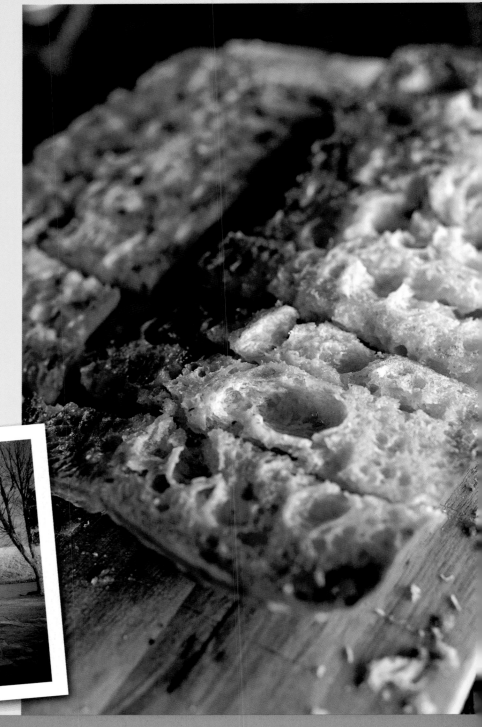

"Whee! Life is fun!"

1. Put an oven rack on the lower level and preheat the oven to 325°F.

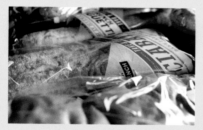

2. Pick the loaf of bread you want.

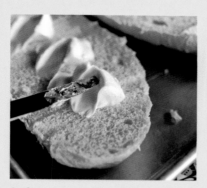

3. Slice it in half lengthwise and lay the halves, cut side up, on a rimmed baking sheet. Smear 1 stick of butter on each half. Yes, I said 1 stick per half.

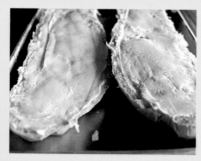

4. Then use a knife to smear it over the entire surface of the bread, covering every last inch.

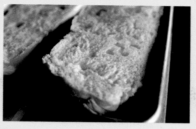

5. Bake for 5 to 10 minutes, until the butter melts and the bread has a chance to warm up . . .

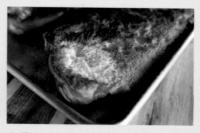

6. Then crank up the broiler, return the pan to the oven, and let it broil until the butter turns deep golden brown and almost starts to blacken. (The key is "almost!" Watch it the entire time; the second you turn your back, it will burn.)

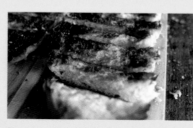

7. Immediately cut The Bread into strips . . .

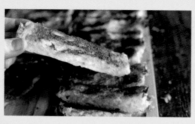

8. And enjoy every bite!

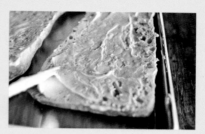

1. That was French bread, but a crustier ciabatta is also good: Smear with butter.

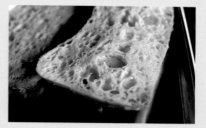

2. 325°F for 5 to 10 minutes . . .

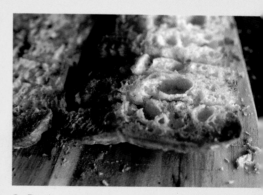

3. Broiler until deep golden and starting to burn. Cut into strips.

This is heaven!

V VARIATION

There is no variation except changing the variety of bread. The recipe is as good as it gets!

S SERVE WITH

Soups

Salads

Pastas

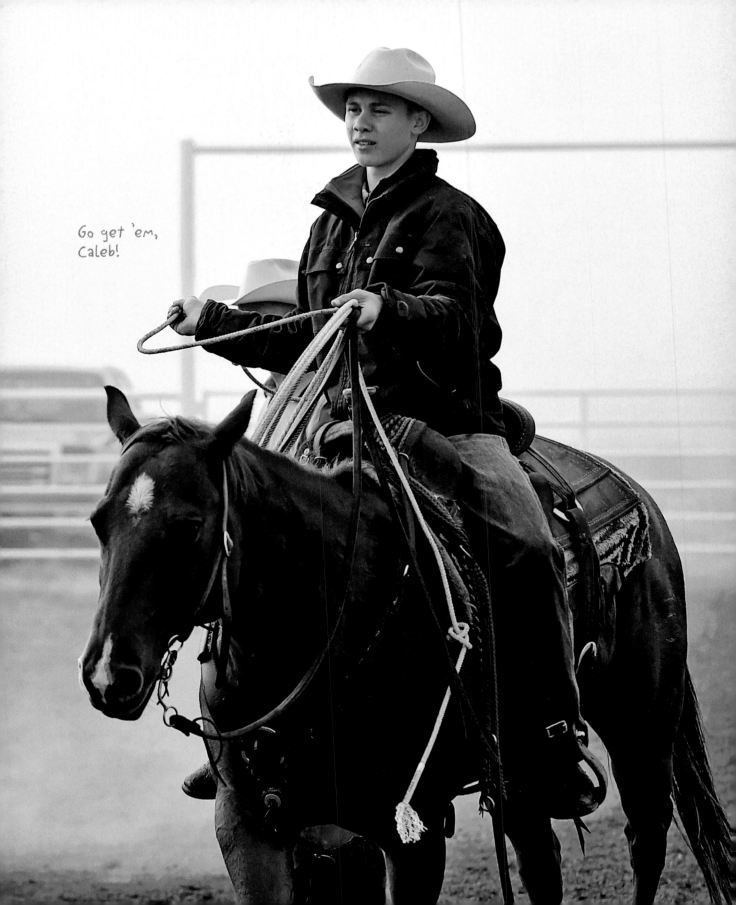

Go get 'em,
Caleb!

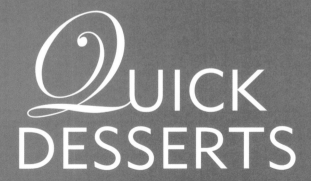

QUICK DESSERTS

I couldn't write a cookbook about dinnertime and not include the most important part! Anyone who tells you they don't crave at least a small bite of something sweet after a satisfying dinner is either (a) talkin' crazy or (b) talkin' crazy. Still, dessert doesn't have to be a seven-layer torte with artisan ganache in order to fill that role! So here are some time-tested, sweet-tooth-approved dessert recipes that hardly take any time to whip up, which allows more time for Monopoly!

VANILLA PUDDING

MAKES 6 TO 8 SERVINGS

I've always found it interesting that there's such a thing as cook-and-serve pudding you can buy in a box. I'm all for convenience items (you'll never get any judgment from me in that realm!), but making pudding from scratch on the stovetop is pretty much just as fast as using the boxed stuff. Make this basic vanilla bean version if you want to be transported back to childhood.

1½ cups sugar

¼ cornstarch

¼ teaspoon salt

3 cups whole milk

4 large egg yolks

2 vanilla beans (or 1½ teaspoons vanilla extract)

2 tablespoons salted butter

Unsweetened whipped cream, for serving (optional)

Grated semisweet chocolate, for serving (optional)

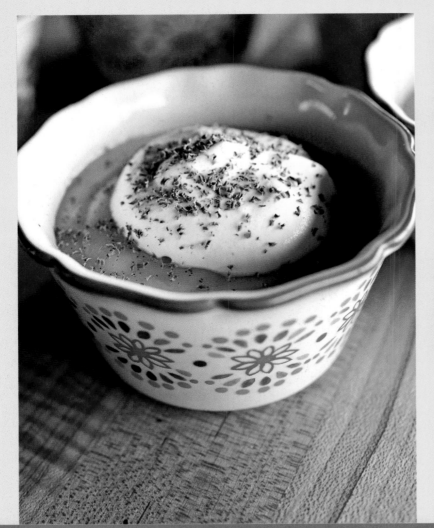

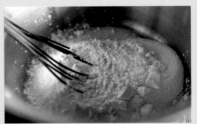

1. In a medium saucepan, gently whisk together the sugar, cornstarch, and salt. (I say "gently" because if you stir cornstarch too quickly, you'll have a cloud in your kitchen!)

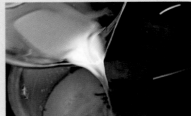

2. Pour in the milk . . .

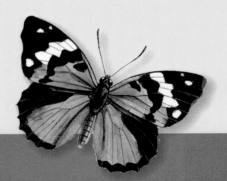

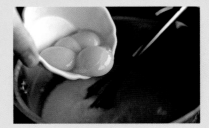

3. And the egg yolks, then whisk until it's all combined.

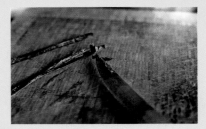

4. Using a small knife, split the vanilla beans down the middle and use the backside of the knife to scrape out the seeds.

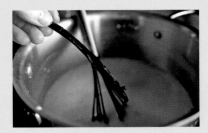

5. Place the seeds in the pan, along with the scraped-out pods (they add extra flavor!). (If you're using vanilla extract, just pour it in.)

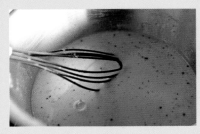

6. Turn the heat to medium and stir gently as the mixture starts to heat up.

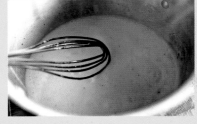

7. It will look like nothing is happening for a good 3 to 4 minutes, but before long . . .

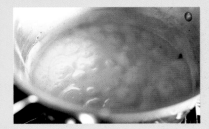

8. It will be bubbling away! Let it bubble up for about 1 minute or so (this is what makes the pudding thicken), then remove the pan from the heat.

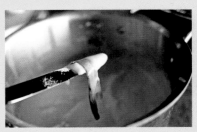

9. Fish out and discard the empty vanilla pods, then stir in the butter.

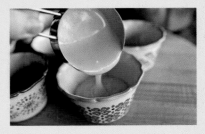

10. Then immediately transfer the pudding to individual dishes.

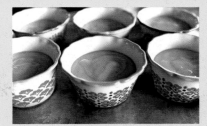

11. You may serve them warm, but I'm a cold pudding gal . . . so I cover them with plastic wrap and pop them in the fridge for a good 2 to 3 hours to chill.

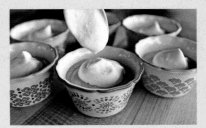

12. Once chilled, the pudding is perfect on its own, but it's even better with some unsweetened whipped cream . . .

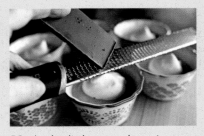

13. And a little grated semisweet chocolate.

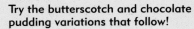

V VARIATIONS

Try the butterscotch and chocolate pudding variations that follow!

Pour the vanilla pudding into a chocolate cookie crust, then chill to make a pie.

Pour into ice pop molds and freeze. Pudding pops!

BUTTERSCOTCH PUDDING

MAKES 6 TO 8 SERVINGS

To make butterscotch pudding, just leave out the vanilla and substitute brown sugar for regular sugar!

1½ cups brown sugar

¼ cup cornstarch

½ teaspoon salt

3 cups whole milk

4 large egg yolks

2 tablespoons butter

Unsweetened whipped cream, for serving

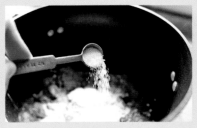

1. Follow the standard pudding procedure: In a medium saucepan, combine the brown sugar, cornstarch, and salt . . .

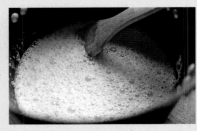

2. Add the milk and egg yolks and stir them together over medium heat . . .

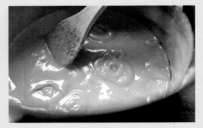

3. Cook, stirring, while the mixture thickens . . .

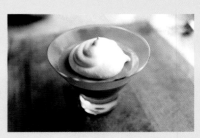

4. And stir in the butter.

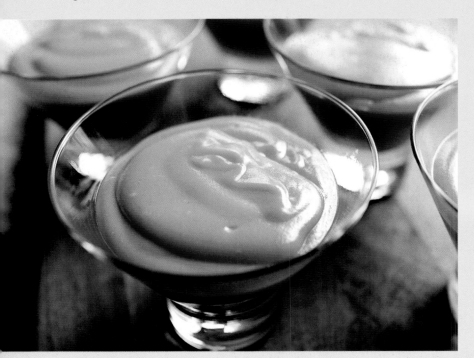

5. Spoon it into glasses or bowls, chill for at least 2 hours, and top with whipped cream. Yum!

CHOCOLATE PUDDING

MAKES 6 TO 8 SERVINGS

Turning vanilla pudding into chocolate pudding is just a matter of throwing in a little chocolate at the end! It's a favorite quick dessert in our house, so I love to whip up a batch at the beginning of the week and watch the smiles unfold.

1 recipe Vanilla Pudding (page 340)

6½ ounces bittersweet chocolate, chopped fine

Unsweetened whipped cream, for serving

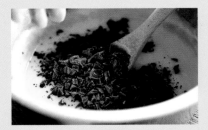

1. When the vanilla pudding is done, turn off the heat and add the chocolate.

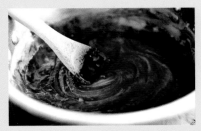

2. Stir it around . . .

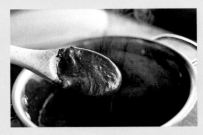

3. Until the chocolate is totally melted and the pudding is smooth and you pretty much want to dive into the saucepan!

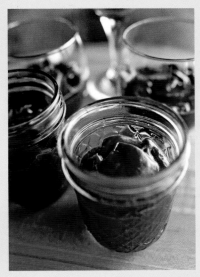

4. Transfer the pudding to jars and glasses and serve immediately, or chill it for at least 2 hours.

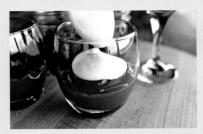

5. Top it with whipped cream, and go for it!

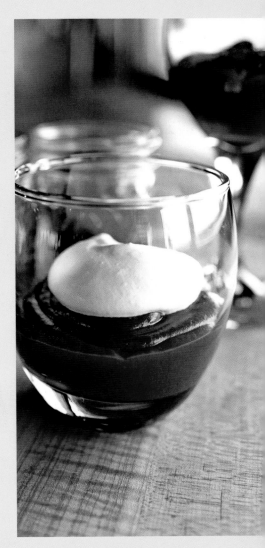

QUICK AND EASY APPLE TART

MAKES 2 TARTS, TO SERVE 6

If you want to make a very quick (well, except for the thawing time!), very easy dessert that also happens to yield impressive results, look no farther than the freezer section of your grocery store, where you can find frozen sheets of ready-made puff pastry. Puff pastry is a magical ingredient—it looks like nothing in the package, but bakes into a puffy, golden, flaky masterpiece that makes the perfect crust for fruit tarts, chocolate pastries, hors d'oeuvres . . . the list goes on.

This simple apple tart is my favorite way to use it.

1 sheet frozen puff pastry

3 Gala or Granny Smith apples, cored, halved, and very thinly sliced

¾ cup packed brown sugar

¼ teaspoon salt

Juice of half a lemon

Quick Caramel Sauce (page 350) or store-bought caramel sauce

¼ cup chopped pecans

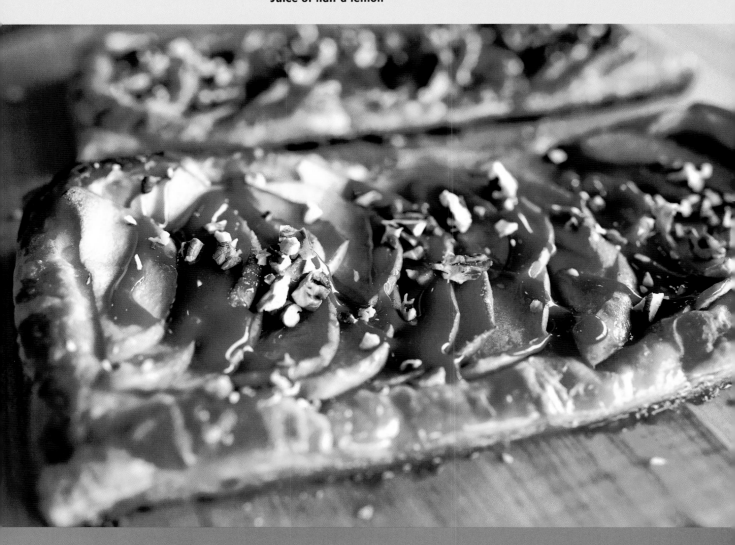

1. Set a rack in the lower third of the oven and preheat the oven to 425°F.

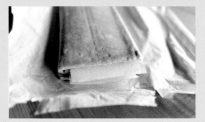

2. 24 hours before making the tart, open a package of frozen puff pastry and remove one sheet. Wrap them in separate plastic bags, return one to the freezer for a later use, and place one in the fridge to thaw.

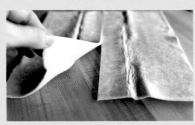

3. When the sheet is thawed, slice it in half down the middle to form two rectangles.

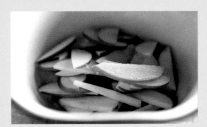

4. Add the apples to a bowl . . .

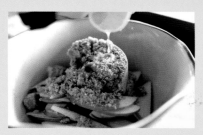

5. Then add the brown sugar, salt, and lemon juice.

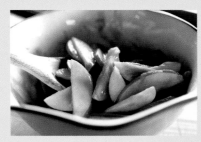

6. Stir to coat the apples in the amazing sugar mixture.

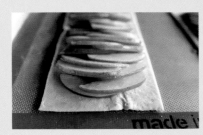

7. Lay the puff pastry rectangles sideways on a rimmed baking sheet lined with a baking mat or parchment. Arrange the apples in a line down the center of each puffed pastry rectangle, leaving at least a ¼-inch border on either side.

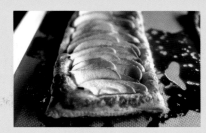

8. Bake them in the lower half of the oven for about 20 minutes, until the pastry is golden and puffed on all sides. Don't worry if a little juice escapes and browns on the pan; this is totally normal! At least for me.

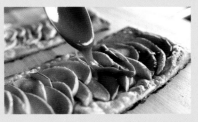

9. Remove the tarts to a cutting board and drizzle them with caramel sauce.

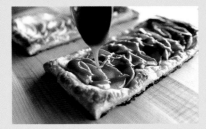

10. Go big or go home!

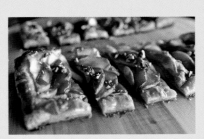

11. Sprinkle with pecans, then slice the tarts into thin pieces and serve warm.

V VARIATIONS

Use pears instead of apples.

Add a little cinnamon and nutmeg to the fruit mixture to give it some nice flavor.

S SERVE WITH

Vanilla or cinnamon ice cream!

A sprinkling of powdered sugar

Whipped cream

RASPBERRY FOOL

MAKES 8 SERVINGS

Fruit Fool is such an easy dessert to make, whether on a weeknight (you can just plop it into a chipped bowl and enjoy every bite) or for company (you can delicately spoon it into pretty glasses and call it fancy).

This traditional English dessert—similar to Eton Mess—is basically just berries and cream, but what's different about it is the presentation. I love the raspberry version, but you can use any berry you want for fool—blackberries are also lovely—and you can soak the berries in booze as I do here . . . but you don't have to.

3 cups raspberries, plus a few more for serving

¼ cup sugar

3 tablespoons raspberry liqueur (or you may just use water)

2 cups cold heavy cream

½ cup powdered sugar

8 vanilla wafers, lady fingers, or similar cookie

 VARIATIONS

Use different berries instead of raspberries: blueberries, blackberries, strawberries, and so on. Substitute different flavors or liqueur, or just use a little rum!

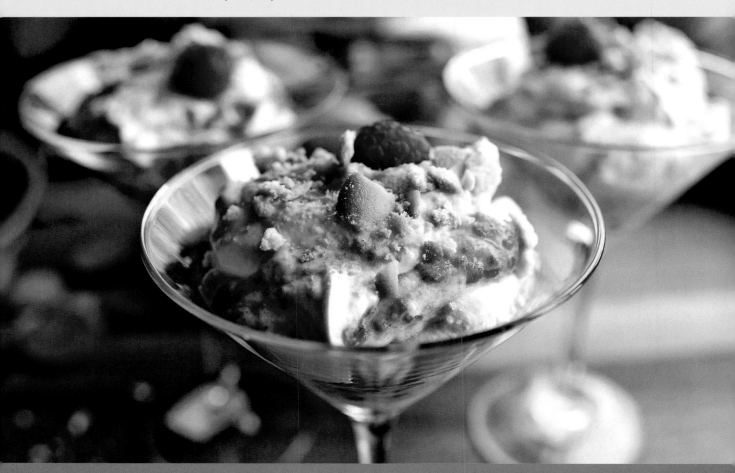

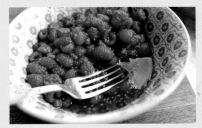

1. In a bowl, combine the raspberries, sugar, and liqueur (or water).

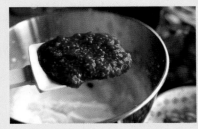

5. Back to the berries: Look at all that glorious syrup! Use a fork. . .

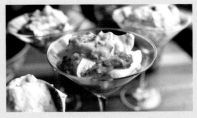

9. Add half of the remaining fruit and fold once or twice. If you want more fruit, add the rest; if not, use the remaining fruit puree as a garnish on top of the individual portions!

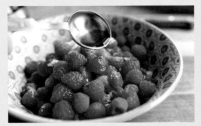

2. Stir and let the berries sit for 10 to 15 minutes.

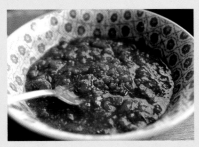

6. And mash them until you have a juicy, mushy mess.

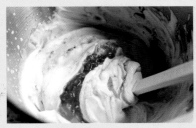

10. Spoon the mixture into pretty glasses . . .

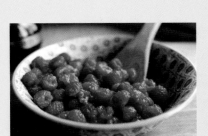

3. Meanwhile, whip the cream: In the bowl of an electric mixer, combine the heavy cream with the powdered sugar . . .

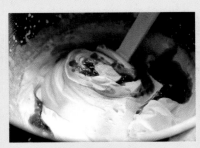

7. Spoon half the fruit into the cream . . .

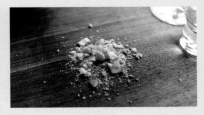

11. Crush up the cookies . . .

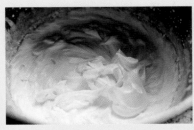

4. And whip it until soft, billowy peaks form.

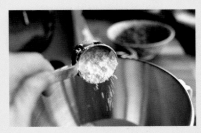

8. And fold once or twice with a rubber spatula—do not overmix! You want to see beautiful streaks of berries in the gorgeous white cream.

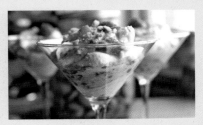

12. And sprinkle the crumbs all over the top.

 NOTE

It's best to make the fool right before serving.

HOT FUDGE SAUCE

MAKES 1 PINT

Homemade ice cream sauces are one of the most brilliant ways to dress up store-bought ice cream, and the possibilities for drippy, decadent dessert sauces are endless. I have to start with the King of All Sweet Sauces, hot fudge, because it's my favorite and because, let's face it . . . it's everyone else's favorite, too.

    Keep a jar of this in the fridge and reheat portions as you need them. You'll be sold on homemade hot fudge forever!

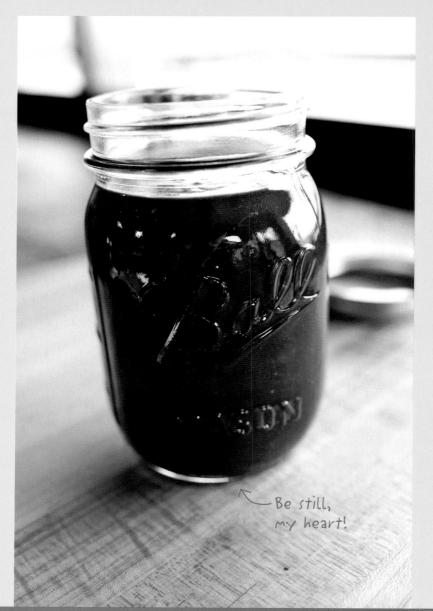

Be still, my heart!

1 cup unsweetened cocoa powder

1 cup sugar

1 cup heavy cream

1 stick (½ cup) salted butter, cut into pieces

3 teaspoons vanilla extract

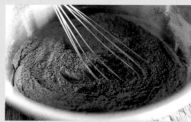

1. In a medium saucepan, gently whisk together the cocoa powder and sugar.

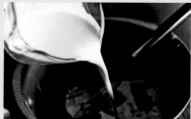

2. Whisk in the cream, then turn the heat to medium and whisk it as it warms up.

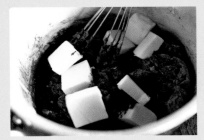

3. When the mixture starts to heat up, add the butter and stir it in to melt.

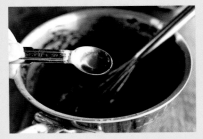

4. Then, when the mixture is nice and hot, add the vanilla and stir it to combine.

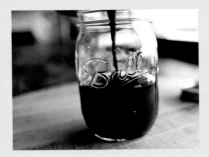

5. Let the sauce cool in the pan for 5 minutes, then transfer it to a mason jar. Store it in the fridge (it will become more solid as it chills). To serve, scoop out the amount you need and place it in a microwave-safe bowl. Heat it for 20 seconds, or until melted and warm.

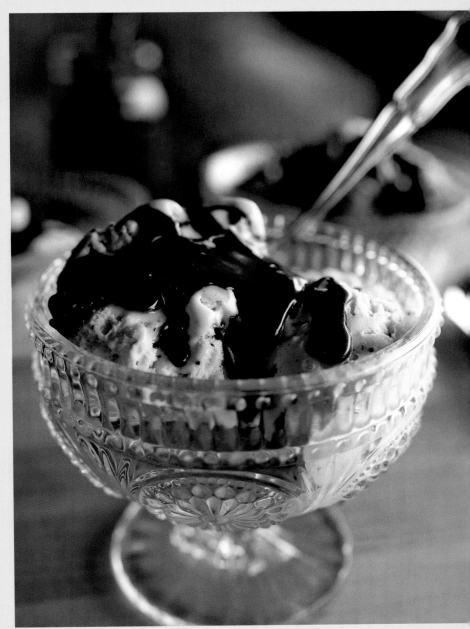

6. Drizzle over your favorite ice cream!

V VARIATIONS

Add ½ teaspoon ground cinnamon to the cocoa-sugar mixture for a nice flavor.

This sauce is very rich and chocolaty, which I love. If you'd like a little more sweetness, add an additional ¼ cup sugar to the sauce.

QUICK CARAMEL SAUCE

MAKES 1½ CUPS

I could drink caramel sauce with a straw. And I have! This is a super-simple version that's no fuss at all. You'll make it time and time again.

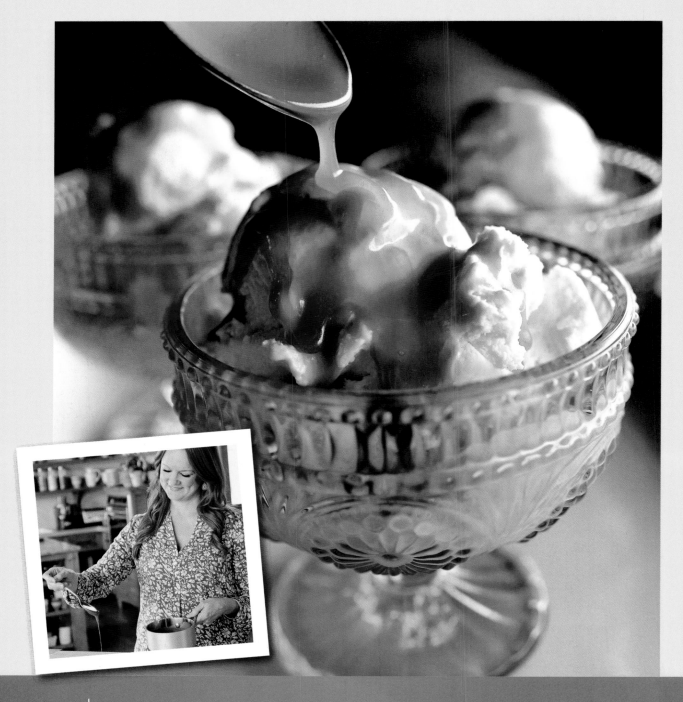

1 cup packed brown sugar
½ cup heavy cream

4 tablespoons (½ stick) butter
1 tablespoon vanilla extract

Pinch of salt

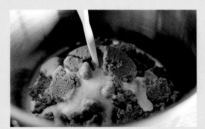

1. Combine the brown sugar and cream in a medium saucepan . . .

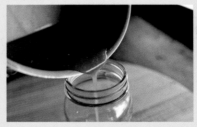

5. Let the sauce cool in the pan 5 minutes, then transfer it to a jar.

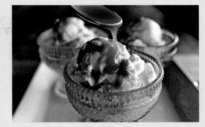

7. Drizzle it over your favorite ice cream.

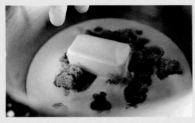

2. Then add the butter, vanilla, and salt.

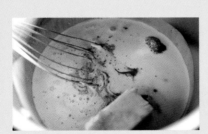

3. Stir the mixture over medium heat as it melts . . .

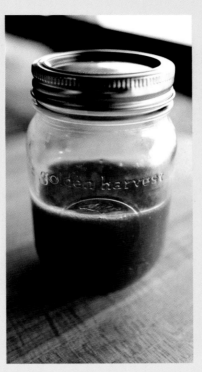

6. Store it in the fridge; it will become more solid as it chills. To serve, scoop out the amount you need and place it in a microwave-safe bowl. Heat it for 20 seconds, or until melted and warm. (Or you can serve it warm, straight out of the saucepan!)

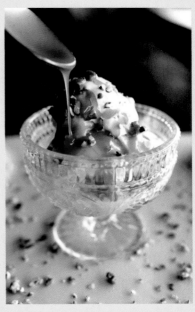

8. Add whipped cream and chopped nuts if you want to be a rebel.

Ⓥ VARIATIONS

Add the seeds from 1 vanilla bean instead of the vanilla extract if you'd like little flecks throughout.

Add a little extra salt for salted caramel sauce—try it out and taste before adding more.

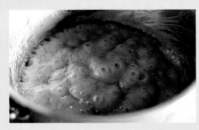

4. Then let it come to a gentle boil and bubble up for 2 to 3 minutes.

STRAWBERRY SAUCE

MAKES 1 PINT

I love ice cream. And I'm *particularly* partial to this strawberry ice cream sauce. Totally simple, extremely basic . . . and that's exactly what I love about it. This sauce is perfect over vanilla, strawberry, or chocolate ice cream . . . but it's also positively yummy over waffles, pancakes, and crepes.

2 pounds strawberries, hulled
1 cup sugar

1 teaspoon vanilla extract
Juice of ½ lemon

A couple drops of red food coloring, optional

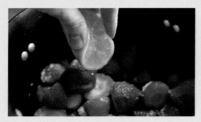

1. Place the strawberries, sugar, vanilla, and lemon juice in a medium saucepan over medium-high heat.

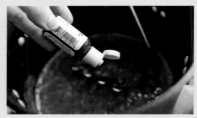

4. If you'd like to bump up the red color a bit, add a teeny bit of red food coloring!

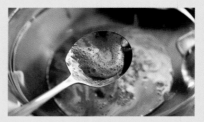

7. Skim as much foam off the sauce as you can . . .

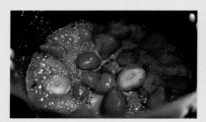

2. Bring to a gentle boil, stirring constantly, and let the strawberries cook for a good 5 minutes, or until they're very soft.

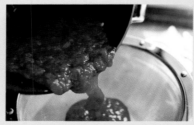

5. Pour the mixture into a fine-mesh strainer placed over a bowl.

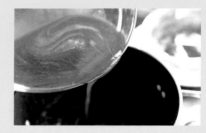

8. Then pour the skimmed sauce back into the same saucepan.

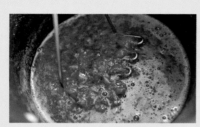

3. Turn off the heat and use a potato masher to completely smush them to smithereens.

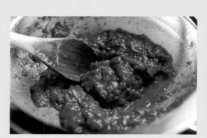

6. Use a spoon to stir the fruit so the liquid is forced through. Set the pulp aside in case you want to add some of it back to the finished sauce.

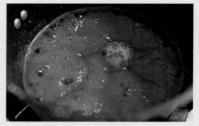

9. Bring it to a boil for 3 minutes over medium-high heat, then turn off the heat and let it cool for 5 minutes.

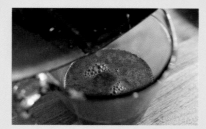

10. Pour it into a pitcher . . .

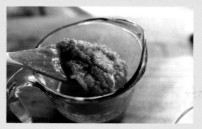

11. And to give the sauce a little texture, add in a spoonful of the pulp and stir. Store it in the fridge until you need it!

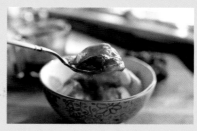

12. Serve it cold straight out of the fridge over vanilla ice cream . . . or reheat the sauce in the microwave and serve it warm!

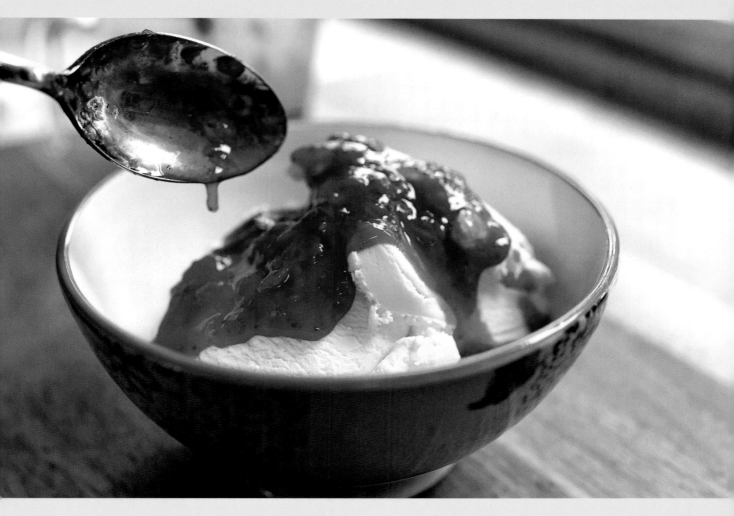

 VARIATION

Add a little rum to the sauce for some yummy flavor.

MINI BLUEBERRY GALETTES

MAKES 8 MINI-PIES

The ease and convenience of store-bought pie crust makes these beautiful little pies an irresistibly quick dessert for any night of the week.

You won't believe how delicious these are!

2 heaping cups fresh or frozen blueberries

¼ cup sugar, plus extra for sprinkling

2 tablespoons cornstarch

1 teaspoon vanilla extract

Pinch of salt

Zest and juice of 1 lemon

1 package store-bought pie crust (2 rounds of dough), or 1 recipe All-Butter Pie Crust (page 140)

1 egg

Sweetened whipped cream, for serving (optional)

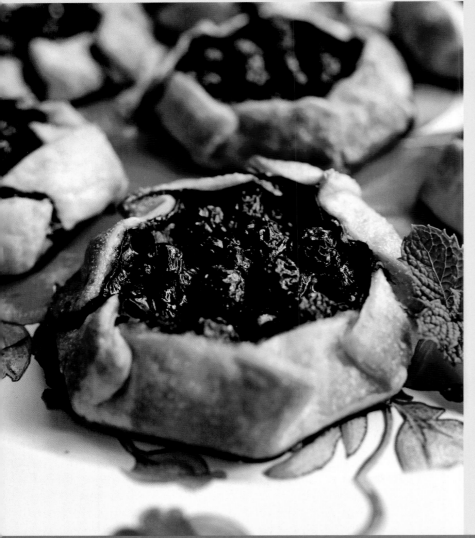

1. Preheat the oven to 425°F.

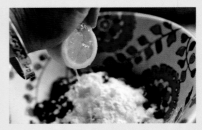

2. In a large bowl, combine the blueberries, sugar, cornstarch, vanilla, salt, and lemon zest and juice.

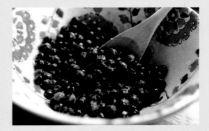

3. Stir it all together and let it sit while you prepare the crusts.

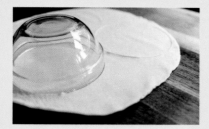

4. Roll out the two discs of dough. Use a 5-inch round bowl or pastry cutter to trace around and/or cut 3 rounds of pastry from each disc.

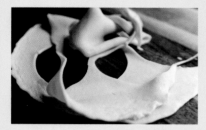

5. Gather up the excess dough scraps, reroll them, and cut out 2 more pastry rounds.

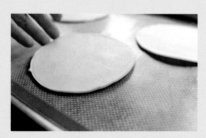

6. Place the dough rounds onto 2 baking sheets lined with baking mats or parchment.

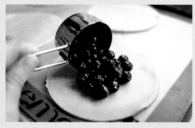

7. Carefully pour ¼ cup of the berry mixture on the center of each round . . .

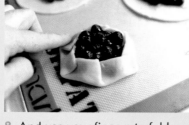

8. And use your fingers to fold up the edges.

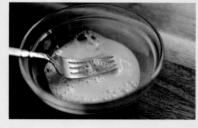

9. Mix the egg with 1 tablespoon water . . .

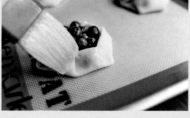

10. Brush the egg wash on the edges of the galettes . . .

V VARIATIONS

Make this recipe even easier by using blueberry, apple, or cherry pie filling.

S SERVE WITH

Sweetened whipped cream

Vanilla ice cream

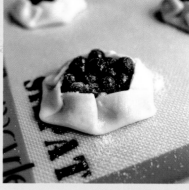

11. And sprinkle the edges lightly with sugar.

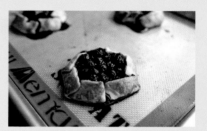

12. Bake the galettes for 15 minutes, until the crust is golden and the filling is bubbly. Let the pies sit on the baking sheet (they will leak a little juice while baking, but this is fine!) for 5 minutes, then remove them to a platter to cool. Serve warm or at room temperature.

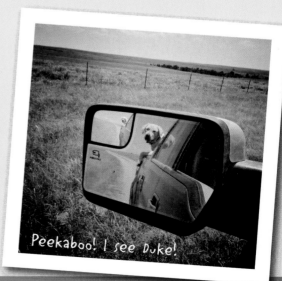

Peekaboo! I see Duke!

SLICE-AND-BAKE COOKIES

EACH RECIPE MAKES 24 LARGE COOKIES

It's hard to get warm, gooey, homemade cookies any faster than this. I love to make double, even triple batches of my family's favorite cookie dough and keep several rolls in the freezer. That way I just pull out the variety we want, slice off what we need, and bake them. Get all the dough-making work done ahead of time, then enjoy the benefits one, two, three, or a dozen cookies at a time. Wrapped well, the dough keeps up to 6 months in the freezer! (Not that it would ever, ever last that long . . .)

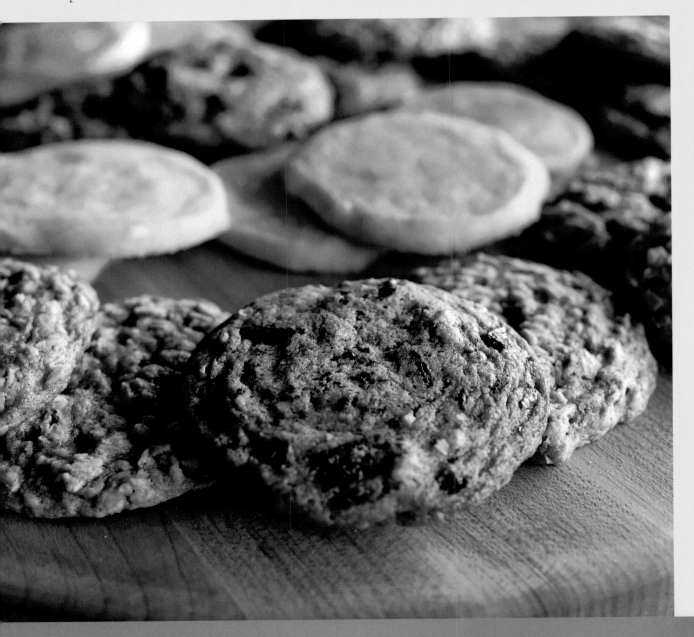

CHOCOLATE CHUNK COOKIES

Undeniably the best chocolate chip cookies I've ever eaten, and that's largely due to browned butter that's swirled into the dough. The cookies are even better when you bake the dough from the frozen state—something magical must happen in that freezer!

1 cup (2 sticks) butter, softened
1 cup brown sugar, packed
½ cup sugar
2 large eggs
1 tablespoon vanilla extract

2 cups plus 2 rounded tablespoons all-purpose flour
1 teaspoon baking soda
1 teaspoon salt
2 heaping teaspoons instant coffee granules

8 ounces good-quality semisweet chocolate
½ cup finely chopped pecans (optional)

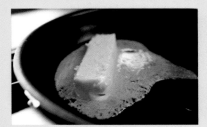

1. First, brown the butter: melt 1 stick of butter in a medium skillet over medium heat.

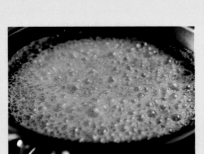

2. Keep a close watch on it, and swirl the pan around regularly! It will bubble up and sizzle . . .

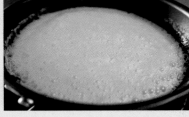

3. Then, a minute or two later, the foam will appear. When the foam appears, it isn't long before the butter is nice and brown. Take the pan off the heat when it gets to this light golden stage, because it'll keep browning even after you take it off the stove.

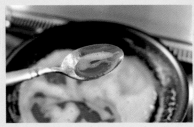

4. When it's nice and deep brown, but definitely not burned or black . . .

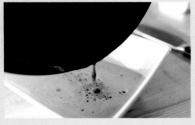

5. Pour it into a dish and let it cool completely. This is difficult to do when you have a hankering for warm chocolate chip cookies . . . but it's a necessity!

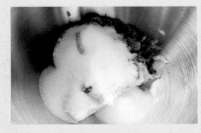

6. When the browned butter has totally cooled, start making the cookie dough! Add the remaining stick of butter, brown sugar, and sugar to the bowl of an electric mixer . . .

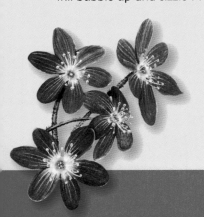

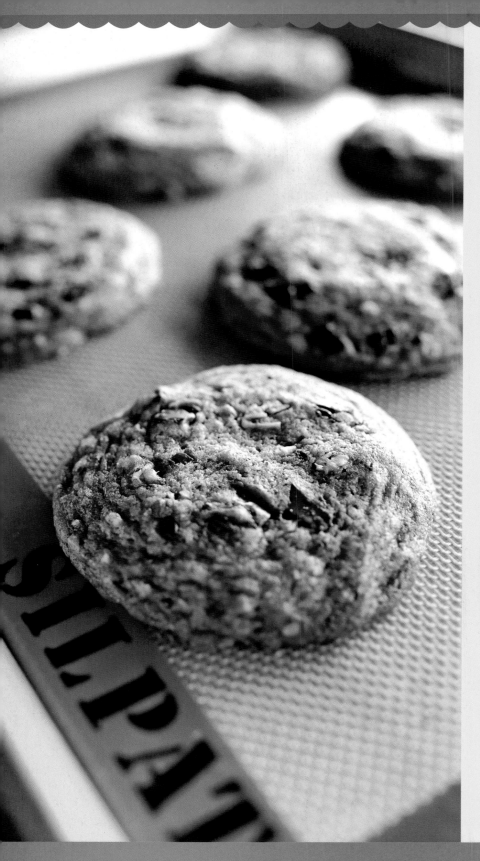

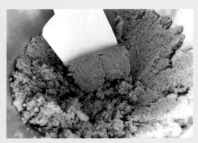

7. Then mix it until it's all combined, scraping the sides of the bowl at least once to make sure it's totally mixed together.

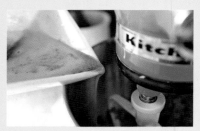

8. Now it's time to add the browned butter! The mixer should be on low, and I can't emphasize enough how important it is to add the butter *very, very slowly and gradually.* If you add it too fast, the mixture will be wet and soupy. So just take your time . . .

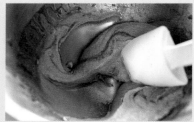

9. Stopping halfway through to scrape the bowl and make sure it mixes in nice and slow. (And be sure to get *all* the dark brown, beautiful solids in there. That's where the flavor is!)

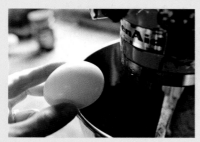

10. Add the eggs, one at a time . . .

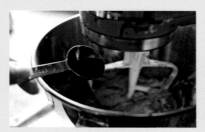

11. And the vanilla . . .

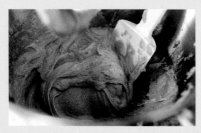

12. And mix until smooth.

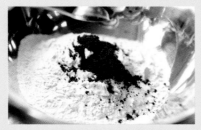

13. In a bowl, combine the flour, baking soda, salt, and instant coffee granules. (If you're coffee-averse, don't worry: You'll hardly know it's there! It just adds a great richness of flavor.)

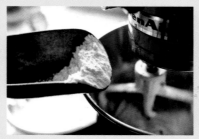

14. Turn the mixer on low and add scoops of the dry ingredients so they mix in gradually, scraping the bowl once to make sure it's all combined.

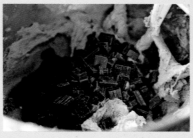

15. Chop the chocolate into small chunks (and the pecans, if you're using them) . . .

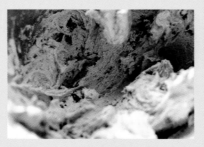

16. And mix them evenly in the dough. Form the dough into a large cylinder on top of a long piece of plastic wrap, wrap it tightly, then freeze it until you need it.

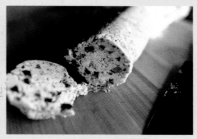

17. When you're ready to bake the cookies, preheat the oven to 375°F and slice off ¾- to 1-inch-thick rounds of dough.

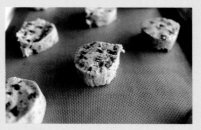

18. Bake the cookies for 14 to 15 minutes . . .

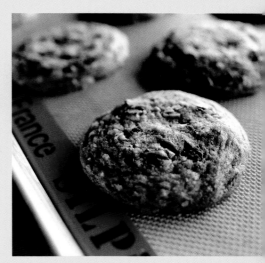

19. Until they're golden brown and slightly puffed. Serve with a nice cold glass of milk!

SUGAR COOKIES

These are the frozen, slice-and-bake version of the Angel Sugar Cookies I've made for years. They're chewy and soft when they first come out of the oven, or you can allow them to cool and enjoy their light, crisp, melt-in-your mouth texture. Decorate them with sanding sugar, ice them with buttercream, or eat them plain! I love having this dough in the freezer.

1 cup (2 sticks) butter, softened
1 cup sugar
1 cup canola oil
2 large eggs

1 cup powdered sugar
1 teaspoon vanilla extract
4 cups plus 2 tablespoons all-purpose flour

1 teaspoon salt
1 teaspoon baking soda
1 teaspoon cream of tartar

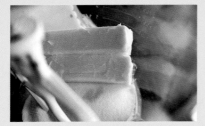

1. Place the butter and sugar in the bowl of an electric mixer.

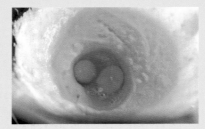

4. Add the eggs and mix them in well . . .

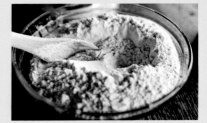

7. In a bowl, stir together the flour, salt, baking soda, and cream of tartar.

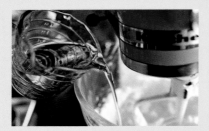

2. With the mixer on medium-low, slowly drizzle in the oil until it's combined.

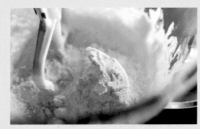

5. Then add the powdered sugar and mix well.

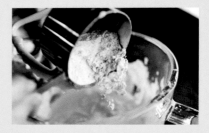

8. Then add the flour mixture to the mixing bowl in two batches, mixing gently after each batch . . .

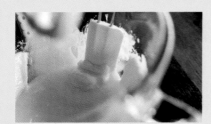

3. Scrape the sides of the bowl and mix again to make sure it's smooth.

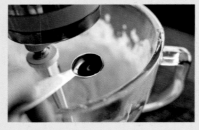

6. Finally, add the vanilla and mix it in.

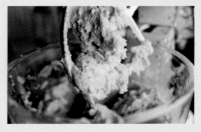

9. Until it's all combined.

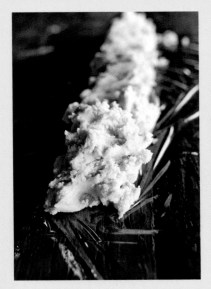

10. Place a long sheet of plastic wrap on the counter and lay out the dough in a rough cylinder.

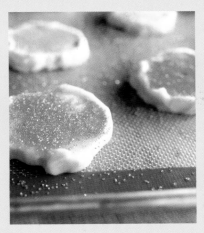

13. To bake the cookies, preheat the oven to 350°F and cut the dough into ½- to ¾-inch slices. Sprinkle them with sanding sugar if desired.

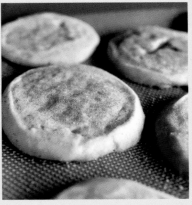

14. Bake the cookies for 13 to 15 minutes, or until they're just starting to turn golden around the edges. Serve them warm right out of the oven or let them cool to room temperature before serving.

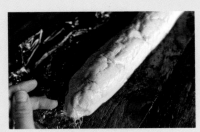

11. Wrap it up in the plastic wrap, forming it into a neat cylinder as you go.

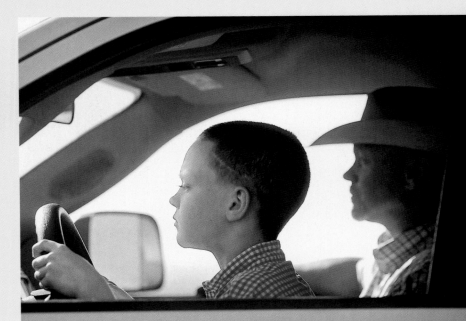

Todd's driving lesson. He had to learn how to drive a stick!

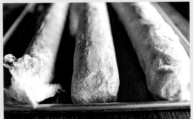

12. Make sure it's wrapped very tightly, then pop it in the freezer with all the other kinds of dough you made!

QUICK FUDGE

MAKES 30 SQUARES

Sometimes all you need after a big, satisfying dinner is a quick little bite of chocolate, and these squares of quick and easy fudge are perfect for that. There's no candy thermometer required with this fudge, and it's pretty much foolproof! Leave it plain (my favorite) or top it with any decoration you'd like.

Nonstick cooking spray

3 cups good-quality semisweet chocolate chips

One 14-ounce can sweetened condensed milk

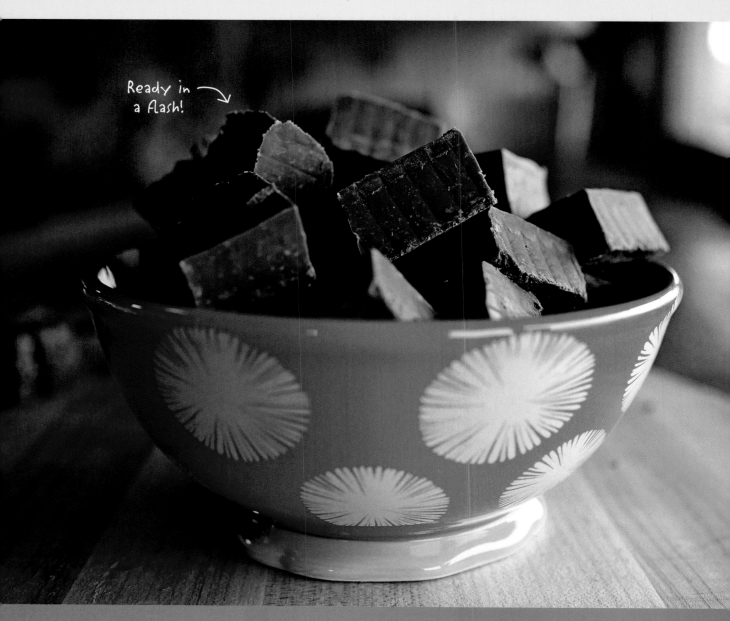

Ready in a flash!

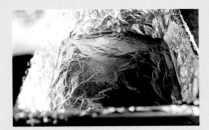

1. Before you begin, line a square 8 x 8-inch pan with aluminum foil and spray it with nonstick cooking spray.

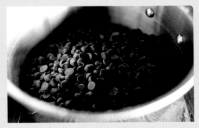

2. In a medium saucepan or double boiler over medium heat, place the chocolate chips . . .

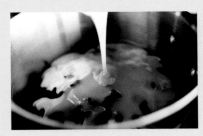

3. And pour in the sweetened condensed milk.

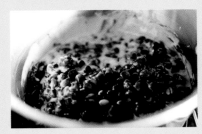

4. Stir them as they melt, taking care to scrape along the bottom of the pan with a spatula to avoid sticking and burning.

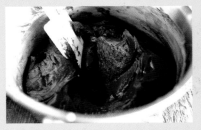

5. Once you can no longer see bits of solid chocolate chip, remove the mixture from the heat . . .

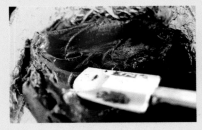

6. And immediately transfer it to the prepared pan, pressing it into a single layer.

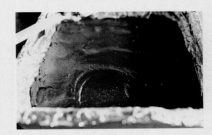

7. Cover the pan with foil or plastic wrap and refrigerate it for at least 2 hours.

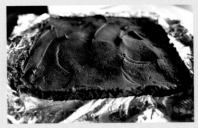

8. Once it's all set, pull the edges of the foil to remove the whole thing from the pan, then peel off the foil.

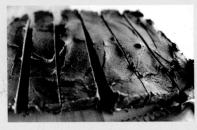

9. Use a long, serrated knife to slice the fudge first into long strips . . .

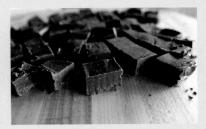

10. Then into squares.

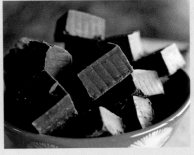

11. Store these in plastic bags at room temperature and pop 'em in your mouth after a yummy dinner!

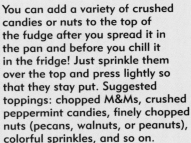

Ⓥ VARIATION

You can add a variety of crushed candies or nuts to the top of the fudge after you spread it in the pan and before you chill it in the fridge! Just sprinkle them over the top and press lightly so that they stay put. Suggested toppings: chopped M&Ms, crushed peppermint candies, finely chopped nuts (pecans, walnuts, or peanuts), colorful sprinkles, and so on.

RICE PUDDING

MAKES 8 SERVINGS

I don't make rice pudding very often, but whenever I do, I always stop dead in my tracks and confront myself with the same question:

"Ree! Why don't you make rice pudding more often?!?"

I mean . . . rice pudding. *Rice pudding.* It's sublime! It's just one of those things that causes you to roll your eyes and sigh when you eat it. Like you've finally come home again. Like the world finally, at long last, makes sense. Like all the questions of life are now answered. And a bonus: It also happens to be one of the easiest desserts in the world to make!

C'mon . . . I'll show ya.

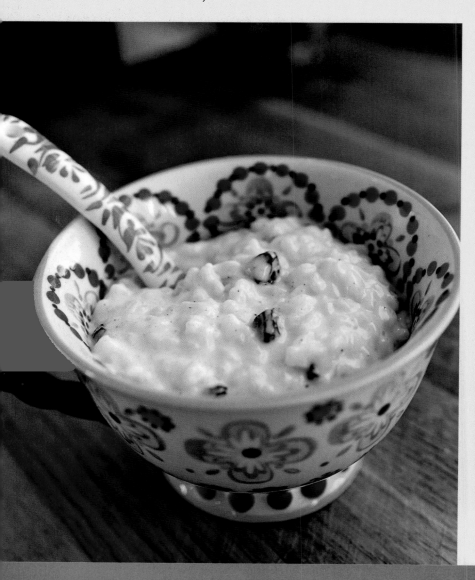

1 cup uncooked medium-grain white rice

2 cups milk

2 tablespoons heavy cream

1 tablespoon salted butter

Pinch of salt

One 8-ounce can sweetened condensed milk

1 tablespoon vanilla extract

Dash of ground cinnamon

Dash of ground nutmeg

1 egg, beaten

½ cup raisins

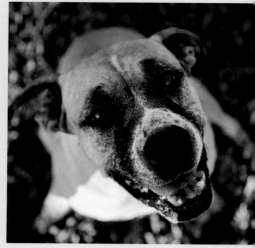

Sweet little Hooker.

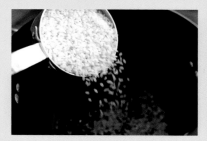

1. Pour the rice into a medium saucepan (nonstick works well!)

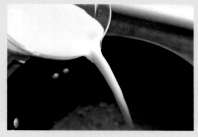

2. Add the milk, cream, butter, salt, and 2 cups water. Stir to combine.

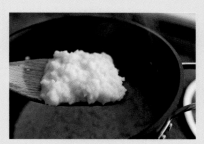

3. Bring the mixture to a gentle boil over medium-high heat, then cover the pan, reduce the heat to low, and simmer for 20 to 25 minutes, stirring twice as it cooks. Note: The rice should be almost fully cooked, but there should still be visible creamy liquid; it should not all be absorbed. If the liquid looks as if it's being absorbed too fast, you can cut this stage to 18 to 20 minutes.

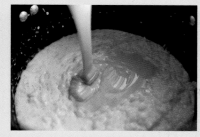

4. Turn off the heat and add the sweetened condensed milk . . .

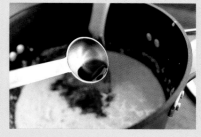

5. The vanilla . . .

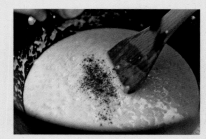

6. And the cinnamon and nutmeg.

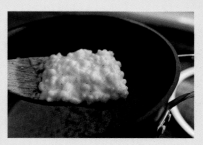

7. Return it to the heat and let it cook for 5 more minutes, then turn off the heat again.

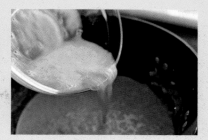

8. Stir in the egg, stirring constantly . . .

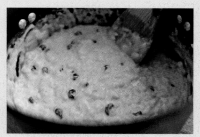

9. And finally, stir in the raisins. Let it sit in the pan for an additional couple of minutes . . .

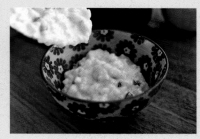

10. Then serve it nice and warm!

V VARIATIONS

Use dried cranberries, cherries, or currants instead of raisins.

Drizzle on a little maple syrup.

Soak the raisins in ½ cup bourbon or other whiskey for 1 hour before adding them to the rice pudding.

DESSERT PANINI

MAKES 2 SERVINGS

I think the concept of a sweet panini is just brilliant. Just use whatever bread you want, whatever drippy, gooey, sinful (or fruity!) filling you want, then grill it, sprinkle it with powdered sugar, and call it a day. The possibilities are deliciously endless.

2 slices bread, any variety
(I used a grainy sandwich loaf)

2 tablespoons Nutella

2 tablespoons marshmallow crème

3 strawberries, hulled and sliced thin

1 tablespoon sliced almonds, plus more for sprinkling

2 tablespoons softened butter

Powdered sugar, for dusting

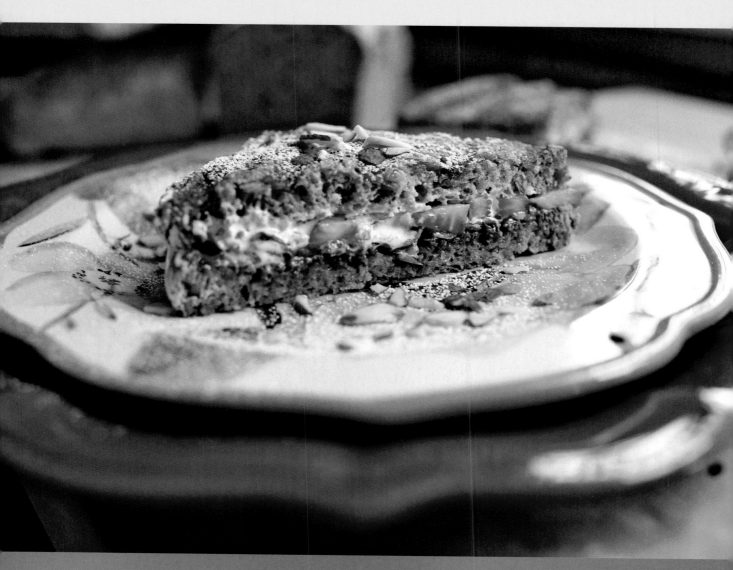

1. Preheat a panini maker to medium heat.

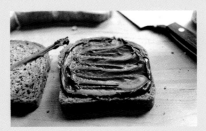

2. Spread one slice of bread with the Nutella . . .

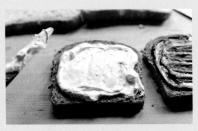

3. And the other slice with the marshmallow crème.

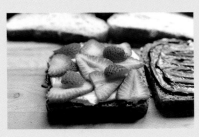

4. Press the strawberries onto the marshmallow crème . . .

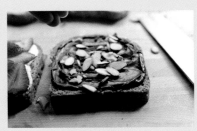

5. And sprinkle the almonds on the Nutella.

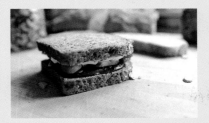

6. Put the two pieces together . . .

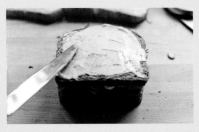

7. Then spread 1 tablespoon of the butter on one side of the sandwich.

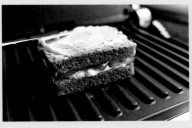

8. Place it, butter side down, on the panini maker and spread the remaining 1 tablespoon of butter on the top.

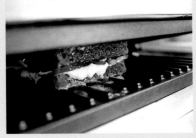

9. Grill the sandwich for 2 to 4 minutes . . .

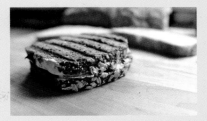

10. Until the bread is crisp and the filling is gooey and warm.

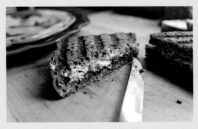

11. Let it sit for a couple of minutes to cool slightly, then slice it in half.

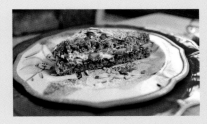

12. Place half the sandwich on each plate and sprinkle with powdered sugar and remaining sliced almonds.

Ⓥ VARIATIONS

Peanut butter, sliced bananas, and chopped walnuts

Peanut butter, marshmallow crème, and sliced bananas

Cream cheese, thinly sliced apples, cinnamon sugar, and chopped pecans

Marshmallow crème and chocolate chips

Use wheat, French, cinnamon-raisin, sourdough, or any kind of bread you have!

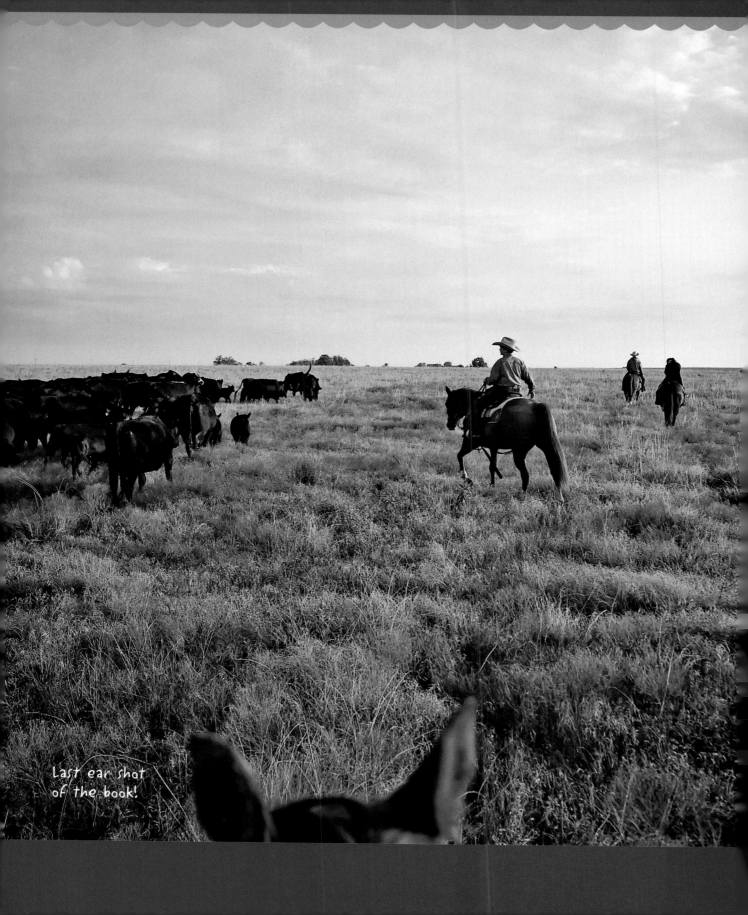

Last ear shot
of the book!

ACKNOWLEDGMENTS

To the tremendous Tiffany Poe, the dauntless David Domedion, and the amazing Andy Fusco, for your over-the-top awesome help with this cookbook. Simply put, I couldn't have done it without you. Love you guys.

To Cassie Jones Morgan, my incredible (and incomparable) editor. I'm so grateful we crossed paths. If you ever leave me, I'm coming with you.

To Kris Tobiassen, for your dedication in designing this cookbook. Your talent knows no bounds, and neither does your patience. (Do we still have time to move that one photo to the left just half a centimeter? Just kidding! I think . . .)

To Susanna Einstein, Sharyn Rosenblum, Liate Stehlik, and Lynn Grady, for your continued support. Thank you!

To the kind people at Walmart, Food Network, Land O' Lakes, Pacific UK, and Gibson, for being so wonderful to work with and for always letting me do my thing. I appreciate you so much.

To Haley, Erika, Lindy, Morgan, and Jennifer. Thank you for all you do!

To Hyacinth, you're my touchstone.

To Beccus, you're my spirit animal.

To Connell, you're my sister from another mister.

To Bets, you're my sister in the literal sense. And for that I thank God every day.

To Jenn, Jules, Sarah, and Ang. Take my hand. We'll make it. I swear.

To my parents, Gerre and Bill, thank you for always cheering me on. And for loving me through those teenage years. (I feel I should publicly thank you at least once every couple of years for that . . .) ☺

To Nan, Chuck, Edna Mae, Missy, Tim, Caleb, Halle, Nicholas, Stuart, Reagan, Elliot, and Patsy. Thank you for being an important part of my life!

To Doug and Mike, thank you for being the best brothers ever.

To my family, Ladd, Alex, Paige, Bryce, and Todd, I love you so much.

And to *you*. Whether you stop by my website, watch my TV show, or enjoy my cookbooks, I can't thank you enough for believing in me and supporting me through the years. I started blogging in 2006, and never could have imagined how much good I would experience as a result. Thank you for being such a huge, essential part of what I do. My cup runneth over. I love you all.

RECIPES FOR EVERYONE!

I love making lists, even though I don't always remember to look at them. In case you're a list lover, too, here are some suggested recipes for the various humans (and occasions) in your life.

Kid-Friendly

I wouldn't call 'em picky . . . just particular! Here are some of the most kid-friendly dishes in this cookbook.

Beef with Snow Peas, 163
Broccoli with Cheese Sauce, 286
Chicken Milanese, 266
Dessert Panini, 366
Greek Yogurt Pancakes, 2
Grilled Chicken and Strawberry
    Salad, 43
Hamburger Soup, 71
Individual Chicken Pot Pies, 138
Peas and Carrots, 293
Quick Shells and Cheese, 214
Sweet Potato Fries, 308
Tortellini Primavera, 204

Cowgirl-Friendly

This is a list of recipes my sister and I would eat if we were locked in a house together, just the two of us, with no kids and responsibilities.

The Carb Buster, 32
Cashew Chicken, 167
Coconut Curry Shrimp, 255
Kale Citrus Salad, 40
Pasta Puttanesca, 178
Polenta, 322
Quinoa Caprese, 64
Spinach Soup, 80
Tuna Noodle Casserole, 222
Vanilla Ice Cream with
    Strawberry Sauce, 352

Cowboy-Friendly

Cowboys are a different breed in more ways than one. One peek at their list of faves and you'll immediately have them figured out.

Breakfast Quesadillas, 21
Buffalo Chicken Salad, 59
Chicken Soup, 94
Chicken Taco Salad, 53
Colorful Coleslaw, 294
Lasagna Roll-Ups, 141
Pan-Fried Pork Chops, 156
Pawhuska Cheesesteaks, 269
Supreme Pizza Burgers, 154
Quick and Easy Apple Tart, 344
Refrigerator Rolls, 334
Skillet Lasagna, 194
Thin Fries, 318
Waffles, 4

Meatless Wonders

It's probably illegal for me, the wife of a cattle rancher, to even write the word "meatless." But I like to walk on the wild side every once in a while.

Black Bean Burger, 149
Huevos Rancheros, 6
Mediterranean Orzo Salad, 62
Panzanella, 46
Red, White, and Green Stuffed
    Shells, 134
Roasted Butternut Squash
    Salad, 56
Roasted Red Pepper Pasta, 206
Spicy Cauliflower Stir-Fry, 170
Breakfast Hash, 28
Tofu Lettuce Wraps, 264
Tomato Tart, 258
Veggie Chili, 96
Veggie Stir-Fry, 172
Wild Rice Pancakes, 30
(and more!)

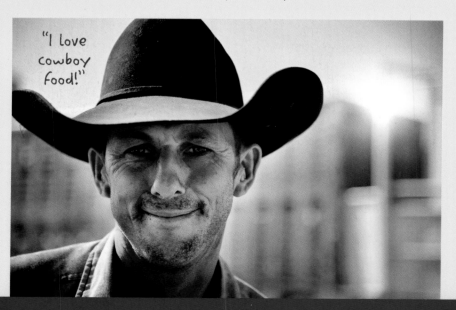

"I love cowboy food!"

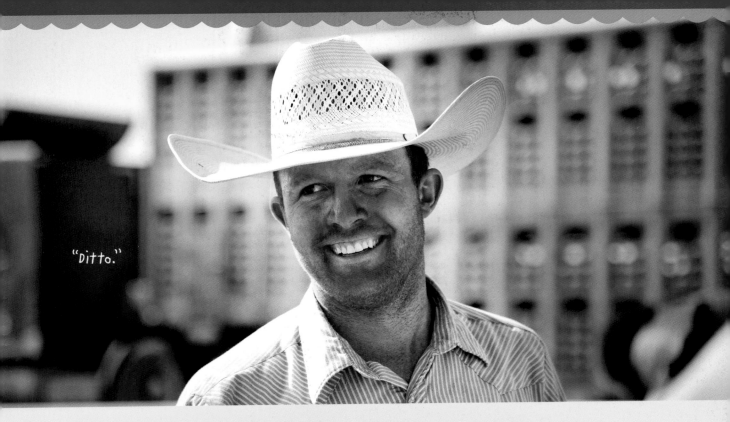

"Ditto."

Casual Company

If your brother or sister or uncle drops by for dinner, you don't really need to go to any trouble. They're family! They're stuck with you! (Make one of these for 'em, though, and they'll get you an extra-special gift this Christmas.)

Fancy Friends

Here are some options for those times your boss comes over for dinner, you're trying to impress a potential in-law, or you want to make your family feel extra-special on a Tuesday.

Neighbors in Need

We all have neighbors and/or friends who face challenging (or just super-busy) times. Here are some good and useful dishes to take them if they could use a little extra help.

UNIVERSAL CONVERSION CHART

Oven temperature equivalents

250°F = 120°C
275°F = 135°C
300°F = 150°C
325°F = 160°C
350°F = 180°C
375°F = 190°C
400°F = 200°C
425°F = 220°C
450°F = 230°C
475°F = 240°C
500°F = 260°C

Measurement equivalents

Measurements should always be level unless directed otherwise

⅛ teaspoon = 0.5 ml
¼ teaspoon = 1 ml
½ teaspoon = 2 ml
1 teaspoon = 5 ml
1 tablespoon = 3 teaspoons = ½ fluid ounce = 15 ml
2 tablespoons = ⅓ cup = 1 fluid ounce = 30 ml
4 tablespoons = ¼ cup = 2 fluid ounces = 60 ml
5⅓ tablespoons = ⅓ cup = 3 fluid ounces = 80 ml
8 tablespoons = ½ cup = 4 fluid ounces = 120 ml
10⅔ tablespoons = ⅔ cup = 5 fluid ounces = 160 ml
12 tablespoons = ¾ cup = 6 fluid ounces = 180 ml
16 tablespoons = 1 cup = 8 fluid ounces = 240 ml

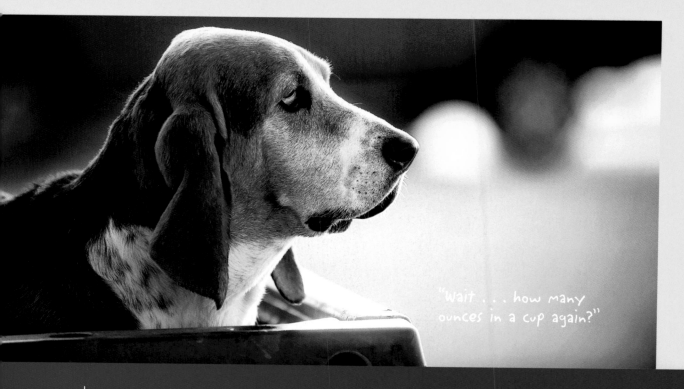

"Wait . . . how many ounces in a cup again?"

INDEX

C

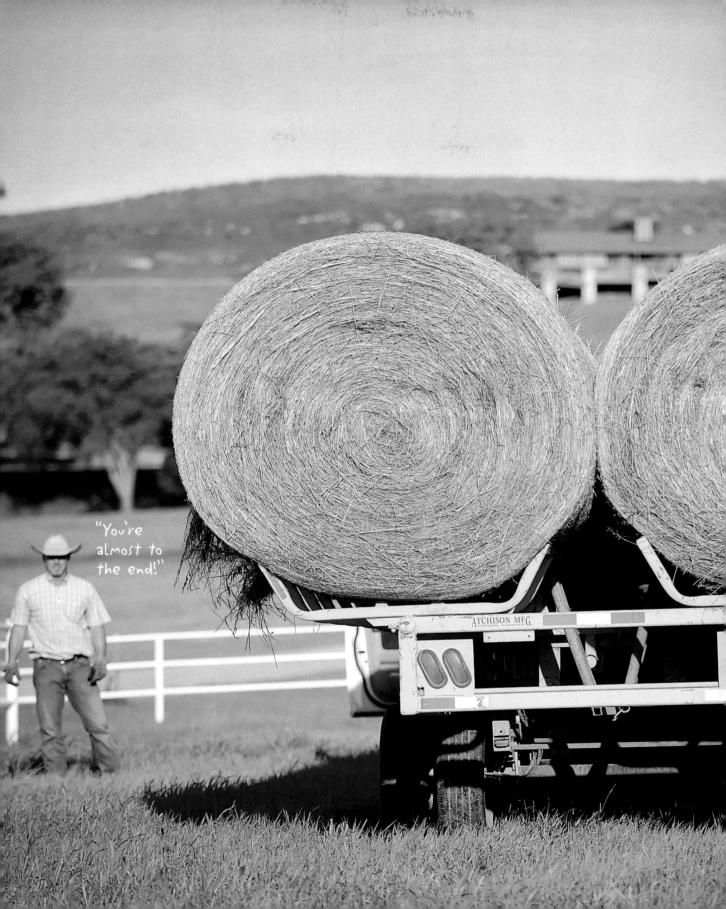

"You're almost to the end!"

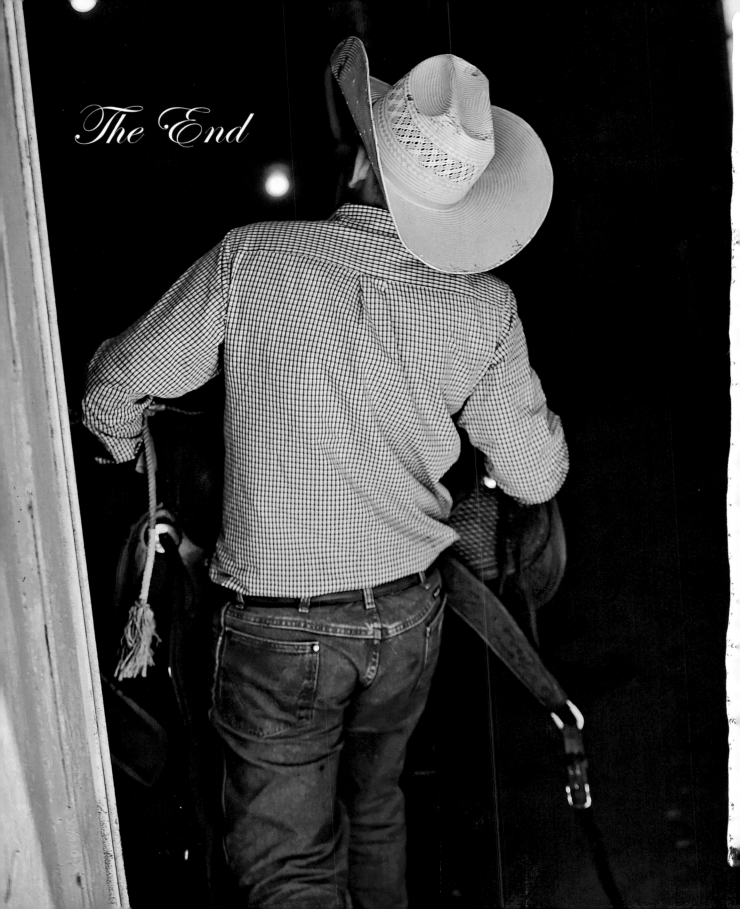

The End